W9-DHH-719

MENTAL HEALTH NURSING:

A Socio-Psychological Approach

MENTAL HEALTH NURSING:

A Socio-Psychological Approach

Helen K. Grace, R.N., PH.D.
Professor of Psychiatric Nursing
College of Nursing
University of Illinois at the Medical Center

Janice Layton, R.N., M.S.N.

Dorothy Camilleri, R.N., M.S.N.

WM. C. BROWN COMPANY PUBLISHERS   Dubuque, Iowa

Copyright © 1977 by Wm. C. Brown Company Publishers

Library of Congress Catalog Card Number: 76-7135

ISBN 0-697-05515-9

All rights reserved. No part of this publication
may be reproduced, stored in a retrieval system,
or transmitted, in any form or by any means, electronic,
mechanical, photocopying, recording, or otherwise,
without the prior written permission of the publisher.

Third Printing, 1978

Printed in the United States of America

CONTENTS

Preface   *x*

Acknowledgments   *xvi*

SECTION 1   **A SOCIO-PSYCHOLOGICAL VIEW OF BEHAVIOR**

Introduction   *1*

Chapter 1   **The Patterning of Behavior: A Societal Perspective   *3***

Social Systems **4**

Socialization **8**

Social Roles **12**

Social Position **16**

Social Norms **17**

Social Mobility **19**

Discontinuity in Social Roles **22**

Summary **24**

Chapter 2   **The Patterning of Behavior: A Developmental Model   *26***

Erikson's Life Stages *29*

Trust vs. Mistrust *31*

Autonomy vs. Shame and Doubt *33*

Initiative vs. Guilt *36*

Industry vs. Inferiority *39*

Identity vs. Role Diffusion *41*

Intimacy vs. Isolation *45*

Generativity vs. Stagnation *47*

Ego Integrity vs. Despair *49*

Summary *50*

Chapter 3   **Life Crises, Defensive Mechanisms,
and the Evolution of Coping Styles   52**

Anxiety 57

Defensive Mechanisms 63

Coping Styles 68

A Socio-Psychological Model of Mental Illness 73

Psychiatric/Mental Health Nursing 78

Summary 80

Chapter 4   **Psychosomatic and Neurotic Coping Styles   86**

Psychosomatic Coping Styles 88

Neurotic Coping Styles 93

Treatment Issues 107

Summary 108

Chapter 5   **Drug Dependence   111**

Definition of Terms 115

Types of Drugs 117

Treatment Issues 142

The Nurse's Role in Treatment of Drug Dependence 152

Summary 154

Chapter 6   **Depressive Coping Styles   157**

The Concepts of Grief and Loss 160

Types of Depression 163

Depressive Reactions 174

Involutional Depression 176

Suicide 177

Summary 191

Chapter 7   **Retreat as a Form of Coping**   *194*

Deviant Life Styles *198*
Schizophrenic Life Styles *200*
Descriptive View of Schizophrenia *202*
Theories About the Origin of Schizophrenia *212*
Treatment Issues *234*
Summary *238*

SECTION 2   INTERVENTIONS

Introduction   *241*

Goals of Therapy   *244*
Methods of Intervention   *245*

Chapter 8   **Types of Treatment Intervention**   *247*

"Talking" Therapies *250*
Behavior Modification *265*
Chemotherapy *267*
Somatic Therapies *274*
Summary *276*

Chapter 9   **The Nurse in the Treatment Process**   *278*

Nature of the Nurse-Patient Relationship *282*
The Nursing Process *293*
Phases of the Nurse-Patient Relationship *297*
Summary *304*

Chapter 10   **Anticipatory Counseling and Crisis Intervention**   *307*

Typical Life Crises *310*
Anticipatory Counseling *311*
Crisis Intervention *319*
Problematic Situations: Aging, Death, and Dying *335*
Summary *339*

Chapter 11   **The Family System: Normality, Disturbance,
and Intervention**   *341*

The Family as a Social System *342*
Disturbances in Family Systems *350*
Principles of Intervention *356*
Summary *362*

Chapter 12   **The Group: Dynamics, Therapeutic Potential,
and Intervention**   *364*

The Dynamics of Small Groups *365*
Therapeutic Potential of Group Interaction *374*
Intervention Techniques *378*
Summary *387*

Chapter 13   **The Therapeutic Community**   *390*

Hospitalization as a Crisis Experience *393*
The Milieu as an Agent of Change *406*
Patient Government *417*
Preparation for Re-entering the Community *423*
Principles of Relating *425*
Summary *432*

Chapter 14   **Ethical Issues**   *434*

What Should Be Treated? *437*
Who Should Be Treated? *438*
Who Shall Treat? *441*
How Shall Treatment Be Financed? *444*
Summary *447*

Glossary   *449*

LEARNING ACTIVITY PLANS   *457*

Index   *538*

PREFACE

A basic premise underlying the development of this book is that psychiatric nursing is currently in a transitional state. This book is explicitly designed to make bridges between the traditional models of the past and those of the future.

Psychiatric nursing practice was initially built on the same medical model that predominated in the practice of psychiatry. This medical model is based on a disease orientation emphasizing the etiological origins, diagnosis, and treatment of specific disease entities. Although this model works very well in many areas of medicine, the situation is problematic in psychiatry where the set of circumstances commonly designated "mental illness" does not meet the usual criteria. There are no precise definitions of the "illness," no predictable sequence of events by which it progresses, and no agreement within the scientific community about common etiological factors. Matters related to treatment are similarly controversial and vague. Of course, modern practice, even in psychiatry, has modified this strict medical model. Many of the current controversies in the field concern not only the usual questions of genetic and biological factors related to specific types of mental problems, but also matters extending far into the social and psychological realms of living. Views about "mental illness" extend from those of medical purists who rigidly hold to a disease model of mental illness, at one end of the continuum, to those of the social scientists who argue that "mental illness" is not an illness at all but rather a state of disaffection created by society; that persons labeled as having mental problems have violated social norms and therefore are excluded from any of the more acceptable roles in society and allowed only the role of a deviant. Another position on the continuum defines the problem as a moral one, surrounding the relationship of an individual to the social order. This, in contrast to the medical point of view, holds that the individual is ill and needs treatment so that his behavior will be within acceptable limits in a given societal context.

While psychiatric nursing traditionally has been developed within the framework of the medical model, recent years have evidenced an increasing movement toward a more socio-psychological perspective. Psychiatric nursing is in a state of transformation to mental health nursing, a focus that encompasses all areas of nursing practice and emphasizes the promotion of mental health, whatever the person's current state. This transformation poses a whole new set of dilemmas that relate to the function of nurses in this confusing and often conflictual field.

Mental health nursing has as its goal *prevention* as well as *intervention;* it focuses on both individuals and larger social groups; and it is not only practiced in conjunction with a defined psychiatric population but extends to all areas of nursing practice, in both traditional institutional settings and the community at large. A practice of this extensive scope requires an amalgam of the best features of the past plus an imaginative projection into new and uncharted areas. Although it would be possible to emphasize the divergencies between the medical and socio-psychological models, it seems currently more appropriate to stress ways in which the gaps might be bridged.

Nurses currently practice in a wide variety of settings; ultimately they will determine the future development of mental health nursing. To do this, they need an appreciation of their historical base as well as some links to a broader socio-psychological realm that will help them move forward in more futuristic directions.

This book includes elements of the medical model, particularly in the categorization and description of certain problems. These elements are linked to a broader social reality, requiring that the categorizations be regarded in a different light than has been usual in the past. For example, while medical terminology is used in describing certain human dilemmas such as neurotic reactions, the discussions center on the network of social relationships and forces as they interact with the individual. This approach has been taken so that nurses practicing in more traditional settings may fit this experience into a wider context, which emphasizes a functional or socio-psychological view of the difficulties in living with which we all cope with greater or lesser success.

It is proposed that instead of relying solely on the illness model, we view people as occupying certain positions or roles (such as sister, daughter, student, classmate) in their relationships to one another and in their society at large. These positions play an integral part in determining the quality of life that an individual can, and does, secure for himself or her self. They are instrumental, that is useful in achieving goals; through these positions, a person has greater or lesser access to the resources and experiences that shape his or her personal characteristics, coping potential, and general life style. Each person, throughout a lifetime, faces a myriad of problems in daily living—some great and some small. One faces these problems with whatever degree of problem-solving competence or coping ability one has been able to acquire up to that point, and each episode renders the individual either more or less able to succeed at the next inevitable episode and so influences subsequent role performances; thus, a circular pattern is set up.

Using this perspective, mental health nursing is concerned with exerting a favorable influence on the network of factors that bear so directly on each person's capacity for successfully solving problems of living. Nurses work with individuals, families, groups, and communities at all levels of problem-solving. Within the community, nurses gain knowledge of the types of problems confronting people in their particular cultural milieu. They participate in working with individuals, families, or groups in developing supportive networks to cope more adequately with common problems. At times they may assist individuals, families, and groups in their efforts toward changing currently unsuccessful coping patterns. The scope of mental health nursing is expanded to encompass all levels of difficulties, real and potential, ranging from those of the "normal" individual within the community to those of the person identified as psychiatrically disabled and seen in the psychiatric hospital.

The format of this book lends itself to a variety of uses, depending on varying curricular patterns and on particular emphases that the faculty may wish to implement. It can be used both with the more traditionally organized experiences usually found in standard psychiatric nursing courses and with some of the more innovative approaches currently being tested. The first section of the book presents a conceptual base for transforming psychiatric nursing into mental health nursing. This conceptual framework, drawn from theories concerning social systems, growth and development, and crisis, is pertinent to an understanding of human behavior generally and as such could be used as part of a core or foundational curriculum. From this base, a theoretical model is drawn that integrates social systems, social-psychological perspectives, growth and development models, and crisis concepts.

It is recognized that in some curricula these building blocks may be provided elsewhere. For example, courses in sociology, psychology, and growth and development may provide some of this basic framework. In this case, faculty may choose to skip some of the repetitive content or to use it to review some basic social science concepts and integrate them into a view of mental health nursing. In any case, the discussions of the bases for our overall theoretical model are necessarily limited, relating only to the model developed within this book. The discussions of these theoretical perspectives are not meant to be exhaustive or all-inclusive; if these topics are to be pursued in greater depth, the investigation of original source material is suggested.

The basic theoretical model underlying the organization of this book is one in which the individual is considered to have a greater or lesser capacity to cope with situations. This coping ability waxes or wanes with the effectiveness of a person's problem-solving. Each time one meets a situation that requires novel problem-solving, one may either rise to the occasion, thus adding to or strengthening his or her problem-solving skills; or one may experience defeat, thus having to narrow his or her range of activity to avoid meeting with failure again. The network of resources that surround a person, and his or her willingness or ability to make use of them, have a significant impact on the person's ability to solve problems effectively. They provide the impetus for the person to resynthesize elements from the skills he or she already possesses and to reach into areas not yet mastered to develop more extensive problem-solving. If the necessary resources are lacking, the enabling spark is missing; the person frequently cannot produce the novel solution required and so experiences failure. Such failures lead to a restrictive range of activity, since the person attempts to protect himself or herself from further difficulties of that nature. The very severe restrictions resulting from frequent episodes of failure are commonly labeled as one or another form of "mental illness."

Nurses concerned about mental health may be effective resources in helping people reach successful resolutions of their problems. Many problems encountered by people involve health-related issues. Nurses working in the areas of maternal and child health may be resources for people as they work through naturally occurring crises of growth and development.

Community nurses, in their concern for a diversity of issues that affect people's health and well-being, are another immediately available resource to people as they encounter a wide range of problematic situations. Medical-surgical nurses deal constantly with crises that are an outcome of physical illness; they are in a strategic position to help people in their attempts to cope with crisis situations. Psychiatric or mental health nurses in some instances work with persons in "normal" crisis situations in community and general hospital settings. In other instances, the people they deal with reflect repeated failure in their problem-solving endeavors. Their coping styles have become so restricted and inhibiting that the goal of nursing interaction is to help them envision and experiment with new forms of problem-solving behavior.

Mental health nursing is not confined to any one specialty group, nor does it occur only in specified settings. The basic concept and the models developed in this book are appropriate to both hospital and community settings. Nurses in all areas of practice need to be sensitive to the types of problems their patients face, the types of coping styles characteristically employed, and ways in which they can assist people to manage their problems more successfully.

To accomplish these ends, the instructor can use this book in a flexible manner. Parts may be used in combination and integrated into an overall curricular format. Other parts are more specific, for an in-depth investigation of problems commonly within the realm of psychiatric nursing. For example, Chapter 3, which develops the basic "crisis and coping" model, may be effectively used in combination with Chapter 11, "Anticipatory Counseling and Crisis Intervention," and could also be integrated into the overall curricular plan or taught as part of a core curriculum component. Other chapters, while on the surface more pertinent to psychiatric nursing (such as Chapter 14), present material directly applicable to the organization of all hospital settings. Chapters 4 through 8, which present materials related to characteristic coping styles, may be applied to a wide range of persons, from those who have mild difficulties in coping all the way to the so-called psychiatric casualties.

The book is organized in two parts, the first providing the basic conceptual framework coupled with a discussion of characteristic coping styles, the second dealing with varying forms of intervention. Intervention is discussed separately from the characteristic coping styles in the interest of strengthening students' awareness of the overarching nature of these techniques. They apply not only with all of these coping styles, but also in varying contexts of nursing practice, both community and institutional. For this reason, no distinction has been made between institutional and community practice; it is our premise that sound mental health practice extends across institutional and community boundaries. Neither setting should be pigeonholed as requiring a different base of knowledge or techniques of intervention. It is our hope that, with these areas clearly identified in the text, instructors will be able to find the material needed to fit with their particular format. We recommend that supplemental material related to particular ethnic groups, communities, and settings in which students practice be selected to facilitate application and provide a more holistic view.

In Section One a sociological perspective of mental illness is presented first. Then (Chapter 2) a growth and development model drawn from Erikson is summarized and discussed within a broader social network framework. In Chapter 3 the focus is on crisis theory and the development of coping styles of individuals as they confront problems of living. Anxiety and loss are considered to be central in the development of coping styles. A conceptual model is developed for understanding the processes underlying development of a person's coping style. Chapters 4 through 8 center on commonly identified forms of maladaptive coping, such as neurotic and psychosomatic coping styles, addictive responses, depressive responses, and retreatism. Prominent in these discussions is the perspective of a society that produces a set of anxiety-producing pressures with which the individual attempts to cope in his or her own unique ways. Section Two of the book centers on treatment issues. Types of treatment are discussed first, followed by an exploration of the nurse's part in treatment counseling and crisis intervention, family therapy, group interventions, and the use of the therapeutic community. The final chapter makes explicit some of the ethical considerations underlying the practice of mental health nursing.

Following the text are Learning Activity Plans related specifically to chapters in the text. These Learning Activity Plans offer an optional approach to guiding the learning process through directed activities and self-testing.

ACKNOWLEDGMENTS

In the course of writing a book such as this, many debts are incurred. It is probably impossible to acknowledge the many ways in which people have helped by sharing ideas, providing support, and in general putting up with the authors as they proceeded with this task. To many colleagues and friends who have offered intellectual stimulation and helpful suggestions when this book was in the germinating state, we offer our heartfelt thanks. Gratitude is also expressed to the University of Illinois College of Nursing for providing the organizational climate where ideas such as those developed in this book could be fostered. Particularly, we would like to acknowledge Dr. Gertrude Stokes, Head of the Department of Psychiatric-Mental Health Nursing, and Dr. Joan King, Professor of Psychiatric Nursing, for their helpful support. Among other people we wish to specifically acknowledge are our reviewers. This manuscript has benefited from critical reading and review by a number of people, several of whom have read it more than once. The final draft of this book has been reviewed by and reflects the input of Phyllis S. Moore, Elaine Mansfield, and Sharon Dimmer. Earlier drafts of this manuscript were reviewed by Barbara A. Munjas, Janet Rodgers, and Lorene Fischer.

Crystal Lange, Director of the Division of Nursing and Allied Health Services, Saginaw Valley (Mich.) State College, has played a particularly key role as a consultant for the Learning Activity Plans. She has toiled long and hard throughout the whole process of developing this material.

A project of this nature could never be completed without the participation of a committed and competent secretarial staff. We thank Rubye Hill for translating our hieroglyphics into a readable manuscript, and Joan Kapsimalis, who constantly updated the manuscript as changes were made. Special thanks to Linnea Walch, who provided the artistic skill to translate our ideas into graphic illustrations. Finally, our thanks to our families, who experience the greatest cost, since they must cushion the highs and lows that authors inevitably experience in the course of an undertaking of this nature. Our families have been remarkably cheerful throughout this long ordeal. The authors have tolerated a considerable amount of peanut butter on the typewriter keys in exchange for which our families have tolerated a certain degree of preoccupation and a number of TV dinners.

January, 1977

Helen K. Grace
Janice Layton
Dorothy Camilleri

SECTION 1

A SOCIO-PSYCHOLOGICAL VIEW OF BEHAVIOR

INTRODUCTION

Section One of this book is designed to give nurses the information they need in developing an imaginative frame of reference appropriate to their expanded role in mental health nursing. What is required of the nurse is the ability to view any piece of behavior from several points of view. A child's performance in school, a mother's interaction with her infant, a person's delusional statements—all need to be understood within both a social and a psychological framework. These behaviors represent, at one level, the influence that society has exerted upon an individual. They also represent that person's carrying out his or her piece of the social action and reflect such things as positions in society, expectations held, number of alternative courses of action available, and access to needed resources, both physical and psychological. All these factors are social forces expressed through individual behavior.

This same behavior must also be seen in terms of the position it occupies in the development of the individual's personality and psychological structure. All social forces do not produce the same results for all people. There is some unique interaction in which an individual molds, processes, and creates his or her own responses to the inputs received within his or her social networks. These responses always depend on the person's past experiences and the meaning they have in guiding his or her behavior. Thus the person has a unique psychological structure. Any behavior has meaning in terms of his or her particular psychological makeup. For example, certain people leap into a difficult stressful situation and take direct aggressive action, while others retreat and find some way to evade the problem.

Mental health nursing requires the nurse to be able to shift from one view to the other in looking at all behavior and all people. Each perspective adds dimensions of understanding that would not be forthcoming if either one or the other were the sole frame of reference. Taking solely a sociological view, one risks losing the unique creative individual component of behavior; while with only a psychological perspective, one risks missing an understanding of the social forces that make the person's particular psychological stance at any particular time viable in a situational context. If the nurse is able to make an amalgam of these two perspectives, she or he is in a better position to take the medical model and cast it in a broader frame of reference. The nurse can make use of some of the advantages of the medical model without getting sidetracked by its limitations.

With these ends in view, Chapter 1 outlines some of the relevant sociological factors to be considered in viewing human behavior. Social factors that converge upon the individual to shape behavior are identified and discussed. The psychological-developmental framework presented in Chapter 2 is that of Erikson. This framework was chosen because it is commonly used in Growth and Development courses and forms a natural bridge between the two perspectives. Erikson has based his model on Freud's personality theory but has changed the emphasis to consider the individual's social experiences which influence development, a view somewhat neglected in early psychoanalytic formulations. In addition, this model includes the entire life cycle, instead of being limited to early life. Chapter 3 describes crises as critical juncture points in a person's life history. Whether they occur naturally or accidentally, they are points where major behavioral changes are possible, changes that would be difficult to achieve during more quiescent periods. Taken together, integrating sociological, psychological, and crisis models, a socio-psychological model of mental illness is presented. The remaining chapters of this section are organized around particular coping styles: psychosomatic and neurotic coping styles in Chapter 4, addictive patterns in Chapter 5, and depressive coping styles in Chapter 6. Chapter 7 depicts two patterns of retreat: acting out and schizophrenic life styles. In all these discussions the coping model serves as a basic framework, combining sociological, psychological, and medical models.

CHAPTER ONE:

THE PATTERNING OF BEHAVIOR: A SOCIETAL PERSPECTIVE

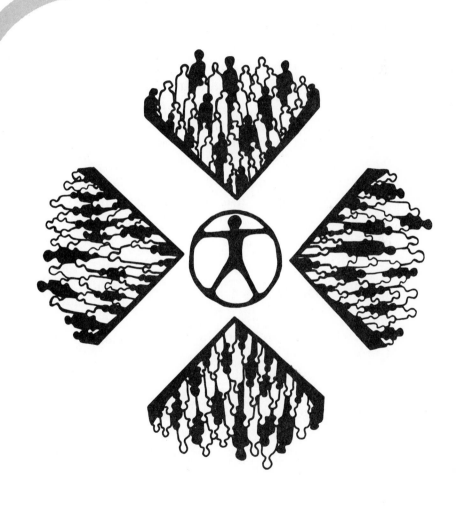

Behavior is never a solitary affair stemming solely from an individual untainted by a social network. Rather, it reflects people in relationship to one another. In fact, each person's uniquely individual personality is formed out of a complex series of interactions between the person and his or her social groups. Because of this "group-rootedness" of people, a social systems perspective is useful in viewing behavior. The group, then, is seen as the major holistic unit, with individuals and individual behavior being seen as attributes of the unit or expressions of some aspect of group interaction. George Herbert Mead argues that

> ... the behavior of an individual can be understood only in terms of the behavior of the whole social group of which he is a member, since his individual acts are involved in large, social acts which go beyond himself, and which implicate other members of that group.[1]

The individual must always be viewed in the context of a broader social system, a social system that does not negate his or her individuality but instead serves as a backdrop to complement and influence the social roles he or she enacts.

SOCIAL SYSTEMS

Each person's relationships throughout his or her lifetime are embedded in groups of various kinds. Life begins within the context of the family. Play groups, neighborhoods, classes at school, peer groups such as Girl Scouts, and work groups are added as time goes on. Each one of these groups exerts its own influence on the person's developing behavior. In each group, he or she is in some ways the same person and in other ways different. The individual is something like a juggler—managing to engage

---

1. Anselm Strauss, ed., *The Social Psychology of George Herbert Mead* (Chicago: Phoenix Books, 1964), p. 120.

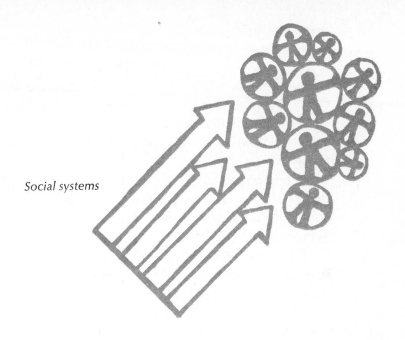

Social systems

in many and differing relationships and keeping all of them in some sort of coherent order. The person does this by identifying his or her place within each and every social group and by placing each group experience in turn within the broader context of all his or her social groups. A student, for example, develops a place for himself in the classroom. But in addition to viewing this immediate situation, he must be able to mesh the experience with other roles, such as that of family member. Further, he needs to be able to imagine the future and how he is going to find his way. He has to see himself as a lawyer, for example, by trying on the role, imagining the steps he must take to get there, and picturing himself within the context of social groups that are significant in terms of attaining this long-term goal.

In any given role performance, the person places that particular group experience within a broader context, much as a thread is woven into a piece of cloth. Lack of congruence between groups may make it difficult for the individual to define his or her place within any particular group. For example, a child who is a member of a rigid authoritarian family structure in which her father's word is law may find it difficult to know how to play her role in a laissez-faire or democratic class situation. Incongruent role performances may be required in different social groups, thereby creating difficult adjustive problems for the individual. The child in the authoritarian family structure is expected to follow orders, while in the democratic classroom the expected behavior is for her to be self-directed and active.

The juggling act for this child is fraught with difficulty. One can view the "self" as the result of the feedback one receives from varying performances, and the feedback this child receives is likely to be contradictory. While adults with well-defined identities could, in such a situation, make the necessary shifts in role performance to achieve positive feedback, children, lacking such a secure identity, are frequently blocked in the development of a healthy identity by such incongruence.

Any social system develops an elaborate complex of communication networks, both within that system and with the larger world outside. Through an exchange of information within the group, the individual can decipher what kind of group this is and therefore decide what type of person he or she is to be within it. Some of this information is processed as feedback; that is, a commentary by other people on the behavior the person is exhibiting. If one does not know what type of group he or she is in, one does not know how to enact his or her role and is likely to elicit considerable negative feedback. An individual may then either withdraw from group interaction or engage in random trial-and-error behavior in an attempt to gain enough response and information to define his or her role in more mutually agreeable terms.

The nature of the work (both expressive and instrumental) of any particular group becomes defined through the members' exchanging information, both overt and covert. Each group has both expressive and instrumental facets. The instrumental functions are most frequently known. A classroom teacher, for instance, knows that he is going to have students do six problems in subtraction in a given session as a means of instilling the skill of subtraction, but he may or may not know about the expressive components of a given group activity. The teacher conveys his view of the values surrounding the work and of each student's capacity to perform at an acceptable level. In turn, he receives from students their views of his performance as a teacher. Using the classroom for a further example, on the first day of class the teacher generally defines what type of class this will be, and the students, wittingly or unwittingly, disclose a great deal of information about themselves and their expectations of the teacher. The teacher's opening statement includes the name of the class, the content that will be included, and the requirements of the course, but this communication also conveys a sense of his or her own values and how he or she hopes the class will progress. Students similarly communicate their own values and expectations, and this process of informational exchange continues throughout the course.

Through the interactive process, a group develops a repertoire of shared meanings which constitutes the group's culture and includes norms that govern behavior of group members. Each group develops a language of its own and consequently establishes boundaries for its system. For example, the discussion of a surgical team involves a unique language or jargon; others entering the surgical suite would not understand what was being said and would consequently perceive themselves and be perceived as outsiders.

Each group similarly defines certain individuals as members and others as nonmembers. In adolescent groups, membership may be defined by the types of clothes worn. Other groups define membership on the basis of occupation, while still others are based upon common interests, such as music, art, or political orientation. In some groups it may be difficult for an outsider to discern the basis of commonality; for instance, a group of bored housewives who share critical views of their husbands, similar feelings about the latest school board hassle, and other such attitudes that serve to bond them together. Every group develops rules about who is an insider and who is an outsider, with accompanying criteria for membership.

Each group establishes limits as to the degree of variance of individual behavior it will tolerate. Take, for example, differences in religious groups: there are variations in religious groups both about what one is to believe and about rules of conduct. Unitarians are likely to tolerate a variety of definitions as to the nature of an all-powerful being, while more conservative religious groups demand precise definitions of "God." Similarly, a wide range of behavior is accepted in more liberal groups, while extremely conservative groups are concerned with manner of dress, recreational activities, and a host of rules governing all aspects of life. Other groups, while on the surface progressive and liberal, have in fact very rigid rules of conformity; for example, groups of "swingers" who will not tolerate the concept of monogamy. In all groups, the values and norms are developed through a complex interactive process that also sets limits as to the amount of behavior variation that will be tolerated. A certain balance is achieved, and through this intricate process the individual learns to play out appropriate social roles within the group context.

SOCIALIZATION

The individual learns appropriate social roles through the process of socialization, which may be defined as "the acquisition of interactional competence."[2] To accomplish this, children need to learn to relate to their world from a frame of reference similar to that of the significant figures in their lives. These definitions and requirements vary widely from culture to culture. Children use information received from others to interpret their world so that their behavior may be appropriately "fitted" into the social context. The person learns the behavior appropriate within the group.

This training process begins at the earliest stages of life. From the day a child is born, he or she is being socialized, in the sense that the child's behavior is influenced to fit into the patterns of significant adults; for example, parents who try to get the child to sleep through the night. Some children learn to sleep amid the uproar created by a houseful of other children, while others learn that they can only sleep in a quiet room with shades drawn and no outside noise. Certain aspects of early socialization stand out as more recognizable than others. For example, in toilet training the child is clearly perceived as being capable of learning some of the rules of society, and efforts are expended to get him or her to conform. Therefore, the child is faced with having to channel actions into appropriate places and to control impulses so as not to behave inappropriately. Life consists of a series of similar hurdles, some not so apparent as others, in which the person must find ways of adjusting his or her behavior so that it is appropriate in a given time and place. This does not imply a conscious effort to decide what behavior one is going to employ at a particular time;

---

2. Matthew Spiers, "The Everyday World of the Child," in *Understanding Everyday Life,* ed. Jack D. Douglas (Chicago: Aldine Publishing Co., 1970), p. 189.

Socialization

rather the person is continuously—and automatically—sorting the cues he or she receives. It becomes a conscious effort only when the person encounters some strange cue that calls attention to the fact that he or she is not performing as expected. As part of this process, the child encounters a hierarchy of values held by parents and other socializing agents.

Socialization involves several interconnected processes. "First the child must learn proper *performance behavior*—that is, he must discover what kind of behavior is approved by the social group and shape his behavior accordingly."[3] A child learns, for instance, that her mother approves when she urinates in the potty chair rather than in her diapers. The reward of her mother's approval becomes a motivating factor in the infant's beginning to learn to control her behavior. Similarly, in the school setting the child faces a series of performance expectations. Meeting these performance expectations elicits the approval of parents and teachers, while not measuring up to them results in censure. In the process of learning about desired performance behavior, the child also begins to sort out values that have meaning to "significant others."

Second, the person learns to play a variety of social roles.[4] This is a building process: In the first stage one tries out a behavior and then observes the response of others to these actions. Largely as a reflection of the responses of others, the person begins to develop an idea of himself or herself as a person. For the first few years of life, the family is the primary

---

3. Robert M. Goldenson, *The Encyclopedia of Human Behavior,* vol. 2 (New York: Doubleday and Co., 1970), p. 1228.
4. Ibid.

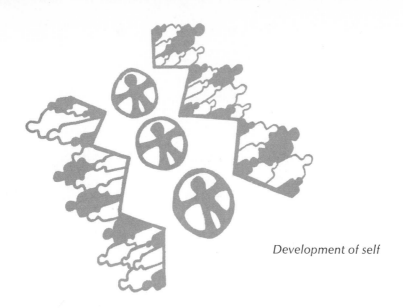

Development of self

group that stimulates this process. However, as the child matures, his or her base of operation enlarges from the family to the community, school, and other networks. The process is undertaken in each of the groups in which the child participates, becoming increasingly complex as he or she deals with larger numbers of people.

Remember that accurate location of oneself within a social system is dependent upon the ability to infer the role of the "other."[5] At each stage of life the individual develops against a background of other people; the determination of "self" at each of these stages hinges on the ability to make these definitions based on interactions with significant others. A circular process, frequently referred to as "reciprocity," governs most social relationships. For an infant to master successfully the developmental tasks of infancy, the mother must simultaneously be mastering the developmental tasks of motherhood. For example, early in life, the child who experiences the feeling of hunger cries. A mother who is able to respond to the child's cries does so by feeding and caring for the baby. The child experiences relief through the ministrations of the mother and realizes that he or she

5. Theodore R. Sarbin, "The Scientific Status of the Mental Illness Metaphor," in *Changing Perspectives in Mental Illness,* ed. Stanley G. Plog and Robert Edgerton (New York: Holt, Rinehart & Winston, 1969), p. 23.

is able to evoke a response from another, in this case, the mother. Through this process of action and reaction, the child learns that certain acts evoke certain responses and so begins to imagine the role of the "other," and to predict his or her world.[6] If his or her behavior evokes responses directed toward fulfilling his or her needs, the child begins to develop a sense that the world may be trusted and to regard himself or herself as an individual who has the capabilities to command the attention of another. Reciprocally the mother feels equally powerful; she has the ability to quell the tears and produce instant satisfactions through her ministrations to her baby. Through this form of reciprocal interaction, both mother and child reinforce one another in their developing social roles.

As people mature, they confront increasingly complex and diversified situations that call for a complicated repertoire of role behavior. Children first learn to play appropriate roles within the family; when they go to school they must devise appropriate behavior in that context. Relationships with peer groups, marital partners, and within an occupational world are but some of the multiple roles that most individuals master within a lifetime. Ability to move successfully from one group to another depends upon the individual's having a wide repertoire of behaviors; the fewer behaviors the person has at his or her disposal, the more vulnerable he or she may be should these behaviors not fit a particular setting. Additionally, successful transitions from group to group depend on some degree of continuity and congruity between social groups.

Although an individual constantly devises role performances to meet the expectations of certain groups, this does not imply that he or she lacks individuality. As a chameleon looks different in different settings, so the individual appears different in the context of different relevant social groups. Yet the individual brings his or her uniqueness and individuality into each role performance. Through a complex interactive process, an individual becomes sensitized to cues that serve as stimuli for him or her to perceive a situation in a particular light. For example, a student seeing a room filled with desks, a lectern in front of the room, and a blackboard is likely to assume that this is a classroom. Because of prior experiences in other classrooms, the student has developed an idea of the type of behavior appropriate in this context. Through a review of past experiences, the

---

6. Ibid., p. 24.

person has a repertoire of behaviors that he or she may choose to display. From prior personal experiences as well as through observations of others, he or she can imagine the types of responses various types of behavior are likely to elicit. From this backlog of experiences, the person attempts to locate himself or herself within a particular setting and tests out a familiar pattern of behavior. If, in the case of the student, for instance, it elicits a response similar to prior experiences, the individual can then play out the role of student as he or she has learned it. However, if the teacher changes the rules of the game and, say, expects a high degree of learner involvement, the person must then find ways of developing a new type of role performance appropriate to the changed situation. If the student has not done the homework and is unable to demonstrate the expected mastery of the content, he or she cannot successfully manage his or her expected "role performance." In other instances, the person misperceives the situation and behaves inappropriately. In such instances the group either attempts to correct these perceptions or isolates the individual from the group, through either overt or covert communication.

A common classroom problem concerns the student who attempts to dominate any discussion. In many instances, the student who performs in this way believes that the teacher and the other students will be impressed by his or her wide grasp of the subject matter. Instead of approving, however, the group usually will go to work correcting the student and pointing out errors in his or her thinking. Over time, many of these overtalkative students become the silent members. In other instances, the extent and nature of their contributions become shaped to approximate that of other students. If such students are isolated in response to their overperformance, it is likely that they will experience being in such a classroom setting as exceedingly stressful and uncomfortable.

Through repeated interactions such as those described, a set of reciprocal expectations and obligations develops. On this basis, individuals develop social roles that they play out within their particular social networks.

SOCIAL ROLES

Spiegel defines a social role as "a goal-directed configuration of transactions patterned within a culture or subculture for the functions people

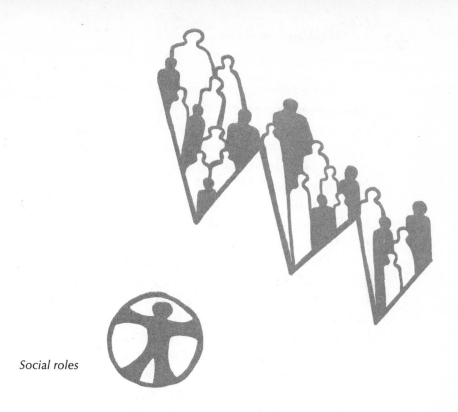

Social roles

carry out with respect to one another in a social group or situation."[7] For example, let us look at the role of the nursing student. With the end goal of becoming a nurse, the student engages in role behavior directed toward that goal. His or her role behavior ranges from technical aspects of performance to the types of social interactions expected in the role of "nurse." To perform successfully duties expected of a nurse, she or he needs to know how to give injections and turn patients on a Stryker frame and is also expected to relate to patients, visitors, doctors, and head nurses in role-specific interactions. Even friends who are not students in the nursing program begin to perceive the nursing student in a different light and to seek out information about their own health. While on one level these significant others still relate to the person in familiar ways, a new dimension is added to their expectations.

---

7. John Spiegel, *Transactions: The Interplay Between Individual, Family, and Society* (New York: Science House, 1971), p. 95.

Another point to note is that social roles arise always out of inter-active situations. For the nurse to perform his or her social role success-fully, someone—in most cases a patient—must play the reciprocal role of acquiescing to nursing ministrations. Although on the surface this may appear to be a rather clear-cut arrangement, an intricate set of interactive behaviors is involved.

A further factor to consider is that any social role develops within a particular cultural context and that the expectations for appropriate role behavior will vary from culture to culture. Being a nursing student in the United States is probably different from being in that position in a coun-try such as the Soviet Union. This is because the culture or subculture dictates the kinds of behaviors specific to particular roles—in this instance, nursing student. Role-taking is tied to an overall culture context.

Role-taking ability, in Heiss's framework, is "the ability to imagine oneself in the place of another and to see things as he sees them."[8] Role-taking in this framework involves guessing; the person guesses the attitude of the other. It is, however, informed rather than blind guessing. Essen-tially, the person bases his or her guesses on information gathered in the past and applies this to the present situation. If the information and the individual's ability to generalize are adequate, he or she will accurately take the role of the other.[9] Much of nursing education concerns itself with helping the nursing student imagine herself or himself in the place of the patient. Basic nursing procedures are frequently learned with students playing the role of patients. Although ostensibly the goal is that of teach-ing nursing procedures, learning the role of the patient accompanies it. First experiences in the clinical area are generally constructed so that the actual work to be performed is relatively simple, allowing the nursing stu-dent an opportunity to observe directly both patients and nurses playing out their roles. With this type of socialization into appropriate role behav-ior, all usually goes well until a nursing student encounters a patient who does not play out the appropriate "patient" role, or a case in which mes-sages conflict as to what the appropriate nurse's behavior is.

Consider a student caught in the middle of a conflict between a nurs-ing instructor and the head nurse about what she or he should be doing

---

8. Jerold Heiss, *Family Roles and Interaction* (Chicago: Rand McNally, 1968), p. 6.
9. Ibid.

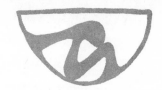

on the unit. A typical situation might be one in which the head nurse wishes the nursing student to assume responsibility for the total care of five patients on the unit. The nursing instructor, on the other hand, may assign the student to only one patient, to whom he or she is to give "in-depth" care: developing a nursing care plan and relating to the patient's social and psychological needs in addition to physical care. The head nurse is concerned with the total unit and "getting the work done," while the nursing instructor is concerned with the quality of the educational experience. Faced with these conflicting messages and contrasting role models, the nursing student finds it difficult to develop a sense of self in the situation in defining herself or himself as a "good" nurse. According to Heiss, three choices are available to the person faced with such a conflictual situation:

> One of these would be to withdraw from the situation and thereby put to rest the potential conflict. . . . Another alternative would be to attempt to define oneself with both identities. A third way in which he can attempt to avoid a decision between identities is to compartmentalize, to try to separate the others who are causing the conflict so that he may utilize the two identities at different times and thereby, at least partially, avoid the conflict between them.[10]

The resolution reached will probably vary depending upon the stage in which the nursing student finds herself or himself. It is very likely that in the first year of study the student will follow the dictates of the nursing instructor, while nearer graduation she or he will tend to reconcile the conflict more in line with the dictates of the head nurse. In either case, the central issue is that of attempting to locate oneself within an overall framework of role expectations and role behaviors.

The role-taking process continues at all levels of social interaction for all roles; the definition of self is intimately tied to a definition of the other

---

10. Ibid., p. 17.

person. The individual, because of varied responses encountered throughout his or her lifetime in a wide range of situations, is able to predict possible responses to his or her behavior. For example, the college student who enters a group as a "know-it-all" is likely to be put down. In contrast, the student who enters as "dependent Daisy" is likely to be left alone by all except a bossy, domineering member of the group. The occasional exception to this would be the woman student who adopts this behavior as a ploy in establishing a relationship with a male member of the group.

SOCIAL POSITION

In addition to categorizing social situations as a basis for role performance, individuals sort out positions of people within social groups and develop differential ways of responding to others. Very early in life, children learn to behave differently in relation to different types of people,

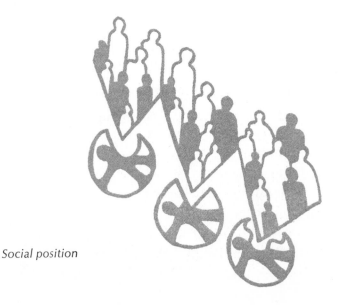

Social position

i.e., they act in certain ways in the company of adults, but behave differently with playmates. In this process children learn that there are those to whom they need pay deference—adults—and those whom they may in turn tyrannize, such as younger children and siblings.

Status differentials are common to all social systems. In the development of the social order, some members gain higher positions in the status hierarchy, while others are identified as lower in the ranking system. Individuals tend to emulate the behavior of those higher in the status hierarchy and to engage in behavior that will elicit approval from those in more powerful positions. At the same time, advancement in the social system is often predicated upon the ability to assign others to lower status positions. For example, a child who wishes to gain the approval of parents will not only do things that will earn their approval but will also point out the deficiencies of another sibling.

SOCIAL NORMS

As individuals vie for position within the social system, they develop certain rules that govern their interactions. An internalized code of "normal" behavior develops, and a hierarchy of values becomes established. For example, one source of power in any social group is the possession of money, but a basic societal rule specifies that one does not openly steal from another group member to gain this type of advantage. For another example, a nursing student tries to develop proficiency in doing such procedures as surgical dressings, but not, it is assumed, at the expense of violating aseptic technique. A multiplicity of rules govern the ways in which individuals are to behave in any given social system.

An additional characteristic of social systems is that those high in the prestige hierarchy have the power to impose rules of behavior on those lower in the structure. Those high in the status structure may violate the rule of not stealing from another, but the manner in which they steal is not considered as rule-breaking. For example, the president of a large corporation may knowingly endorse the production of inferior goods and the selling of this merchandise at inflated prices without being punished for stealing. However, for the poor man who steals a loaf of bread to feed his family, frequently the penalty is severe. General principles governing or dictating behavior are commonly called *rules*. These rules always reflect the values of the whole society or of smaller subgroups. Some authors refer to them as *norms*. The existence of rules or norms usually becomes apparent only when they are broken. For example, the teen-age girl moving to a new school frequently violates the norms of the group relating to standards of dress. She may wear the appropriate blue jeans, but with a blouse, not the usual tank top. This type of a rule is rarely overt, and she becomes aware of it through overhearing remarks or laughter and observing she is the only one dressed in that style.

Some form of penalty is a frequent consequence of rule-breaking. The penalty for breaking certain rules is clear-cut. One who steals or murders is defined as a criminal and sent to jail. But in other instances people break rules that do not violate the rights of others; they simply violate a sense of propriety. For example, one rule in our society is that people act as though they hear someone talking only when they are actually in the presence of a person who is talking or are listening to a radio, telephone, or some other auditory device. Someone who acts as though he or she hears voices and responds to stimuli others cannot hear is pointed out as being strange. Behavior also is considered appropriate or inappropriate depending on the context in which it occurs. Laughter itself is not inappropriate, but a person who laughs uncontrollably at a funeral violates a societal norm and is considered strange. A large number of societal rules, usually not apparent until they are violated, govern the full range of human behavior.

When a person acts in an unexpected fashion that is in violation of the expected norms or rules of a group, other group members try to correct him or her in an attempt to restore the social order. These attempts take varying forms. The first level is to attempt to get the person to go along with the norms: the effeminate boy may be given a football or enrolled in military school to get him to "shape up." If the person responds by conforming, then all is well. If he or she does not conform, the corrective attempts continue.

The attempts at correction vary according to the social status of the norm violator. For example, if a very wealthy person engages in bizarre behavior, it is generally categorized as an eccentricity to which he or she is somehow entitled. Wealthy people may engage in a wide variety of eccentric behavior and still not be derogated. However, for those who are not wealthy or renowned, different adjustments are made in response to rule-breaking. The first attempt is to find some explanation that will make the behavior appropriate. A plausible explanation is first sought in the immediate situation; for example, in the case of the person laughing at the funeral, others first attempt to discern if there is something in the situation that might trigger laughter. If there is nothing, other explanations are sought. If no plausible explanations can be found, the social group attempts to ostracize the individual who violates the rules. One of the ways of dealing with the problematic individual is to define him or her as "mentally ill." By so labeling, one no longer has responsibility for the outcast's behavior; his or her position in the group has been established. A mentally ill person is judged to be incapable of governing his or her behavior and so is excused from adhering to the norm.

SOCIAL MOBILITY

Most people attempt to maintain their status position within the social structure. Moreover, in this society, not only do they seek to maintain their position, but must also attempt to advance and rise within the hierarchy of their social groups. Commonly both father and son, for example, expect that the son will advance farther on the social scale than did his father. Generally, such advances are made in an orderly progression and do not upset the status quo. For example, the son of a business executive may be expected to become a company president, but not the poor boy from the ghetto. For the poor boy to become company president would be noted as an exceptional case, as would also be true if it were the executive's daughter rather than his son who aspired to this position. In making unexpected advances, the person proceeds with caution and usually gauges his or her performance carefully according to the expectations others in the group have about the roles he or she plays, as well as those to which he or she aspires. Those who overplay their position are likely to be "put down" as were the overtalkative students.

Another problem arises when the person is a member of more than one group, which hold opposing expectations. Consider the position of the young college graduate seeking his first job in the early '70s and trying to make a decision about shaving off his beard. To do so would indicate that he

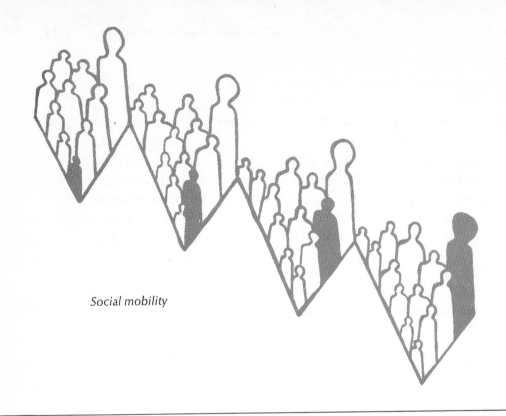

Social mobility

is a traitor to his peers and is obviously knuckling under to the Establishment. But if he does not, his family may consider him an embarrassment with no respect for propriety and no real wish to get a job, as evidenced by his appearance. In making a decision as to what course to take, he weighs the relative power in each of these groups and charts his course of action.

Other sources of conflict arise when the person exceeds the expectations of the group and thus poses a threat to the status quo. Conversely, the demands placed upon the individual in some settings exceed his or her potential. He or she cannot measure up to others' expectations, and the end result is a threat to his or her self-esteem.[11] In either case, penalties are imposed to bring the individual "into line." The individual's position within the status hierarchy and the protection that comes from that position are significant elements determining the strength and nature of censure as well as his or her vulnerability. Some statuses are ascribed; that is, they are granted by society. Common ascribed statuses are related to such

11. John Lofland, *Deviance and Identity* (Englewood Cliffs, N.J.: Prentice Hall, 1969).

things as age and sex, like "mother," "old maid," and "teen-ager." Achieved positions are those the individual earns by acquiring skills necessary to a role performance, for example, the mechanic or the concert pianist. In our society, penalties imposed for nonperformance in achieved status positions are not so great as those for nonperformance of ascribed roles. If an individual with a college education chooses to work in some form of unskilled labor, he or she may be viewed as eccentric, but societal censure is minimal. However, if a man does not perform in accordance with societal expectations for male behavior, he is severely censured, as is the mother who fails to care for her children. Pejorative labels, such as "homosexual" or "unfit mother," are commonly attached to such individuals, and they begin to be treated as nonpersons.[12] Attempts are made to transform them.

Persons lowest on the socioeconomic scale have identities composed primarily of ascribed roles, with little opportunity for attaining achieved roles. Their niche in society is rigidly and carefully circumscribed. The more limited one's repertoire of role behaviors, the more vulnerable one is to threats to his or her self-esteem, the reason being that the individual's identity is based on a limited number of roles. Inability to perform these limited roles, with the accompanying negative valuation, results in the individual's accepting the negative views of society as his or her self-image. Thus, the individual occupying the lower strata of society is faced with a dual problem: (a) available roles are primarily granted by society and are limited; and (b) nonperformance of these granted roles is negatively sanctioned to a greater extent than if a wider range of roles were available.

The first phase in the process that may result in behavior characterized as "mentally ill" usually involves an incident in which the person's self-esteem is severely threatened. As has been pointed out, there is a wide range of variability in one's vulnerability to stress. Whether one succumbs to the threat to his or her self-esteem depends on many factors. The person who has a many-faceted role identity may not be as vulnerable as the person who has only limited role identifications. A person high on the status hierarchy is more protected than others at lower levels. For example, to an individual who has a high level of educational credentials and the potential to find another job easily, loss of a job may not be as threatening as it

---

12. Sarbin, "Scientific Status of Mental Illness Metaphor," p. 27.

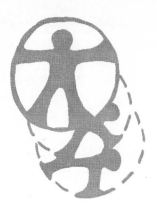

Discontinuity in social roles

is to an individual whose main identity is formed through being a bread-winner for the family and whose capabilities for finding another job are limited. The crucial variable is the degree to which one identifies his or her "self" with his or her position. If an individual's only identity is tied up with his or her occupational position, loss of a job is severely threatening. Similarly, a child with very few role options is extremely vulnerable to threats to his or her self-identification. A woman whose sole identity is built around being a wife and mother is most vulnerable when her children are grown and her husband divorces her. Thus a number of social factors serve to make a person more or less vulnerable to stressful situations.

DISCONTINUITY IN SOCIAL ROLES

In addition to individual differences that determine one's vulnerability to life stresses, there are particular turning points in the life cycle that are more stressful than others. Usually any situation causing major discontinuities in social roles creates a problematic situation. An obvious discontinuity surrounds the sudden loss of a role. For example, the widow not only loses a husband but also loses her role as a wife and the status that accompanies this role in our society. In her social groups, she confronts the problem of establishing an alternate place from that she shared with her husband. Other types of stressful situations involving role loss include loss of a job, separation or divorce, death of a child, and birth of a premature child. In each instance the person must redefine his or her role.

Secondly, a person experiences difficulties when he or she cannot meet the role expectations that significant others hold. An extreme example of this is the retarded child whose parents cannot accept retardation as a reality and instead interpret the child's inability to learn as an act of defiance against them. In the context of the developmental sequences outlined in the next chapter, most persons are able to move with relative ease through these stages. However, some experience difficulty when there is an incongruity between role expectations and their capacities to meet them. A similar process occurs when a person loses the physical capacity to engage in usual role performances. He or she is then faced with having to redefine role relationships vis-à-vis others who are not incapacitated; a new set of reciprocal role expectations and performances must be worked out.

A third type of difficulty may arise when one cannot accurately define a place for herself or himself within a given social structure. This may occur when one cannot play the expected role. For instance, a person cannot play the role of doctor until he or she has learned the necessary skills attendant on the role. Persons who enter a group totally dissimilar from their prior experiences or relationships are likely to find it difficult to ascertain their place within it. Role expectations that are markedly different and contradictory in varying social systems may also pose problems. For example, the unmarried pregnant adolescent encounters conflicts between the role expectations held for an adolescent within a family, for a student in school, and for an expectant mother.

Fourth, if individuals are unable to acquire necessary information to orient themselves to the group, they may experience stress. Someone who is blind or deaf, or those from a foreign country who do not speak the language, may be unable to understand what is going on within a group and therefore may be unable to define a role for themselves.

Finally, inability to fit individual behavior into the norms of a group may be problematic. In all these situations the person is in a dilemma. The usual definitions of his or her social role do not fit in the altered situation. He or she must make role transitions and in so doing risk the potential loss of self-esteem.

These situations will frequently usher in a crisis. Whether or not they do depends upon the meaning that the particular situation has for the person. For example, the loss of a job may have many different meanings.

For some men, loss of a job may mean loss of male identity and their status in the family. For others, loss of a job may provide a welcome opportunity to explore new avenues of employment or to experiment with new social roles, such as staying home and taking care of the children while their wives go out to work. In any event, life entails a series of changes, precipitated in some cases by naturally occurring developmental processes and in others by a series of accidental occurrences. In all instances, an individual is constantly adjusting and readjusting his or her position vis-à-vis the social groups in which he or she holds membership. The ease with which one makes these necessary adjustments, and the flexibility of significant social groups in accommodating to the individual, are a primary force in determining how well or how poorly the person fares as he or she moves through life.

SUMMARY

All behavior is rooted in and grows out of group interaction; it is never a solitary affair. Human behavior must therefore always be considered from the viewpoint of the person's connections within a social network. The individual is a member of multiple groups and sometimes has difficulty in meshing behavior if the appropriate social roles in these varying group contexts are contradictory.

Some of the more salient factors influencing the way people can form and enact their roles are communication networks that involve the kind of information and the way in which it is transmitted between members of the group; shared meanings developed within groups; ways in which the group defines its boundaries; and the degree of variation among members tolerated within the group.

Socialization is the process by which people learn to fit their behavior into the framework of the groups in which they participate. This fitting of behavior into a group framework consists of learning appropriate social roles and developing reciprocity between members of any social network. As part of the process in any social group, differential status of group members and a series of norms governing behavior are developed. Violation of these norms or status differences is considered "rulebreaking" and is dealt with by the group.

People sometimes experience difficulties in meeting the role expectations of multiple, sometimes conflicting, group demands, or cannot adjust their behavior to fit appropriately into particular group contexts. When this happens, they are faced with having to develop a whole new set of role behaviors.

FURTHER READINGS

Becker, Howard S. *Outsiders: Studies in the Sociology of Deviance.* New York: The Free Press, 1963.

Goffman, Irving. *The Presentation of Self in Everyday Life.* New York: Doubleday, Anchor Books, 1959.

Laing, R. D., and Esterson, A. *Families of Schizophrenics.* Sanity, Madness, and the Family, vol. 1. New York: Basic Books, Inc.

Lofland, John. *Deviance and Identity.* Englewood Cliffs, N.J.: Prentice Hall, 1969.

Moore, Bernice. "Education for Family Living—What is It?" *Nursing Clinics of North America* 4 (June 1969): 359-370.

Robischon, Paulette, and Scott, Diane. "Role Theory, the Family, and the Nurse." *Nursing Outlook* 17 (July 1969): 52-57.

Scheff, Thomas. *Being Mentally Ill: A Sociological Theory.* Chicago: Aldine Publishing Co., 1966.

Smoyak, Shirley. "The Confrontation Process." *American Journal of Nursing* 74 (Sept. 1974): 1632-1635.

CHAPTER TWO:

THE PATTERNING OF BEHAVIOR: A DEVELOPMENTAL MODEL

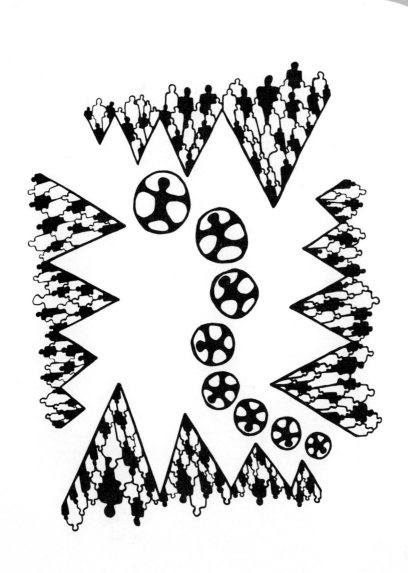

Any human behavior is a result of patterning at multiple levels ranging from the intrapsychic to the broad sociological. These levels may be viewed separately, but in understanding the behavior of any individual it is important to recognize that there is a constant interplay between them. To illustrate this interplay of factors, let us consider a period of time in the life of Peggy, a healthy two-month-old child who lives with her mother, father, and older brother Michael, age four.

Peggy awakens from a two-hour nap, studies her hand for a period of time, cooing, and then begins to cry. She continues to cry for a period of time until finally her mother comes, picks her up, and says, "My what a pair of lungs. I'm sorry, Peg, but Michael skinned his knee. He picked a bad time, didn't he, just when you couldn't wait for that bottle! Poor little pumpkin . . . ." She cuddles Peg and continues the sweet talk as she takes her to the changing table for a diaper change. Peggy has stopped crying and focuses on her mother's face.

"And now where's a bottle for my girl?" She turns on the TV to her favorite soap opera, settles into the rocking chair, and gives Peg her bottle. They both seem to be enjoying the situation. Michael dashes through on the way to the cookie jar on the kitchen counter. "Michael, only two—your dad will be home in half an hour and we're having an early dinner. Mike, before you go out, you know you shouldn't have that jacket on—your denim one is on the hook behind the door, so get it." Michael responds disgustedly, "Ah, Mom," gets the proper jacket, and goes out. After this disruption, Mother and Peg again settle down.

A few minutes later Dad comes in. "Oh, Jim, I didn't realize it was that time already. I haven't begun dinner." He comes over and picks Peg up: "That's okay. Let's see what you've learned today."

Keeping this piece of interaction between Peg and her mother in mind, what can we say about Peg's personality development? What kind of a person will she be when she is twenty? Well, we cannot say much based on such limited data, but if we take this interaction to be fairly representative of how Peggy is faring during this stage of her life, we can comment on several factors that interweave to form the fabric of her infancy.

We might begin by noting that Peg seems to fare quite well in the "creature comfort" department. She was born into a family where having enough nutritious food is not a problem. Nor does her family engage in a daily struggle with problems such as keeping warm, dry, and free from environmental hazards like rats and lead poisoning. Peg is healthy and likely to be protected by immunizations, routine checkups, and medical attention before illnesses become catastrophic or chronic. In short, Peg's family is both able and willing to care for her physical needs.

Peggy's good fortune so far as physical needs are concerned spurs her development in direct and indirect ways. Directly, Peggy can count on the material supplies she needs being available. Her body does not have to undergo stresses such as insufficient and unreliable feedings or discomfort due to inadequate shelter or clothing. In contrast with Peg, a child who does live in such deprived circumstances lacks sufficient opportunity to develop the pattern so crucial to infancy of "I cry, significant other comes, something happens, my tension disappears, I am content." The materially deprived child must frequently develop other means of coping with tensions arising from physical need, and the coping patterns he or she has available are usually not so conducive to healthy growth and development. For instance, some children learn not to notice the cues they receive from their bodies, since noticing only focuses their attention on their discomfort and is not reliably successful in diminishing it. Taken to an extreme, this denial or apathy is life-threatening, but it can and does exist in a significantly attenuated version.

The direct benefits accruing to Peggy as a result of her access to physical supplies are impressive; equally impressive is the influence of this favored position on another area of general influence—that of interpersonal involvements with other family members. The most important task confronting a newborn infant is to establish connections with a significant person or persons in his or her interpersonal environment. With luck these early relationships will be stable over time, and their nature will be such that mutual needs of both the child and significant others will be met, rather than the needs of one being exploited in the interest of the others. In the favorable environment surrounding Peg, it is more likely that both her physical and psychological needs will be met, given the resources in the situation.

But imagine for a moment that there were no milk in the house and

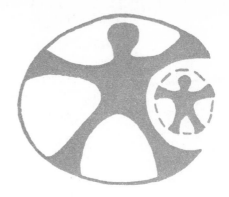

The unattached infant

no money to buy any. As the mother approached Peg, she would certainly be having a reaction, but not the one we originally described. Undoubtedly she would be troubled at having no food for her children and irritable because she herself is hungry and she cannot do anything for Peg. She may have hoped Peg would sleep awhile longer. She may feel depressed and hopeless about her situation and may feel that Peg has to learn the same way she did. Even if she were able to extend herself to Peg and try to comfort her, this would be to lesser avail because she cannot satisfy either the child's physical or psychological needs. If the child's physical needs are not met, she cannot become attached to significant others because she cannot experience the connection between the appearance of an adult and the elimination of tension.

ERIKSON'S LIFE STAGES

It is exactly this sequence of events resulting in attachment of the infant to significant adults that Erikson refers to as he discusses the establishment of trust in the first developmental stage.[1] Erikson has viewed the entire cycle of life from a psychological perspective and has delineated eight developmental stages, outlining the learnings the individual must successfully master at each stage. He views each stage as containing its own nuclear conflict, which, for better or for worse, the individual must resolve

---

1. Erik H. Erikson, *Childhood and Society* (New York: W. W. Norton & Co., 1950).

Table 2-1   Erikson's Eight Life Stages

STAGE (Focal Conflict)	AGE (Approximate)	CENTRAL ISSUE
Trust vs. Mistrust	0 - 18 mo.	Testing out of the trustworthiness of the infant's significant others.
Autonomy vs. Shame and Doubt	18 mo. - 3 yr.	Testing of individual capabilities in relationship to significant others.
Initiative vs. Guilt	3 - 5 yr.	Testing out abilities to compete in outside world.
Industry vs. Inferiority	5 - 12 yr.	Gaining mastery of cultural tools.
Identity vs. Role Diffusion	13 - 19 yr.	Developing a sense of personal identity vis à vis significant others.
Intimacy vs. Isolation	20 - 30 yr.	Merging of identity with another to achieve intimacy.
Generativity vs. Stagnation	30 - 60 yr.	Investing of creative energies in promoting the social welfare.
Ego Integrity vs. Despair	60 - death	Acceptance of the life one has lived as worthwhile.

for himself or herself. The learnings represent an amalgam of physical capacities, psychological readiness, environmental stimulation, life space occupied by significant others, and broader cultural dicta. At each of these junctures, a "developmental crisis" occurs where the new learnings which take place result to some degree in shaking off old ways of being and behaving to give rise to a new, more mature status. Table 2-1 lists Erikson's life stages, the approximate age span covered by each of these stages, and the central theme of these periods.

Each stage is ushered in by a variety of stimuli, among which physical maturation is certainly prominent. Just the pure fact of increased physical capacities and abilities triggers change in the way a person experiences his or her world and is in turn regarded by the people in that world. For instance, when our infant, Peggy, learns to crawl, she will have very different horizons from those she has when she must sit wherever she is placed until someone moves her. As a crawler, she can provide herself with any number of experiences which add to her cognitions, feelings, and mastery of her environment and herself. Never again will she be able to view the world in her earlier, pre-crawling way. She will have matured beyond that point and will have incorporated new behavior and notions about herself and others into her infant role.

Another example of this sort of change is puberty, when physical changes are both numerous and obvious, with the appearance of the secondary sexual characteristics. The endocrine activity associated with sexual maturation results in the adolescent's regarding his or her body in a different way and experiencing different feelings about peers. The behavior that may have served well during the prior developmental stage no longer fits. The old behavior is out of phase with the new person. A lack of fit such as this, although based on different issues, occurs during each stage of development. It is the struggling through the period of uncertainty, in which old patterns are no longer possible but new ones are just emerging and not yet comfortable, that qualifies the process as a developmental crisis.

TRUST VS. MISTRUST

Before moving to Erikson's stages, a brief word about the chronological factor in most developmental frameworks. Ages are given, but they are always approximate and are best regarded as guides, not rules. Boundaries between stages are not clear-cut and will differ markedly, particularly among children. They do not coincide with exact chronological ages and frequently overlap; not uncommonly, one may still be working on the tasks of one stage while moving into subsequent stages of development. The task associated with a stage assumes focal importance during that stage, but it is always present in some prototypic way before that stage and does not cease to exist once a particular stage passes. In other words, although at certain points in the continuum of life certain tasks predominate, evidence of these same tasks may be found at other points.

Returning to our example, let us examine Erikson's psychological stages of development as Peg and the others in her family may experience them. Peg, for all of her first year of life and then some, will be in the infancy stage. Erikson characterizes this stage as being primarily concerned with the central conflict of trust vs. mistrust. All of the experiences of an

infant relate to the question of whether or not to develop a trusting attitude toward the world and the people in it. Infants acquire information
about the trustworthiness of their world from the way in which they are
cared for. If their needs are met with sufficient warmth, certainty, and
regularity, they become confident that what they need from the world,
especially from significant others, will be forthcoming. In a corollary vein,
they develop trust in themselves and confidence in being regarded favorably by others.

From the vignette about Peg's family, we have some reason to hope
that the relationship she and her mother share has enabled Peg to feel
quite trusting of the world she has experienced so far. We can notice, for
instance, that she stopped crying when her mother picked her up, not
waiting until she was completely settled and comfortable with a bottle in
her mouth. Peg must have felt that the appearance of her mother meant
that her bottle would be forthcoming. For the baby to make this connection, her mother must have followed this routine fairly consistently. If
food were frequently not available, the connection between the appearance of her mother and the elimination of hunger tension could not have
been made. If the mother's existence makes her troubled and anxious, the
connection will not be made as favorably. The child may have lingering
doubts about the willingness of the significant other to play her role or the
reasonableness of oneself in signaling hunger and so calling forth the
mother's activity.

Peg's mother attends to much more than hunger tension as she cuddles, changes, and coos to the child. Numerous other bodily tensions are
ameliorated by her mother's intrusion into Peg's world at the point where
she was lying crying in her crib. The touching and cuddling provide sensory stimuli and physical satisfaction (or relief from tension) for Peg and
engage her attentiveness on the mother's person. During the first few
months of life, Peg will not be able to differentiate between what is herself and what is external to herself, and she will experience her mother
as just another part of herself. As she matures, she will be increasingly able
to establish her mother as a person different and separate from her own
self. Peg's attentiveness to and absorption in her mother are important at
each point along this continuum, and her mother's dependable presence
is instrumental in providing the predictability and backdrop satisfaction
against which Peg will structure both her internal and her external worlds.

In contrast to Peg's positive experiences, which result in feelings that the world and oneself may be trusted, a child raised in a less favorable psychological and physical milieu may develop feelings of mistrust. These basic attitudes and feelings are then carried over into later life. Without this basic foundation of trustworthy relationships, the individual experiences the world as a potentially lonely place, and himself or herself as isolated within it.

AUTONOMY VS. SHAME AND DOUBT

At some point, usually between 12 and 18 months, Peg will become involved in a major way with matters related to developing autonomy. Erikson states that the central issue at this stage is the testing of individual capabilities in relationship to significant others. At this stage the foundation is laid for the way in which the individual views himself or herself as an able person—a view that will persist, more or less, throughout his or her life. The notions children will acquire in regard to their abilities will depend largely upon the responses of others to their actions. Children at this age are actively exploring their world. If they are constantly confronted with "No, you shouldn't be doing this," they have difficulty in evaluating their abilities in beginning to master their world. In addition, they acquire the idea that aggressiveness in reaching out gets them into trouble and results in others' disapproval. They are left with the conflict of whether to persist with the effort to push forth, which means battling with significant others, or to acquiesce. If they do acquiesce, they never have the opportunity to test out their abilities, and therefore they experience doubt. Furthermore, the disapproval of significant others makes them feel ashamed. This is not to imply that the most productive way for the toddler to proceed through this stage is to experience no limits, since he or she needs to bounce against reasonable reality barriers to arrive at a realistic evaluation of his or her abilities. For example, a child needs to find out that she cannot do the same things at the stove that her mother does, but instead can play with the pots and pans on the floor. She needs to know that if she runs out on the street cars may hit her, but that she may explore freely in the back yard or go to the street if her brother or sister helps her.

Walking, talking, and control of the body are all tasks that the infant begins to master at this stage. Faced with the magnitude of these tasks, the infant meets constant frustration. To accomplish these tasks, the child needs the encouragement and support of significant others. Toilet-training is the culminating event of this developmental stage. Parents are heavily invested in their child's mastery of this task because of wider cultural values. A child who is not toilet-trained is a constant source of embarrassment, and to have a child who has not mastered this task is equated with parental failure. This situation brings into focus both the parents' and the child's attitudes about the child's autonomy. From the child's point of view, the discovery that control of bodily functions is in his or her domain, not that of the parents, provides a powerful tool for pleasing or displeasing them. If the child has acquired sufficient trust and has developed a sense of personal autonomy through mastery of other areas of the environment and self, he or she finds it unnecessary to use withholding as a weapon against the parents. Parents who foster their child's autonomy are very likely to view accidents and failures as signs that the child is not quite ready rather than viewing them as invitations to battle, as do parents who see the child's failure as evidence of "spitefulness."

Moving back to Peg, what are the clues to how her family and she will go through this next developmental stage? In observing the mother's interaction with Michael, it would appear that she allows him the freedom to be himself while maintaining some boundaries on his behavior. She noted that he was wearing his best jacket for going out to play, that he should know that the rule was "wear your denim jacket for playing." She requires him to stop and change his jacket, although still allowing him to express feelings about this limitation on his behavior, and indicates that she has faith in his ability to manage himself properly outside and to return at the required time.

Relating this type of family interaction to what it portends for Peg as she moves from the dependency of infancy, we would expect favorable growth of autonomy. First, Michael's good development and healthy view of himself will be reflected in his benevolent view of his sister. Since he is secure in his own position, he will be able to tolerate Peg's incursions into his "territory" and will not have to build his own self-esteem at her expense. In the light of all these factors, Peg has a better than average chance of moving successfully through this developmental stage.

A word, also, about this family structure and its mediating influence in regard to broader cultural values: The views of Peg's mother and father toward toilet-training, as an example, will be based on many things, among them their own experiences in being toilet-trained and the generally held feelings about toilet-training in their social network of family and friends and in broader cultural contexts. Generally, parents transmit their feelings to their offspring, and much that they do is a response to signals within themselves rather than to those given off by the offspring. In some instances, parents impose toilet-training at a certain age regardless of any indications from the child as to his or her readiness. Other parents may not respond to the child's signals of readiness because of their own memories of this experience and their resolve never to engage their children in the types of struggles that they experienced.

Ideally, parents separate out the signals that their children are sending from those originating within themselves and thus are able to serve as

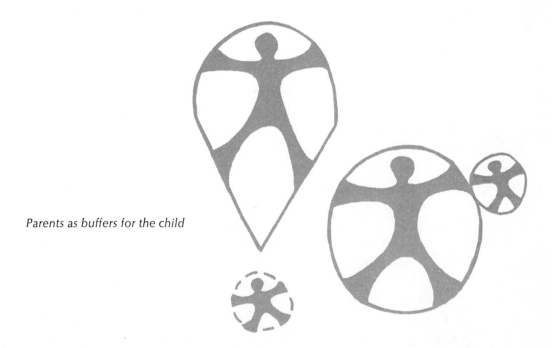

Parents as buffers for the child

a buffer to protect the child from pressure. Therefore, parents may delay toilet-training until the child gives signals of readiness, even though he or she has passed the usual age for training. The abilities of the parents to function as a buffer depend to a large extent on their own sense of security. This sense of security will depend not only on cultural and individual factors already mentioned, but also more general socioeconomic factors. In a sense these general socioeconomic or environmental factors can be a third source of signal influencing family interaction. A mother who must have a child toilet-trained before she or he can go to nursery school, so that the mother can work, is likely to exert pressures upon the child to become toilet-trained. The mother who is concerned about safety in the neighborhood is not likely to encourage the child's free exploration of the environment.

INITIATIVE VS. GUILT

In the next, or third, stage of development, children's focus changes from concerns about mastering their bodies to concerns about their abilities to influence the outside world. Erikson considers this the stage where patterns of initiative are set, and that undue difficulty with abilities to manipulate the outside world successfully will result in guilt. Guilt arises out of the anger and antagonism generated by being thwarted. The guilt arises not only from frustration but from a desire to "push out," if these impulses have had disastrous results in the past. Characteristic of this stage is the child's developing aggressive behavior toward his or her environment. He or she tries to manipulate the environment and people and can sometimes be seen as quite competitive in the sense of wanting to be more powerful than anyone else. For instance, children want to make the biggest house, ride their bikes the fastest, and own the biggest toy truck. This type of vying is directed toward establishing one's superiority in manipulating the environment, along with establishing one's success relative to others.

It is this period that is often referred to as the Oedipal stage. Very briefly, the sense of this has to do with the child's wish to be the most important figure, first, to the mother and later, in the case of girls, to their fathers—a wish which means that the parent of the same sex must be dis-

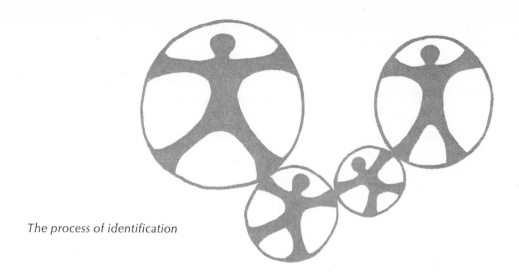

The process of identification

posed of. During the course of this stage, which lasts two or three years, the child feels intense emotions of love, anger, and despair. Eventually the child renounces the competition with the same sex parent, at least in part because of fears of retaliation. As the child has angry feelings about the parent and wishes to annihilate the mother or father, the child in turn feels that that parent has similar feelings about him or her. A noteworthy feature of this Oedipal struggle is its sexual nature. The child both pretends the sexuality in his parents' relationship and experiences physical pleasure at the manipulation of his or her own genitals. He or she connects genital activity with the special status relationship and wishes to engage the favored parent in such a relationship, however immature and warped his or her notion of such a relationship may be. Typically, the child resolves the conflict by identifying with the same sex parent and becoming like the mother or father rather than striving to compete. This identification involves incorporation of parental values. This, then, is the stage at which sex patterns become most noticeable. A considerable group of scholars hold that definite sexual behavior patterning occurs at this stage, although there is controversy about whether the patterning is culturally or biologically based. Erikson points out that the play of children at this age has characteristic variations. He notes that, when building with blocks, girls tend to make round, enclosing structures while boys tend to build tall, intrusive structures. Generally, girls are felt to be more passive and nurturing than boys, and boys are considered more aggressive and venture-some than girls. Again note that there is controversy over whether these traits are inherent or culturally induced.

Instead of again turning to Peg, let us now consider Michael, her four-year-old brother. Michael's boundless energy is characteristic of children of this age, and it is the quality Erikson refers to when he talks about children at this stage having consolidated their prior learnings so that they may now attack the outside world. Michael can be expected to venture forth confidently into the neighborhood, in contrast to his earlier confinement to the boundaries of the home. In Michael's circle of friends, there is likely to be a considerable amount of testing. In their play one will hear such things as: "Mine is better than yours," "I can do it better than you," "I can build a bigger house than you can," and similar boasts. Characteristically, adults, on hearing such claims, may intervene on the basis of good manners, the golden rule, or some such thing, and take it much more seriously than do the children, who seem unconcerned about the competitive boasts of their playmates.

Within the family this same theme is reworked in concerns about "Who is best?" To Michael, his status compared with Peg's would be of particular concern. Parents with children of this age are frequently bombarded with statements like "I can dress myself and Peg can't," "I don't make a mess when I eat, and she spits up all over," or "I can help you clean the house, but the baby can't." Children at this age actively seek recognition from their parents for things they are able to accomplish and repeatedly make the case that they should have first place in their parents' affection. The converse situation—with the same goal—occurs in some families, where an older child will copy the baby's behavior, hoping, of course, that a measure of the baby's favored position will thus become his or hers.

Continuing our vignette, picture the following scene:

> Father goes to call Michael for dinner and finds him playing with two neighbor boys in the driveway. He overhears Michael saying, "No, you didn't, I did it better the last time, and anyway I'd have mowed you down before you got around the corner." He sees his father and says, "Hey, Dad, Fred thinks he can be a better Indian Scout than me. He thinks he'd have captured my fort, but did you see me? I saw him before he took ten steps." Father responds, "I'd surely hate to be the one you boys were trying to get; you certainly play a tough game. Maybe

you boys could come back after dinner because Michael has to come in for dinner." Michael says, "Oh, no, Dad, Mom said not for another half hour yet. I can stay here and finish my game." Father responds, "I know, son, but I came home a little early and we are going to eat a little earlier than your mother thought. . . . Mom said I'd better call you while she was getting things ready because she knew you wouldn't know we were going to eat so early." "Gee, guys, I guess I'll have to go, but I'll see you later, and this time I get first pick."

Notice the options that the father had in responding. He could have corrected Michael's grammar, or insisted that he play nicely with his friends, or conveyed to Michael that he certainly expected him to be the best. Now each of these things might indicate an underlying attitude that would also be expressed in other ways in his relationship with Michael. What Jim, the father, did do, probably without thinking, was to respond to the boys' need for approval and reinforce that what they were expressing was all right. If he were concerned with Michael's meeting some standards of perfection that came from his own background, then he might have corrected the boy's grammar, pointing out how Mike was not meeting his expectations. Jim might have been upset by Michael's supposed lack of kindness to his friends, if he himself had not come to terms with his own competitiveness. Similarly, a statement that he expected Michael always to be the best would be another manifestation of the same problem. In any case, Jim's approach to his son served to reinforce and encourage Michael in mastering the tasks of this developmental stage.

INDUSTRY VS. INFERIORITY

The fourth phase of development, paralleling the primary school years, is characterized by the development of pride in industry. Attention is focused on gaining mastery of cultural tools; in the case of our culture, this involves intellectual and technical skills. In this culture, a crucial part of a child's developing identity is composed of an awareness of the things one can do. A school-age child very quickly develops an awareness of whether he or she is a "good" or "bad" student, and both adults and children relate to the child on the basis of this identification. For example, children who are identified as good readers are regarded as capable and

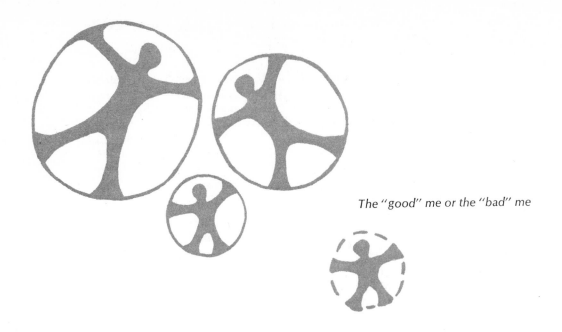

The "good" me or the "bad" me

dealt with as people who can do things. This, in turn, reinforces their desire and accompanying ability to do them.

Conversely, children who do not have good experiences in setting up a reading pattern frequently come to view themselves as not bright or not good in schoolwork. Frequently, other areas of competence, such as art or mathematics, are overlooked as everyone becomes more involved in the child's failures than in his or her successes. It is easy for children to incorporate more of the notions of failure into their views of themselves and carry over these negative valuations into areas in which they have a natural competence. A pervasive sense of inferiority governs their lives, and they may start into a career of being a failure. Some children may attempt to compensate by becoming the class clown or instigator, which affords them a certain measure of esteem with their classmates and gets them recognition from adults, even though it may be negative.

It is of interest to note the cultural values that are transmitted at this stage. In a highly urbanized culture, intellectual skills tend to be rewarded while manual skills are of secondary importance. In a rural area, the converse might be true. In the past in this culture, it was considered more important for a girl to develop the qualities that would make her a good wife and mother than to accomplish much intellectually. In any setting, there is a tendency to place greater value on certain skills while paying relatively little attention to other skill areas.

Imagine a family picnic celebrating Peg's grandparents' 40th wedding anniversary. Jim's two brothers, Bill and Roger, and his sister, Ann, are there with all of their families. Peg's mother, Lora, and Ann are engaged in a conversation:

> *Ann:* My, Michael seems to be really growing up to be a fine boy. I hope he does well in school and isn't like my Johnnie; he just can't seem to do anything right. We're thinking of making him repeat the second grade so he can learn to read better. If you can't read, you just aren't going to make it. All he does is get into mischief in school; the teacher says he just doesn't concentrate.
>
> *Betty (Roger's wife):* You know, that's an interesting idea. I wish we had done that with our Jack. Maybe if we had, he would have learned to do better at school. As it is now, all he likes to do is tinker with things; he's always building things or working with old cars. Roger gets awfully upset about it, because he wants him to go to college and get a good education so he won't be a mechanic like him.
>
> *Jill (Bill's wife):* I've never had that trouble with my children; they've been straight-A students.
>
> *Lora:* If this is what I have to look forward to when the children get to school, I don't know if we'll make it.

As is obvious from this typical form of interaction, this stage of life involves the child's mastering the necessary tools to equip him or her to fill projected roles in society. Success in achieving at this developmental stage is contingent on the child's capacities and interests in fitting into roles prescribed for him or her both by parents and in the wider cultural milieu.

IDENTITY VS. ROLE DIFFUSION

The fifth stage, corresponding to the adolescent years, is one that, in this culture, has been given a lot of attention and thought. Our discussion of this stage will necessarily be limited and will emphasize only main trends or themes of adolescence. It is interesting to note that adolescence is not the same in all cultures; in our culture, it is like an hiatus in which one is neither a child nor an adult. It is an ambiguous status fraught with contradictions. We give adolescents many mixed messages which other cultures do not. An eighteen-year-old freshman college student is not expected to be a responsible contributing adult in the economic sphere, and he or she is still very much dependent upon decisions made by others. On the other hand, he or she is supposed to be a responsible person, to vote wisely, to go to war if necessary. If the young adult is out in public and acts like a child, he or she reaps the censure of adults who expect "responsible behavior." In the sexual sphere, there is great discontinuity. In this culture, it is still considered that actual sexual intercourse is something that should be delayed until one is an adult. But in our culture one is not viewed as an "adult" until one is established in a work role and in a stable heterosexual relationship; in many instances, this situation is not achieved until the late twenties or even the early thirties for those entering professions requiring long-term higher education. Adolescence tends to be a never-never land, not circumscribed by age limits, but related to the establishment of adult work roles; it may sometimes extend from age twelve to the mid- or late twenties—a lengthy period of time in which one is neither a child nor an adult.

In other cultures, and on certain socioeconomic levels of American culture, a child goes immediately into adult status at the point of puberty. In certain situations, in our culture, the period of adolescence may be circumscribed. A thirteen-year-old girl may marry, have children, and immediately be perceived as an adult without any identifiable adolescent stage. Similarly, a boy may terminate school at an early age, be employed in a laborer role, and not experience a prolonged period between being a child and being an adult. Adolescence in our culture is a middle- and upper-class phenomenon, and its length is closely related to position in a socioeconomic and class structure.

Erikson views adolescence from a middle-class perspective and sees as its primary task the establishment of identity. Identity, in his framework, consists of all of the attributes that one might think of in answering the question "Who am I?" To answer this question the individual must have settled the following issues: How is he or she similar to and different from his or her parents? What is his or her position vis-à-vis significant

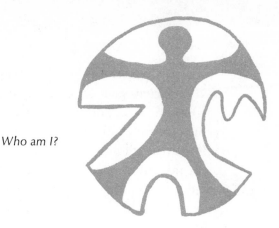

Who am I?

social groups? In reviewing the ideologies learned through the years, is he or she going to accept these basic values as a guide for living his or her life? If not, what will replace them? What vocation is he or she going to choose? And who is he or she going to select as friends or sexual partners? Biologically, the adolescent's body is developed and he or she may experience the sexual drives of an adult while still vacillating between childhood and adult status.

As adolescents seek a resolution of these questions, they no longer view their parents in the same way they did as children. Instead of viewing parents as the prime source of information and guidance, adolescents vacillate. At one time they seem to be seeking the parents' direction, while at another they go in an entirely different direction, usually that of a significant peer or reference group. The major conflict of this period surrounds the issue of dependence vs. independence. At some points adolescents revert to being their parents' child, while at other times they strive to establish themselves as individuals in their own right. This conflict is enacted through patterns of behavior in which on some days the adolescent associates with peers that his or her parents approve of, while on other days he or she chooses to associate with those of whom his or her parents strongly disapprove. The peer group is of particular importance during this time and serves as an anchoring point in the adolescent's attempt to free himself or herself from the parents' primacy.

Since so many of the tasks of adolescents are achieved within the context of various peer groups, it is important to note the parents' reactions to these groups. The parents' reactions are the reciprocal of the adolescent's—parents will vary in the degree to which they react to their children's apparent throwing aside of all the values that they hold dear. In some instances, parents will feel competitive with the groups with whom their child is closely associated and will express this by setting up rigid rules about with whom the adolescent may associate and under what circumstances. A usual response to this type of rule-setting is for the child to act out against it and not follow the rules, which may precipitate further rule-setting by the parents.

An additional problem in this youth-oriented culture is the value placed upon youth and the devaluation of growing older. Many parents are at the point of feeling themselves growing older when their children are adolescents, and complications can arise in several ways: Parents may relive their own youth through the child and not allow the child to be his or her own self; they may resent their child's ascendancy while they perceive themselves as declining and respond by derogating the child's manner of dressing, choice of friends, and abilities. One of the solutions children may reach in the face of these types of conflicts is to ally themselves closely with a gang as a means of achieving an identity separate from that of the parents. It is at this stage that an adolescent can become allied with gangs perceived as delinquent. Depending upon the reactions of parents or significant others at this stage, an adolescent may become "locked into" a deviant self-identity as the only way to achieve independence from the parent.

In Erikson's terminology, role diffusion is the negative outcome of this developmental stage. In this situation the adolescent's identity consists of conflicting bits and pieces instead of an integrated feeling of unity. It is as if the individual cannot experience a feeling of satisfaction in knowing who he or she is as a separate person. The adolescent has failed to find the answer to the question "Who am I?" and instead lives his or her life as a reflection, either positive or negative, of what other people perceive him or her to be. This individual has not internalized his or her ideas and is unable to relate to others as an independent individual, but instead attempts to find an identity in being whatever the group wishes him or her to be at any particular moment. Conversely an individual may maintain his or her identity only through consistently acting out against any ideas of the group.

INTIMACY VS. ISOLATION

As pointed out, the transition between adolescence and adulthood in our society is not as clearly demarcated as it is in other cultures. Achievement of adulthood hinges upon moving into certain adult roles and responsibilities not necessarily associated with a specific age. In our society a number of persons of advanced chronological years are still working on adolescence or earlier developmental tasks. As an example of this, think back to the scene of Michael and his friends playing in the driveway and the competitive, "me first" attitude they expressed. What is appropriate for Michael at age four will not be appropriate at age thirty, but many thirty-year-old men may still relate to others predominantly in this mode. Erikson characterizes the sixth developmental stage as a stage in which the individual, secure in his or her own identity, is able to move into intimate relationships with others. The central issues of young adulthood surround the establishment of intimacy as opposed to isolation; a key issue at this stage revolves around the manner in which one relates to people. Based on the changes in self that are to have been solidified during the adolescent phase, the adult is now expected to get over the hurdle of taking this new self and merging with another. This does not mean that everyone has to get married, in a formalized or legal sense, but an individual should have the capacity for developing deep, meaningful relationships with other human beings.

In the process of becoming intimate with someone else, the individual risks becoming vulnerable, and in so doing, must be secure enough in his or her own identity that he or she will not be destroyed or engulfed by such a close relationship. For instance, the young man who sees himself as athletically inclined, a lover of music, and the life of the party, and who thinks he has the potential to make it in business, must feel fairly definite and secure about these aspects of himself before he risks exposing himself to a woman or another man in an intimate way—only to receive a nonconfirmatory response to his self-image. Traumatic experiences in this realm lead some people to abandon the quest for intimacy and to isolate themselves as a means of protection. The process of establishing stable relationships involves this type of exposure, reaching compromises, and in essence, the fusing of identity with that of someone else. At this stage a common experience is progressively to decrease talking about "I" and increasingly to refer to "we." This fused identity does not indicate that the individuals have lost their individual identities to the relatonship, but that they have found pieces of their identities that merge or complement one another, while other aspects of their identities remain uniquely their own.

At this stage of life, certain events usually take place, such as marriage, establishment of a work career, and development of a stable social network outside of one's own family. Birth of children necessitates establishment of oneself within the context of a newly created family structure. In each of these relationships the individual has to achieve some merging of his or her identity with that of the other, but in the process must maintain a sense of self simultaneously as a separate and unique individual of worth. The danger at this stage of life is for the person to seek to find himself or herself vicariously, through a relationship with another. For example, the young man who questions his abilities to "make it" may seek out a young woman and marry her in the hopes that she will provide the necessary reassurance that will enable him to succeed. Usually these relationships have unanticipated consequences. The clinging vine who adoringly cheers her hero on all too often becomes an emotional parasite drawing strength from him. The two become merged in their mutual inadequacies. A common socially acceptable example for women is the twenty-year-old woman attracted to the highly successful older man because of what he can provide. Her identity becomes that of her husband. In a certain sense, she is a success because of her husband's success.

At this stage, families are started. Success in launching children into the world is related to the appropriate resolution of the dilemma of merging one's identity with another while simultaneously maintaining a sense of one's personal self. A parent who has not achieved a sense of his or her own individuality has difficulty in establishing boundaries between himself or herself and a child. In this instance, the child may play out a part of the parent's existence. At the other extreme, parents who have not been able to merge their individualities successfully and so maintain isolation in marriage tend not to give anything of themselves to their children.

GENERATIVITY VS. STAGNATION

In the seventh stage, nuclear conflict revolves around the issue of generativity vs. stagnation. Generativity, from Erikson's perspective, involves the ability to invest one's creative energies in promoting the social welfare of society at large rather than investing energies solely in the family group. This stage corresponds typically with middle age for most people: the time when children are launched out of the home and parents are confronted by a need to redefine their roles in relationship to one another, to their family, and to a larger world outside the family. Individuals frequently do a major assessment of their accomplishments in life and make peace with dreams that will never be. For example, a man may need to come to grips with the fact that he will never be "chairman of the board" because his career pattern to date has not moved him in this direction. He comes to a realization, "If I haven't made my move by now, I'm never going to make it." A common situation for many women, of course, is when their last child goes off to college or a job away from home or is married; this is a point at which her traditional role as a woman must be redefined. This stage typically is a time when individuals become aware of aging processes and sense that time is moving on. Another generation is moving into the spotlight, particularly in this youth-oriented culture.

This is usually the time also when parents lose their own parents. All these occurrences may represent to the individual that he or she has come to the "end of the line"; on the other hand, it may represent the challenge of assuming leadership in the larger social sphere. The critical factor influencing the outcome is the ability of the individual to redefine his or her role in society as having something of value to offer, even though it may not be what was envisioned as an adolescent dream. For example, the businessman who does not become chairman of the board may come to the realization that, although he has not achieved this dream, he is making a contribution in his work, has a Boy Scout troop, is a leader of a community group, or in some other way is making a societal contribution. This type of resolution provides an opportunity for the individual to rid oneself of constricting dreams and fantasies about the direction of one's life. Achieving this commonly involves a change in orientation from a very materialistic view of "making it" to a more interpersonal orientation. Open communication, making another person feel good, helping someone less for-

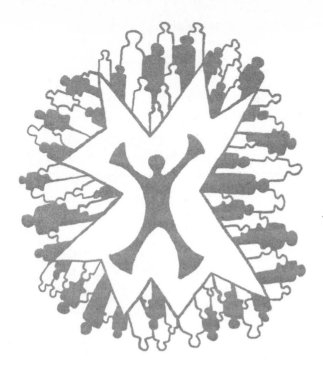

The individual as captive

tunate, trying to be concerned about issues of justice, and broader social issues become predominant themes rather than the earlier preoccupations of providing a living for a growing family. Women who have not followed a career undergo similar types of changes, with the focus in their lives moving away from caring for children. Ideally, they become involved in activities outside of the home; their focus changes from the nuclear family to a greater involvement in broader social issues. For example, the nurse who has been both a mother and a nurse may become increasingly involved in such issues as giving leadership to professional nursing; instead of only running her unit she may become involved in a group that is deciding whether nurses should strike—her attention changes from merely doing her job—being a wife, mother, and nurse—to broader issues of social justice.

Individuals unable to make the transitions of this period are forever captive to their unfulfilled dreams. The prospect of growing old is frightening, rather than a period of growth in which they can realize a new type of fulfillment. Energies are invested in holding back the tide of time. Witness the middle-aged woman who tries to dress as a young girl; the parents who insist on leading their children's lives for them, thus vicariously being that age again; the man who increasingly expands the cocktail hour from lunchtime to bedtime, deluding himself through alcohol that he has fulfilled his youthful fantasies; and the stereotypic man who starts affairs with younger women so he can continue to see himself as young, virile, and attractive to women.

EGO INTEGRITY VS. DESPAIR

Development in the eighth and final stage of life centers on coming to some meaningful harmonious terms with the kind of life one has lived. The nuclear conflict here is that of ego integrity vs. despair. The quality of ego integrity arises out of the elderly person's evaluative review of his or her life, and from the acceptance of that life, with whatever joys and sorrows it held, as a necessary and worthwhile piece of work. This is not to say that one must view one's past through rose-colored glasses or that one must have had, on the whole, a gratifying existence. It does mean that the elderly person must be able to find a sense of order and purpose in his or her life; to feel that the moment in the sun was not wasted; that his or her productions—children, things, ideas—will continue to be valuable to future generations; and that this one life has been lived as well as possible.

The person who has succeeded in achieving a reasonable degree of ego integrity is in a strong position to weather the many depredations that accompany the advancing years. The older person faces declining health—physical powers are diminishing, senses are not as acute—and also the need for turning over the controlling position to the middle-aged succeeding generation. In this culture, with its high value on youth, there are few rewards for growing old. All too often, there is no place for the older person in the surrounding social structure. To his or her children's families, the older person may be a nuisance to be cared for rather than a contributing member of the family constellation. Faced with the loss of friends of the same age, the elderly person has few persons who are able to appreciate his or her reflections on the life of the past. In short, the elderly person experiences many losses that must be worked through with some sense of forbearance. Facing these losses from a backlog of positive experiences of feeling one has been a contributing member of society, an individual may successfully relinquish life with a feeling of accomplishment in serving his or her purpose. Conversely, the individual who has not successfully mastered the tasks of development through the life stages faces this period of life with despair. The despair grows out of a preoccupation with the failures of life and a wish to redo and recapture opportunities that are forever past. The final disappointment is death.

SUMMARY

Erikson views the life cycle as consisting of eight stages, each of which is characterized by its own particular nuclear conflict. The individual is called upon to develop new skills and competencies as he or she rises to the challenge of each stage; how well one succeeds depends on the extent to which one masters the tasks of the stage. The less one achieves, the more one is subject to the negative outcomes for that stage, and the more difficulty one will have during the subsequent stages. For instance, the four-year-old, near the beginning of the stage of initiative, is faced with the world outside his or her immediate home environment. The child transfers some attention away from the self and toward trying to achieve some mastery over that environment, exploring the neighborhood, making friends, competing with playmates, and testing himself or herself in various ways that had not occurred previously. The four-year-old is involved with the nuclear conflict of initiative versus guilt, and failure to achieve mastery results in feelings of guilt over the impulses and feelings he or she has about extending himself or herself into the environment. A similar process occurs at each stage; only the issues constituting the conflict differ according to the stage.

The stages and associated nuclear conflicts cited by Erikson are as follows: (1) trust versus mistrust, (2) autonomy versus shame and doubt, (3) initiative versus guilt, (4) industry versus inferiority, (5) identity versus role diffusion, (6) intimacy versus isolation, (7) generativity versus stagnation, (8) ego integrity versus despair.

In summary, people progress through the life stages always in interaction with others who accommodate and adjust to the alterations in social roles as the individual grows and changes. Success or failure in making the desired progression is a composite of the individual's capabilities, both physical and psychological, in mastering the developmental tasks within a social network that either facilitates or blocks this progression.

FURTHER READINGS

Aug, Robert, and Bright, Thomas. "A Study of Wed and Unwed Motherhood in Adolescents and Young Adults." *Journal of American Academy of Child Psychiatry* 9 (October 1970): 557-594.

Bowlby, John. *Child Care and the Growth of Love.* Baltimore, Md.: Penguin Books, 1953.

Bronfrenbrenner, Urie., ed. *Influences on Human Development.* Hinsdale, Ill.: The Dryden Press, 1972.

Caplan, Gerald., ed. *Prevention of Mental Disorders in Children.* New York: Basic Books, 1961.

Corbett, Jacqueline. "Reclaiming the Infuriated in a Ghetto-Area School." *American Journal of Nursing* 70 (July 1970): 1476.

Duran, Maria. "Family-Centered Care and the Adolescent's Quest for Self-Identity." *Nursing Clinics of North America* 7 (March 1972): 65-73.

Erikson, Erik. *Childhood and Society.* 2d ed. New York: W. W. Norton, 1950.

Group for the Advancement of Psychiatry. *Normal Adolescence.* New York: Charles Scribner & Sons, 1968.

Kimmel, Douglas C. *Adulthood and Aging,* New York: John Wiley & Sons, 1974.

Maas, Henry S., and Kuypers, Joseph A. *From Thirty to Seventy.* San Francisco: Jossey-Bass Publishers, 1974.

Mental Health: From Infancy Through Adolescence. Report of the Joint Commission on Mental Health of Children, pp. 165-66. New York: Harper and Row, Publishers, 1973.

Meyer, Virginia. "The Psychology of the Young Adult." *Nursing Clinics of North America* 8 (March 1973): 5-14.

Diekelman, Nancy, and Galloway, Karen. "The Middle Years."

CHAPTER THREE: LIFE CRISES,
DEFENSIVE MECHANISMS,
AND THE EVOLUTION
OF COPING STYLES

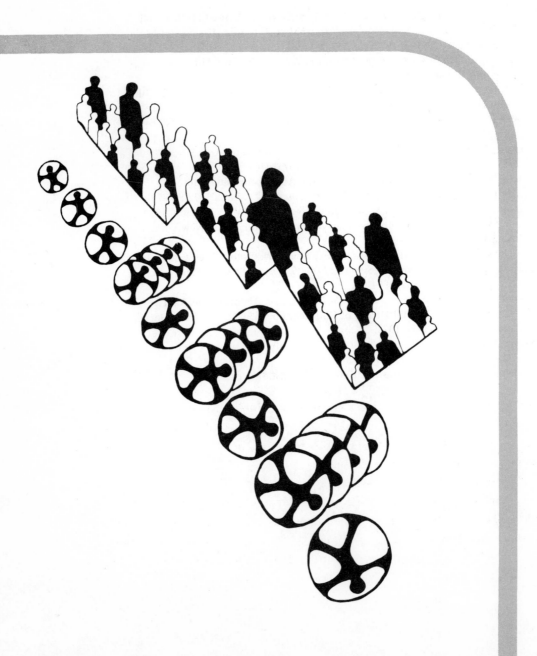

A further element necessary in understanding any one particular person's behavior is the influence of crises on his or her life. Crises have been defined from many different perspectives, but most theorists agree that their essential quality is that of a turning point or upheaval in the usual life pattern. These upheavals are always time limited (6-8 weeks being the most commonly identified outer limit), and they always result in a change (for better or worse) in the coping style of the person. Having weathered a crisis, the person is never exactly the same—he or she is either better or less able to perform effectively with subsequent problems. Crises range from unexpected, highly dramatic, accidental, or situational occurrences to the sequential maturational changes described in Erikson's developmental framework (see Chapter 2).

Typically an individual develops a unique personal style of responding to problems. Some aggressively tackle the problem and will not rest until a solution is attained. Others take a rather passive stance, fully expecting that something will happen to resolve or otherwise ameliorate the problem. Whatever the person's usual problem-solving style, within his or her particular context, it works. Individuals can be said to be in crisis when their usual problem-solving patterns no longer succeed in solving a certain problem, and they are unable to invoke more productive patterns. In effect, they are blocked in attaining some goal. An important characteristic of a crisis is that the goal is one that cannot be given up; the person feels driven to solve the problem that blocks the goal, but remains unable to do so. It is this inability to resolve the problem that throws the person into a state of disequilibrium or imbalance, and a relatively predictable sequence of events ensues.

Before discussing the typical phases of crisis, let us consider some usual problem-solving steps. First, a person encounters a meaningful stimulus that places him or her in a state of disequilibrium—that is, he or she is motivated to take some action toward attaining whatever goal he or she associates with the originating stimulus. Let us identify this state of being

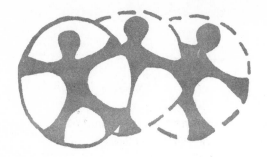

Change as a result of crises

motivated to attain a goal as synonymous with being faced with a problem. The next step in the problem-solving sequence is for the person to categorize the problem. He or she makes judgments about its nature and imagines the actions he or she might take to solve the problem, using any past experience with similar problems in making these judgments and projections. Having chosen a course of action, the person tries it out. Should this particular sequence succeed in attaining the goal, it is stored for future reference. Should it not succeed, this behavior is discarded; the individual continues the process until he or she settles on another solution. When this person next meets a stimulus that produces a similar state of disequilibrium, he or she makes use of the learnings from the prior situation.

Caplan describes four phases in the development of a crisis.[1] In the first phase, the person encounters a problem that he or she cannot solve, although it is felt necessary to do so. All the problem-solving approaches tried have been ineffective in reducing the tension or in re-establishing equilibrium. In the second phase, there is an increase of tension accompanied by an escalating state of upset and ineffectuality, as the person becomes immersed in this problem that he or she is still unable to solve. Experiencing failure at the second stage, the person moves to the third stage, where he or she makes use of internal and external resources which may not have been called on before. An analogy might be made to the long-distance runner and the final spurt of adrenalin that allows him to surpass his usual physical capacities. At this stage, the person tries approaches to problem-solving that have not been in his or her prior coping

---

1. Gerald Caplan, *Principles of Preventive Psychiatry* (New York: Basic Books, 1964), pp. 40-41.

repertoire. Frequently these new approaches will involve some change in definition of the problem. Going back to Peg's family (described in Chapter 2) for an example, let us imagine a crisis in which Jim, her father, is laid off from work for four weeks because of a major reorganization in the company, which has jeopardized his position. One could say that he is redefining the problem if he shifts from viewing himself simply as the breadwinner of the family who is no longer bringing home the bread to seeing himself as the head of the family who is serving many useful functions that are highly valued by all family members. The one function, "breadwinner," is in need of adjustment, but this role is not the only one available to him; he is valued for a far wider range of capacities.

Another way in which Jim might redefine his situation is to begin to identify other companies that would value his skills and then to seek out alternative employment. In the process, he discovers that the company he has worked for is not the whole of his world, a fact he had not noticed before. Still another alternative for Jim would be to give up some of the benefits of his current position and, for the sake of security, take a less rewarding role within the same company. Note that in all these solutions, Jim's change of role will involve accompanying changes vis-à-vis significant social groups. Some solutions would lead to an improved position, while others would diminish the importance of his social role.

In some cases a person, no matter what he or she tries, is unable to solve the problem and then moves to a fourth phase, that of continued and rising tension which may culminate in major personality disorganization. Lofland[2] has noted that the initiating stimulus which we have identified as leading to a crisis usually entails the loss of self-esteem, one way or another, and that a major factor in problem-solving endeavors is an attempt to save face. One reason that some solutions are said to be less productive than others is that they involve settling for lower self-esteem in order to escape tensions. For example, if Jim took a lesser job as a solution and it did not bring him as much satisfaction as his prior job, he would experience a blow to his self-esteem and begin to identify himself as a less capable person.

Frequently, people in situations such as this lash out in a variety of ways and thus begin a vicious cycle that leads to the establishment of a

---

2. John Lofland, *Deviance and Identity* (Englewood Cliffs, N.J.: Prentice Hall, 1969).

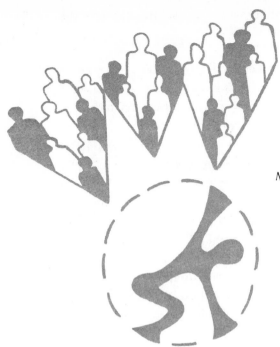

Major personality disorganization

deviant role. A man, for example, might begin to be extremely cantankerous to everyone and become locked into the role of company "crank." Others might then begin to identify him as a "crank" and to isolate him from all warm, positive types of interpersonal exchanges, which in turn would lead to an increasingly lessened self-esteem and another round of lashing out. One reason that people in crises so easily get locked into roles they otherwise would avoid is that the crisis produces a heightened state of vulnerability.

People in crisis are more susceptible to any influence, good or bad, than they are under ordinary circumstances. In some instances, this vulnerability may work to their advantage. For example, if the man who had settled on the role of company "crank" at some earlier time were faced with a new crisis, he might then respond more favorably. Suppose the company "crank" again faces the threat of losing his job. The outcome of this new crisis may be a revamping of his type of coping, so that he relies on people in an increasingly positive way, thus re-establishing a supportive network for himself and abandoning his isolated, "I'll go it myself" attitude.

A word about the time-limited nature of crises: A crisis exists only as long as a solution to the problem has not been reached. As soon as some tension-reducing behavior is adopted, whether it be a productive or non-productive solution, the crisis subsides. Within 6 to 8 weeks the individual usually has settled upon a course of action that serves to reduce the tension and becomes incorporated into his or her typical coping style.

Two types of crises commonly arise: situational or accidental and maturational or developmental. A situational crisis is one that is triggered by some unanticipated event. According to Caplan,[3] such a crisis occurs when a hazardous event threatens the individual. Common examples are amputation of a body part, loss of a loved one, moving to a new home, changing jobs, and accidents. A developmental crisis involves the loosening up of previous personality structure so that the individual may move on to a new maturational stage. For a period of time, the behavior patterns appropriate to an earlier stage of development no longer work, while new patterns of behavior have not as yet been stabilized. During this period, the person is faced with the need to restructure his or her relationships with significant others and in this sense faces a developmental crisis.

In both situational and developmental crises, the person must make a shift in role definitions and relationships with significant others. Individuals who are faced with the necessity of reappraising and readjusting social roles experience anxiety.

ANXIETY

The most generally accepted view of anxiety is that of an uncanny, unpleasant feeling that something is not right, always accompanying some threat to individual security. These threats may take many forms. In some instances, the threat triggering anxiety is easily discernible, while in others the observer would need to understand a great deal about the background of the individual to be able to accurately identify the source of his or her anxiety. For example, an infant may experience anxiety if flooded with stimuli that he or she cannot mediate when the mother is not available to hold the child or provide some type of channeling or relief from tension.

---

3. Caplan, *Preventive Psychiatry*, p. 86.

Another common example is that of the student who must write an essay for class but cannot figure out what the teacher expects. Other examples may not be quite so apparent. For example, in the Japanese culture people stand much closer to one another while they are talking. When a person from Japan engages in conversation with an American who has a different orientation toward territoriality, the American experiences anxiety because his or her personal life space is violated.

May defines anxiety as ". . . the apprehension cued off by a threat to some value which the individual holds essential to his existence as a personality."[4] The values alluded to are unique to the individual. To one person, power and prestige are essential; to another, independence and freedom; while a third's security is based on being loved by others. Whatever the value, it is seen by the person as necessary, and when it is threatened, he or she experiences that discomforting state called anxiety.

When a person experiences anxiety, he or she usually does something to try to reduce the feeling of unpleasantness or uncertainty. Thus, anxiety serves the purpose of focusing the person's attention and behavior so that remedial action can be taken to eliminate anxiety. This focus frequently leads to more effective problem-solving behavior, and in this sense, a manageable amount of anxiety is said to be "growth-producing." For example, in an examination situation most people experience anxiety that is apparent in such physical manifestations as sweaty hands, inability to eat or sleep beforehand, and general restlessness. The examination situation poses a threat to the student's definition of himself or herself. The physical manifestations, which signal the individual that he or she is anxious, may serve to spur a student to concentrate on study and to organize the information presented during the course. During the examination itself, the person may experience a heightened capacity for recall and do better on the exam than he or she had anticipated. In this instance the anxiety experienced has served to motivate the person in ways that are growth-producing.

If the person is unable to handle the anxiety effectively, it escalates and begins to make him or her less productive, rather than stimulating his capacities to respond in a useful fashion. The person becomes consumed by anxiety and is less able to focus on the realities of the situation and

---

4. Rollo May, *The Meaning of Anxiety* (New York: The Ronald Press, 1950), p. 191.

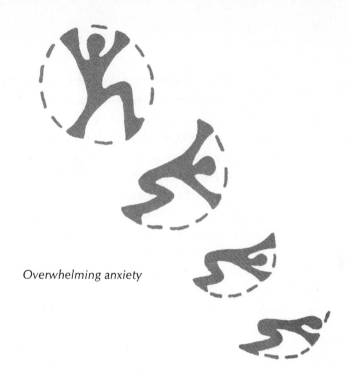

Overwhelming anxiety

productively channel his or her energies. As the anxiety increases, his or her perceptual field becomes narrowed. An example of this is a student who is so anxious about an exam that when he opens the book to study he cannot focus on the words written there, but is totally preoccupied with his fears about the examination.

As the level of anxiety increases further, the usual control mechanisms no longer work; the result may be panic, in which the individual is totally disorganized, consumed with anxiety, and no longer able to perceive his or her situation with accuracy. The person is inundated by stimuli, has a subjective feeling of impending doom or horror of some sort, and feels totally helpless to control his or her destiny at that moment. This is indeed an extremely incapacitated state and is synonymous with the situation described in Caplan's fourth stage of crisis, that is, the stage in which continued and rising tension from the unresolved problem situation can culminate in major personality disorganization. At the height of the upset, when the usual controls are not functioning, people are frequently flooded with memories from their past lives which are either painful or unaccept-

able to them in their usual state of functioning and so have been completely walled off. This situation is untenable and calls forth emergency
measures to reduce the anxiety and re-establish control. While the person
seeks to regain control, he or she is at a point of openness where major
personality changes occur. Sometimes these changes result in behavior that
in our culture is frequently identified as evidence of "mental illness," but
in other cases the changes may bring about the development of increased
potentialities for dealing with problematic situations. Whatever the individual does in his or her attempts to regain control, coupled with the responses of significant others to these attempts, has long-range implications
in his or her life.

R. D. Laing,[5] in his description of the schizophrenogenic condition,
describes the individual who goes through life playing out the roles others
choose rather than becoming a person in his or her own right. Panic, for
this person, occurs when he or she can no longer live in the pattern established by others; and at this point he or she breaks out of these bonds in
the interests of becoming a person in his or her own right.

Take, for example, Alice, a girl who chose nursing not because of any
consideration for the kind of person she felt herself to be, but because of
obligations to, and expectations of, others. Alice proceeds along this road
until she meets a crucial event, a traumatic first day in the delivery room,
where a mother delivers a stillborn child; there is some question about
why the doctor was not notified of the diminished fetal heart tone. Alice
returns to her room in the student residence, broods about this occurrence,
and wonders if she should have done something. As she attempts to go to
sleep that night, she ponders the situations more and more, begins to question her capabilities, and finds her anxiety mounting. Thinking about
having to go back the next day, Alice goes into a panic state.

One could say that this experience stimulated some concern about
herself that Alice has kept out of her awareness, such as a wish that she
were having a baby; or that she finds the whole nursing experience most
distasteful, dislikes the regimented life of being a nursing student, hates
taking care of people, gets no personal satisfaction from ever feeling she
has done a good job; or that she is really not adept at nursing techniques
and can never do anything satisfactorily. These are not thoughts available

---

5. R. D. Laing, *The Divided Self* (New York: Pantheon Press, 1960).

to her under ordinary circumstances, although she recalls that at the beginning of her sophomore year she wondered if she were cut out for nursing and suggested to her parents that she wanted to leave college and try something different. Her parents were adamant about her making the most of this opportunity (one which they had never had) and assured her that she would certainly make a good nurse and that the family was counting on her to succeed.

During the night after the incident with the stillborn baby, which has confirmed (in her own eyes) Alice's feelings of incompetence and inability to function, these unacceptable thoughts break through and can no longer be denied. Faced with this situation, a student who had legitimately chosen nursing as an expression of the kind of person she wanted to be would simply conclude that her decision to become a nurse was unwise and that the solution would be for her to leave. However, a girl like Alice, who is in the situation out of obligation to her parents and who has not developed any feeling of being a person in her own right but is playing out the roles that her parents have decided are appropriate, cannot reach such a straightforward solution. She becomes entangled in denying her own perceptions, trying to keep her feelings under control, hating her parents for imposing their will on her, and hating herself, both for buckling under and for not being able to live up to their expectations. In short, she ends up in a position in which there are no moves that are satisfactory to her.

Alice, enmeshed in such feelings, experiences anxiety because she can make no satisfactory moves to solve the problem. Faced with a situation in which she can see no solutions, not even denial, and in which loss of identity as a potential nurse is equated with total loss of self-esteem, her anxiety mounts until she is in a state of panic. In this state, she is only too aware of at least some of her denied feelings. There are a number of possible ways Alice may take to resolve her feelings of panic. She may move toward a resolution in which she throws aside all the usual norms and settles for nonperformance of societal roles. In most instances such behavior would be classified as psychotic, in that it is antisocial, disorganized, and impulsive from society's viewpoint. Laing[6] makes the point that in this state a person like Alice has the opportunity to reconstruct a social role that represents her "self" rather than a mirror of what other people insist she be.

---

6. Ibid.

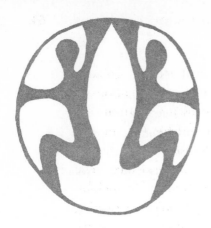

The divided self

There are other ways out of the dilemma than that represented by what is usually called a schizophrenic "break." One other way of throwing aside the roles prescribed by others is attempting suicide, while a third way of getting out of this panic state is a more open resolution of the problems that have led to this extreme anxiety. The most usual way to reach a more open resolution of a problem of this nature is through the assistance of someone else. For instance, Alice may call the counseling service and, with a counselor, engage in exploring the kinds of issues that seem to be involved in her panic. For the first time she may be able to face her true situation—that she never wanted to be a nurse, that it is her parents who wish this for her. She may be able to examine why it is so important for her to meet every expectation of her parents and to understand somewhat the fact that she is angry with her parents and herself over the situation. She might be encouraged to give some thought to what she would have chosen had her parents not been so involved in planning her life, as a beginning step in more clearly appraising what she herself wants to do. She might be encouraged to give some thought to what she might do instead of becoming a nurse. In short, her energies would be transferred to some affirmative action rather than being immobilized by overwhelming feelings of anxiety.

A question can be raised about which of the possible solutions available to the person may be settled on, and what their long-range consequences are; more specifically, which solutions are classified as "mental illness" and which are deemed acceptable from a societal viewpoint. In

Alice's case, if she can get her feelings sufficiently under control to go back to the ward the following day and go through the appropriate motions so that she eventually becomes a nurse, she will have chosen a solution that pleases significant others, namely her parents and perhaps her nursing instructors. But this solution is reached at tremendous cost to Alice as a person. She will forever be bound by feelings that must be denied. The energy required to keep those unacceptable thoughts from her consciousness is energy that is not available to spend on more personally rewarding activities. Alice will go through life playing a role, rather than experiencing the satisfaction of enacting a role she perceives as an expression of her true self.

DEFENSIVE MECHANISMS

Let us now turn to a more detailed explanation of ways in which persons respond to anxiety. First we will discuss the immediate defensive response, commonly called "mechanisms of defense," and then we will consider how these automatic patterns become incorporated into overall styles of coping. We are using "coping" in the sense of the form of mastery a person has developed to handle problematic situations. The word does not imply any positive outcome of the mastery; a particular style of coping may have unfortunate outcomes. Coping as represented here implies a relatively complete sequence of steps in problem-solving that is incorporated into one's readily available repertoire. Some other authors use the term "adaptation" in much the same way as we are using the term "coping," but adaptation has so many divergent meanings that we prefer the term coping.

Remember that anxiety is a signal to the person that something is amiss, and thus serves a useful function in preparing one to ward off threats. It is only when the person encounters constant anxiety-provoking situations that exceed his or her capacities for coping, or if usual coping responses do not lead to a reduction of anxiety through successful problem-solving, that he or she experiences difficulties. Let us first look at the ways in which persons commonly defend themselves against anxiety.

Most theorists consider *repression* to be one of the more central or basic mechanisms for eliminating anxiety. In the simplest terms, repression is automatic forgetting that occurs at times of severe anxiety. Precisely what is forgotten depends upon the details of the anxious circumstance; it usually includes whatever wishes or feelings people perceive as getting them into the trouble, as well as a varying amount of concrete recall of the situation itself. Remember that a concomitant of severe anxiety is that one is unable to organize; one's perceptual field is grossly narrowed, one cannot focus attention well, and therefore one either does not notice or can easily be mistaken about a large number of the details accompanying the anxious situation. In a family in which angry feelings are felt to be unacceptable, probably all the children go through many experiences which result in their repressing anger. If a small boy is in a position of feeling angry toward a parent and acting on it, he meets severe disapproval which leaves him terribly anxious because of fear of retaliation or abandonment. Faced with this threat of abandonment or other retaliation, he automatically wipes out or forgets that he is angry at the parent, and thus the usual caring relationship is restored. Later, if asked about the incident, he not only denies that he was angry but may not even remember a great deal about the situation that caused it. Given this pattern, the boy fails to learn much about the utility of anger, his own or anyone else's. He will simply recognize that when his angry feelings are aroused, he is in trouble, and therefore the presence of anger becomes equated with anxiety and has to be eliminated. He also will have to find some different means of coping with whatever behavior by his parents initially aroused the anger. Because anger is a very common part of life and difficult to avoid, the child will have to expend a share of energy that could better be spent elsewhere in keeping this whole area of living out of his consciousness.

Some theorists consider *suppression* to be a related, but not identical, mechanism. Whereas repression is forgetting that occurs automatically without the person's knowledge or control, suppression is the result of one's voluntary effort to put the disturbing or anxiety-provoking matter out of his or her mind. In both instances, the end result is no longer capable of being recalled. In the example given above, if the boy simply does not pay attention to something that his mother does that inevitably leads to anger, such as always giving his sister special treats while he is not given the same attention, he is using the mechanism of suppression. In this instance, he is choosing not to think about the fact that his mother obviously loves his sister more; by not thinking about it, he avoids feeling angry.

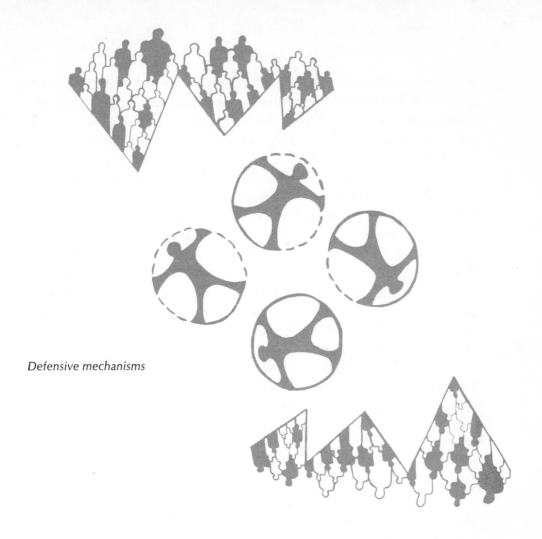

Defensive mechanisms

Denial is a related defensive maneuver. Here the person refuses to admit the existence of unpleasant reality. In the instance of the boy and his mother, if he were to use denial as a mechanism he would simply refuse to acknowledge that his mother favors his sister. This process of denial is automatic and does not imply that the person chooses not to be aware of unpleasant realities.

Intellectualization is another common defensive maneuver, whereby the person achieves a split between the affective and cognitive aspects of a situation. The affective component is frequently repressed, leaving only a cognitive explanation. Referring back to the example given above, the son would be intellectualizing if he adopted the approach of "Yes, my mother does love my sister more, but that is only natural because they are both women and there are many things that they can share."

Rationalization resembles intellectualization in that one again seeks to justify or make an excuse for oneself in the situation, which removes him or her from the anxiety. A common type of expression reflective of this mechanism is "I didn't want it anyway." In the family above, the mother might frequently tell the children and herself that she is disciplining them "for their own good," hiding from the fact that she is angry.

Displacement is one of the better known mechanisms, perhaps because of its frequent illustration in comedy situations, where the hen-pecked husband kicks the dog instead of his wife. Here action involving the original object of the motive or feeling arouses anxiety, and so one substitutes another object as the target in carrying out the same behavior.

A somewhat similar mechanism is *compensation*. Here, when a person is blocked in one avenue of endeavor, and the endeavor is important enough that failure to achieve it causes anxiety, he or she lessens or eliminates the anxiety by moving into an alternative avenue. For example, the boy in the family who is not able to do well in sports may instead become very interested and skilled in fixing bicycles and other suitable masculine activities.

Sublimation is one of the more important mechanisms and is considered by some to be an important basis of learning or progress. The boy in our original example who early learned to repress anger may, as he grows older, make the vocational choice of becoming a surgeon, construction worker, or researcher in biology. In this way he is able to transform raw, naked anger into socially acceptable aggression in such a way that he is highly rewarded, both monetarily and socially, because of the societal need for these services. He never has to notice that there might be other meanings attached to some animal experimentation, the tearing down of buildings or trees, or the aggressive construction of new buildings.

In *reaction-formation,* the wishes or feelings associated with the initial anxiety are transformed to their opposites. Thus the son, in the original example, may become known for his extreme consideration and concern for people, replacements for his original responses of anger. These opposites frequently are incorporated into people's coping styles in a very rigid and all-encompassing manner, so that their life gets organized primarily around these central themes.

Undoing is a phenomenon considered by some to be a mental mechanism and by others as more of a generalized pattern of behaviors with one common motivation. To eliminate the anxiety associated with the forbidden wishes and feelings, the person engages in behavior that makes amends, or atones, for these feelings, thereby neutralizing them. It is sometimes difficult to differentiate, in reality, between reaction-formation and undoing, since both have similar manifestations, although the explanations for what is going on within the individual are somewhat different. One principle to keep in mind is that undoing frequently follows some break in the usual pattern of keeping oneself unaware of the unwanted feelings. The son in our example, for instance, would do something to signify or demonstrate his love for his mother after some incident that allowed, or came close to allowing, him a glimpse of the anger he harbors toward her. A bad dream, for example, or a discussion with a friend about the deficiencies of mothers, might stimulate him to spend extra time with her or praise her cooking more.

When the anxiety associated with some wish or feeling is channeled into physical symptomatology, *conversion* is said to have occurred. The son, in the example given, might become an asthmatic as a means of coping with the anxiety associated with anger at his mother. The person with physical symptoms has no awareness of either anxiety or any unacceptable wishes; his or her attention is focused solely on the physical symptoms.

In *projection*, the person assigns his or her unacceptable wishes or feelings to someone else. As an example, the boy mentioned above may feel that other people are angry with him rather than being aware that angry feelings have been stimulated in himself.

Introjection can be seen as the mirror image of projection. To ward off anxiety, the person adopts certain attitudes and behaviors of other people. Thus the child incorporates parental standards regarding his or her behavior in order to avoid the anxiety of parental disapproval. The child is not necessarily aware that he or she is adopting the parents' standards, but views them as coming from himself or herself. Prisoners who take on the behavior of their guards are another frequently cited example.

It is sometimes difficult to differentiate introjection from another commonly used term, *identification*. Identification has a less specific meaning. While it also refers to a person's adopting or incorporating the attitudes and behaviors of others, the process is not linked exclusively to the reduction of anxiety. The end point of both processes is that a person includes in his or her behavior attributes acquired from significant others in his or her life.

Using the anxiety component of the coping model as our base, let us then consider how these defense mechanisms become incorporated into an overall coping style.

COPING STYLES

First, one can notice the physical manifestations of anxiety. Physiologically, one responds to anxiety by preparing to defend oneself against danger. With stimulation of the autonomic nervous system, especially the sympathetic division, the rate and force of cardiac output increase and the blood vessels supplying the skin and viscera are constricted. These circulatory changes result in an increase in blood pressure and allow a greater blood supply to the heart, muscles, and brain. Salivation and gastrointestinal activity are inhibited. Pupils are dilated to permit greater visual acuity, and bronchial passages are dilated to allow greater air intake. Perspiration is increased on the palmar surfaces of the hands and feet. In addition, the adrenal medulla is stimulated to secrete adrenalin, which helps increase cardiac output, sustains the sympathetic nervous system response, and stimulates the liver to convert glycogen to glucose to meet the body's energy needs. In short, the body diverts its forces to prepare to defend itself.

Under ordinary circumstances, there are emergency measures and are not particularly useful to the individual when the stress is not of a physical nature. Usually, when the stress stops and the person returns to a normal physiological state, there are no permanent bodily changes. However, in situations of chronic anxiety, either physiology or anatomy may undergo permanent physical change.

Focusing upon physical symptomatology, the person deflects his or her attention from the problem that originated the anxiety and also channels the anxiety. For instance, instead of noticing her rage at a teacher, a student can focus on an allergy, an asthma attack, or other physical reaction rather than having to do something about her relationship with the teacher. There are positive and negative aspects to such a maneuver. On the one hand, it does succeed in diminishing the anxiety and providing a course of behavior that seems reasonable and allows the student to carry out a role that is harmonious with other elements of the personality. On the other hand, it does not allow the student to focus on the difficulties with the teacher that stimulated her original anxiety response. In fact, the teacher may never know that there is any interpersonal difficulty and so will tend to define the symptoms according to the student's presentation of them. The true nature of the difficulty between student and teacher remains unclear, and it is likely that further transactions are based upon the teacher's perceptions of the student as someone with a physical problem. If the use of such a symptom has been successful for a person—for instance, if it enabled a student to get over the difficulty in doing a paper or facing a critical evaluation with an instructor—in another time of stress, this pattern of coping is likely to be one of the behaviors called forth from the person's memory bank and put into operation.

There are certain coping styles that, because of the way anxiety is handled, frequently are labeled neurotic. Several steps always are involved in the development of this type of life style. Initially, the person has been faced with a conflict so overwhelming and anxiety-laden that he or she could not go through the usual problem-solving steps; the person thus comes out with neither an accurate assessment of the nature of the conflict nor an effective plan of action to eliminate the source of anxiety. Because of the overwhelming anxiety and the lack of ability to take any action to solve the conflict, the person has to retreat from it; this measure prevents one from having certain types of experience that would have resulted in learning, but it serves to eliminate the anxiety. Retreating from conflict requires that one block out the original experience and avoid future situations that would serve to reactivate the original conflict. These two factors —that one cannot recall the original conflict and that one must avoid all situations that would reawaken it—lead to the behavior that is frequently labeled neurotic. Anxiety is experienced by this person whenever he or she is stimulated by anything associated with the original conflict. But the person is unable to do any reasonable conflict resolution and usually redefines a situation focusing only on the felt anxiety and the mechanisms that succeed in eliminating it for him or her. An extreme example would be the soldier who is unable to return to battle because one arm is suddenly paralyzed for no physical reason. He does not realize that the battle situation stimulates some earlier experiences involving his father. He could tell you about the battle situation being difficult but is at a loss to explain the paralysis of his arm.

A number of persons have difficulty tolerating anxiety experienced at points of disequilibrium and resort to various substances such as cigarettes, alcohol, drugs, and other symbols associated with security. Whatever object is associated with the reduction of anxiety becomes incorporated in their overall life style. The complicating factor in the use of these crutches is that instead of staying a means, they turn into more important end points. For example, a soldier in Vietnam who had ready access to a high grade of drugs may have begun using them as a means to combat boredom, to get enough courage to face the next day of guerilla warfare, or to endure the unexpected occurrences that might arise on the next patrol. After a while the soldier began to take pleasure in the consumption of the drug itself and thus his motivation changed; he no longer sought relief, but the drug.

In thinking about coping styles, it is well to keep in mind that the learnings we spoke of as occurring in each part of the developmental phases are of primary significance. For example, the second stage of development involves conflict about the issue of autonomy. It is possible for people with undue thwarting at this stage to develop doubts about their abilities that result in the development of a general tendency to pull back, as a learned response that then becomes incorporated into their overall life style. This response may be carried over into an adult coping style and will be manifested in the choices they make in responding at points of disequilibrium. At such times they will not choose an open, aggressive attack on a problem, but instead will either pull back, defer to another, or resign some piece of their own interest for the sake of keeping a peaceful, low-key situation. In fact, such people probably will develop a style in which other people are required to step in and take an active role in managing aspects of their lives. Whenever they encounter an anxiety-provoking situation, their choices of action will be limited to those that can be defined as passive. This course will sometimes get them into trouble because it requires them to bottle up feelings rather than express them openly with the people involved. The cost, however, is more than merely being passive. Such persons must allow only one facet of their potential selves to develop. They must spend a certain amount of energy in keeping other potential facets

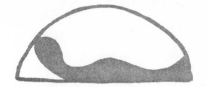

from surfacing lest they have to act on them. It is this quality of limitation of expression, requiring energy to maintain, that is referred to when some theorists talk about certain solutions as being more costly to the individual than others. People who must always keep their feelings under cover spend all their energies in this way rather than having energy to invest in more productive patterns of relating.

People employing such a passive coping style tend to rely heavily upon other people's judgments and seek their approval rather than take a stand based upon their personal opinions. They sacrifice their own individuality rather than risk expressing an opinion or taking a position at variance from those around them. The person with this particular life style experiences any type of impulsivity of his or her own as being equated with the "bad me"[7] that was so disapproved in the earlier stage of development.

In contrast to those who have very strong, though conditional, relationships with people and would be at a loss without significant others around them, there are people who develop much more of a "loner" theme as a predominant characteristic. They avoid putting themselves in a position of getting close to someone else because, in their earlier developmental stages, they have learned to associate such closeness with being hurt or disappointed. Faced with problems, these persons would never choose options involving some intimate emotional exposure to another person, since this renders them vulnerable. On the surface it may appear that these persons relate in a satisfactory manner, but in analyzing the character of their relationships, it is found they tend to be transitory, superficial, and not truly involving the individual in any intimate way with another. Any attempt by another person to get close stimulates the "loner's" underlying anxiety, and he or she responds by withdrawing from the relationship. While avoidance of any close interpersonal involvement with other

7. Harry Stack Sullivan, *The Interpersonal Theory of Psychiatry* (New York: W. W. Norton, 1955).

The isolated position

people serves to protect the person from possible hurt and disappointment, it proves costly in terms of the amount of energy invested in maintaining this social distance. The person always approaches any interpersonal situation in a suspicious manner and must ever be alert to protecting the boundaries so firmly established to maintain his or her isolated position. Further, instead of being able to rely upon the support of other people in working out solutions to the inevitable problems of life, this person must rely solely on himself or herself.

The coping styles described here are prototypic; usually any one person has a mix of coping responses, some of which are growth-producing and some of which are not, in that they are psychologically costly. If a person has too many unhealthy styles, the increasing limitations make him or her ever more vulnerable; that is, he or she moves into a position of solving problems with another round of increasingly more constricting and limiting solutions. Exceeding whatever limit he or she has set as a solution is accompanied by anxiety. Thus the person faces ever increasing anxiety-provoking experiences with a lessened ability to cope adequately, which may eventually lead him or her to a state of complete personality disorganization.

It is important also to keep in mind that as the individual engages in varying forms of coping behavior, he or she is surrounded by a social network of people who are responding to this behavior. As his or her attempts to cope exceed the boundaries of accepted behavior, it is likely that the person will begin to become identified as "not quite right," as someone with a problem, or "peculiar." As this process evolves, he or she becomes set apart as "different," which in turn creates further anxiety; from both a personal and societal point of view, the person is projected into the career of one who is "mentally ill."

A SOCIO-PSYCHOLOGICAL MODEL OF MENTAL ILLNESS

Each person develops his or her own unique coping style based upon the patterns learned as he or she establishes social roles, makes developmental adjustments, and faces crisis situations. Diagram 3-1 schematically represents the development of an individual's life style.

Diagram 3-1
A Socio-Psychological Model: Crises as Turning Points

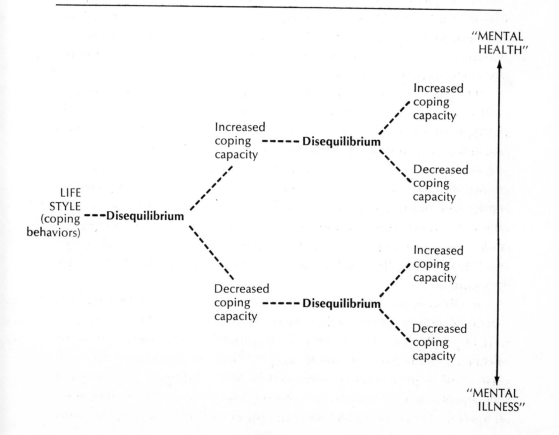

All the things discussed thus far—developmental accomplishments, interactions within a social network, long-term cultural influences, and responses to life crises—culminate in an individual's particular life style. In the life history of any person there are regular points at which disequilibrium occurs. Sometimes because of life crises, sometimes simply because of basic needs, and sometimes because of altered life circumstances to which the person adjusts, he or she is pushed to get himself back into a state of equilibrium. Ideally, the person accomplishes this by enlarging his or her repertoire of coping skills; when one does this, coping capacity is increased (according to the diagram), and one becomes more adept at confronting inevitable subsequent changes. He or she may now have more roles available, more success in modifying roles, and expanded capabilities for problem-solving. But when the re-establishment of equilibrium entails the resignation of some important need, value, status, or role, the individual has essentially decreased his or her capacity. There are more strictures; the person is in a more vulnerable position and has fewer options, less flexibility in the roles he or she plays, and lowered self-esteem. In the diagram, he or she would be at a lower point. The ultimate end point of inadequate problem resolution is personality disorganization.

Note that at each point of disequilibrium, it is possible for the individual to make changes that are not possible when he or she is in equilibrium. Even though the person with the increased capacity has the cards stacked in his or her favor, this person still could come out of a particular situation having resigned some portion of that capacity. Similarly, although the person with a primarily poor capacity does not have as many options or possibilities for successful mastery of disequilibrium experiences, at these points he or she has the chance to renegotiate some prior solutions, add some new skills, increase his or her options, and therefore emerge with an improved capacity for problem-solving. At any time, the person can be located on a continuum from the most optimum organization to total disintegration; this process is continual throughout life, and his or her position on the continuum changes accordingly.

Note the crucial variable of how significant others respond to the altered life style of an individual at any point. Some who respond to an experience of disequilibrium by arriving at an improved life style may encounter considerable resistance from persons who carry out reciprocal roles. For example, a woman may respond to the crisis of giving birth to a defective child by enlarging her ego strengths and increasing her repertoire of roles to involve some activities outside the home, such as a part-time job at a school for retarded children. Her husband, however, may consider her to be abandoning him because of these outside activities and consider it a reflection upon him, indicating that he is not able to provide adequately for the family. Such behavior will probably lead to another situation of disequilibrium, and at this juncture she might resign some of her new-found role options and return to the home, brooding over the loss of her child or becoming an obsessively compulsive housekeeper. On the other hand, it is also possible that this husband and wife will be able to work out another solution, such as her going back to school to prepare for a teaching career, which the husband as well as the wife sees as profitable to the family.

Note also that when someone chooses a role, he or she tends to get locked into this choice by the responses of others. Suppose this wife does become an obsessively compulsive housekeeper. People might accommodate to this and expect orderly behavior of her; she in turn feels compelled to reciprocate. This factor is particularly important in understanding how people get locked into deviant roles arrived at as a result of resolutions that decrease their coping capacity.

It may be helpful to consider in more detail the meaning of the concept of deviance. Sociologists point out that one's behavior becomes defined as deviant when one violates some important social rule. Whether or not a particular behavior becomes identified as deviant is, to a marked degree, dependent on the social network surrounding the individual and the definitions agreed upon within these groups. The Watergate disclosures of the mid-1970s illustrate this point. The same incidents may be considered from two separate points of view: One point of view holds that the men who broke into offices, obviously breaking the law to do so, were really not breaking the law because they were doing this in the interests of national security, and that they therefore should be considered as patriotic servants of their government. Another point of view is that they were clearly breaking the law and should therefore be treated as criminals. Thus, while on the surface an issue may seem to be clear-cut, such as the edict "Thou shalt not steal," when one explores the underlying issues, determination of right or wrong becomes increasingly problematic. Assessment of the intent underlying the act becomes a crucial variable in decid-

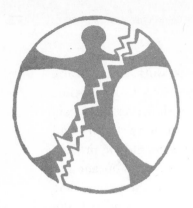

The person perceived as mentally ill

ing whether the person has engaged in deviant behavior and whether he or she should be punished.

On another level, there are certain acts in our society that are clearly examples of rule-breaking. Murder is an outstanding example, though even its definition can become problematic as the underlying circumstances are considered. But there are other behaviors that are not as clearly demarcated. Talking to oneself; seeing visions; weeping; dressing in an unusual manner; screaming at one's children, spouse, or relatives; laughing at the wrong time; or having hair of a certain length are all examples of behaviors that at certain times are identified as examples of rule-breaking. These cues become evidence that this person is not following the same set of rules as everyone else and that therefore something is wrong with him or her. Such an assessment follows from the universal assumption that everyone should follow the same set of rules. Usually the "something wrong" is interpreted in a derogatory fashion. The common response to someone's not following the rules is to search for an explanation, the most frequent of which is that a person is "mentally ill" and therefore incapable of following the rules. There are some noticeable exceptions. Some persons who claim to see visions and foretell the future, instead of being perceived as unable to follow the rules, become identified as persons having special powers. In these instances, the person gets positive recognition for behavior that under other conditions might be taken as a symptom of mental illness. One of the factors resulting in the positive assessment in this situation is that the individual does not wait for someone else to label the behavior, but instead advances a plausible explanation.

Employing this perspective, some sociologists[8] argue that deviance is created by society by the types of rules that it sets up. The "mental illness" category develops as a means of classifying and explaining rule-breaking behavior that is problematic to society.

By calling rule-breaking behavior mental illness, other factors are brought in that maintain this identity. First, the label implies that the person classified as ill is incapacitated and unable to carry out societal roles. What this person *is not* doing becomes identified as something that he or she *cannot* do. Adding the label "mental" further implies that the person's behavior is apt to be erratic and unpredictable. Most people feel that mentally ill people are unable to hold a job, cannot be trusted, are unstable and dangerous, and may even hurt little children. Critics of this view question whether this stereotype has grown out of the actual behavior of people so designated or the reverse: viewing persons as unstable creates an expectation for behavior that they in turn fulfill.

In the discussion of anxiety, it was noted that the behavior of someone in a panic is likely to be disorganized. During this time the person is likely to break societal rules of decorum and reasonable conduct, for instance, by dressing inappropriately or acting in an impulsive manner. Also at this time, a person is more susceptible to outside influence, including the acceptance of someone else's definition of the situation and of himself or herself. Once having accepted the definition "mentally ill," "weird," or "crazy," the individual, too, may begin to define himself or herself in this manner and act accordingly. Thus the vicious cycle is set in motion.

To summarize, each person develops his or her own particular life style which is relatively constant but not immutable. The life style is a result of a myriad of influences including the broad cultural milieu; one's particular place within a societal structure; how well able one is to acquire the necessities of life, both physical and psychosocial; the opportunities afforded within the family and society; and one's abilities to fulfill the accompanying expectations. As a result of upsets or crises, changes occur within this overall life style which force an individual to revamp some aspect of the coping abilities that constitute his or her life style. The responses of others to the person are particularly important during these

---

8. Thomas Scheff, *Being Mentally Ill: A Sociological Theory* (Chicago: Aldine Publishing Co., 1966).

crisis periods in terms of their influence for good or for ill. When people's life styles are such that they are considered deviant by some important segment of society, these persons may acquire the label "mentally ill."

PSYCHIATRIC/MENTAL HEALTH NURSING

The role of the psychiatric nurse may be defined as simply that of fostering each person's ability to develop his or her capacities to cope with life's disruptions. In other words, the nurse's role might be considered to be that of promoting a productive life style for each individual, whether he or she be a socially successful person by society's standards or a psychiatric patient on a long-term unit. In some instances the nurse's primary focus is on the individual, in others on social networks, while in still others the emphasis is on mediating between the individual and some relevant social group. A nurse might help an elderly man face up to the tasks of aging through helping him work through his grief over the losses incurred, thus helping him adjust to his circumstances. This same nurse may also assist in getting him involved in a golden age group in the community and work with the family in negotiating a position for him within the home of one of his children.

In fulfilling this role, the nurse will inevitably become involved in extremely diverse activities, such as assisting someone in negotiating with the social security system, helping a mother get food stamps, trying to understand someone's hallucinations, being with someone experiencing anxiety, supporting someone's ideas about suing the landlord, or conducting family or group therapy.

Sometimes the nurse's work not only encompasses various ways of helping individuals cope, but also includes influencing social networks to reduce the stress-producing factors that overextend coping potentials. The psychiatric nurse faculty member who works as part of a student-faculty group to change the hours that students spend in the clinical unit at night may be doing a great deal to reduce a stressful situation in which nursing students find themselves. The psychiatric nurse working with the family of an adolescent girl who is a chronic runaway may have to help the family look at the rules they have established for their children so that changes allowing for more individuality may be adopted.

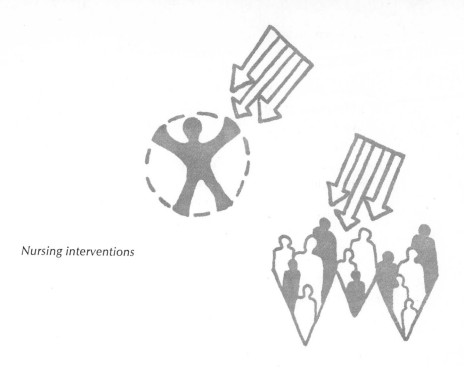

Nursing interventions

In some instances, nurses work within the broader context of a total community, becoming involved in issues that affect the social well-being of community residents. Working with tenant groups to assist them in organizing for better housing, or within community health agencies on issues related to the general health and welfare of the community, such as rat-control, or with the PTA to improve the quality of education are examples of nontraditional activities nurses might profitably pursue. Having accepted tasks such as these as bona fide aspects of their role, nurses can be amazingly resourceful in finding opportunities for entry into the social systems of the community.

The crisis model view of behavior allows the nurse to predict certain junctures of life at which persons are apt to encounter stressful situations. A psychiatric nurse, predicting these life stresses, can organize groups as a way of providing social support to help persons at risk develop adequate coping patterns. Some typical groups might be unwed adolescent mothers, parents in single-parent families who must cope with children at various developmental stages, persons suffering from varying types of physical disorders, victims of natural disasters such as earthquakes, unemployed, and golden age groups.

Although it is possible to anticipate particular crisis situations, plan preventive work accordingly, and thus diffuse the impact of a crisis, the more typical occurrence is for a nurse to encounter people who are already in crisis. These instances provide an excellent opportunity for intervention, since people in crisis are especially susceptible to outside help. The work of the nurse at this point is to help the individual, either singly or within the context of an appropriate group, sort out solutions that are growth-producing rather than constricting.

Concern for those who have limited coping abilities and who are at, or close to, points of disorganization has long been identified as the legitimate domain of psychiatric nursing. The specific activities of psychiatric nurses with these persons do not differ in kind from their activities with other groups. Their overall goal is still to provide experiences that allow for changes to occur in the coping patterns of the individual, no matter what his or her level of functioning. Facilitating these changes entails work with the individual, his or her family, and a wide variety of social networks ranging from the hospital unit to the community.

SUMMARY

In summary, both situational and developmental crises represent turning points in a person's life. At these times a person is facing a situation that he or she cannot master without the development of some new and different skills of coping. As the person struggles with trying to solve these problems, he or she is much more open to influences, good or bad, than he or she would be under other circumstances.

Anxiety is usually thought of as an unpleasant, apprehensive feeling that arises in response to some perceived threat. The sources of anxiety are different for different people, and their responses to dealing with anxiety are similarly different. Anxiety in moderate amounts is felt to be useful because it focuses people's attention on some matter on which they can concentrate their attempts at mastery. In severe amounts, anxiety is disorganizing in the sense that it blocks the person from concentrating on taking remedial action related to the cause of the anxiety.

There are various defense mechanisms that people use in developing their coping styles. These all have the same basic function, or purpose, which is to protect the person using them from the anxiety that would otherwise be experienced. They usually involve some altering in the way the person defines perceived reality, so that it no longer poses a threat. Some of the more commonly identified mechanisms are repression, suppression, intellectualization, rationalization, displacement, compensation, sublimation, reaction-formation, undoing, conversion, projection, introjection, and identification. Although some mechanisms, such as sublimation, are considered more favorably than others, such as reaction-formation, it is generally the extent to which the defense mechanisms are used that is considered healthy or unhealthy.

With the help of these mechanisms, people tend to develop whatever coping behaviors prove successful in managing anxiety for them, and these successful behaviors add together to form their coping style. Although most coping styles represent mixtures of elements, they frequently have a certain identifying characteristic. A coping style with too many elements that limit the person's range of activity places him or her in a vulnerable position, since it is difficult to manage life without exceeding those limits and thus experiencing anxiety. Such a style would be considered unproductive.

FURTHER READINGS

Aguilera, Donna G.; Messick, Janice M.; and Farrell, Marlene S. *Crisis Intervention: Theory and Methodology*. St. Louis: C. V. Mosby Company, 1970.

Angrist, S. "Nursing Care: The Dream and the Reality." In *Changing Patterns of Nursing Practice,* edited by E. Lewis. New York: American Journal of Nursing Co., 1971.

Barrell, Lorna M. "Crisis Intervention: Partnership in Problem-Solving." *The Nursing Clinics of North America* 9, no. 1 (March 1974): 5-16.

Beattie, W. "Matching Services to Individual Needs of the Aging." In *Working With Older People—the Aging Person: Needs and Services*. Bethesda, Md.: U.S. Department of Health, Education, and Welfare, 1970.

Beland, Irene I. *Clinical Nursing: Pathophysiological and Psychosocial Approaches*. New York: The Macmillan Co., 1965.

Bellak, Leopold, and Small, Leonard. *Emergency Psychotherapy and Brief Psychotherapy*. New York: Grune & Stratton, 1965.

Bernstein, Rose. "Are We Still Stereotyping the Unmarried Mother?" In *Crisis Intervention: Selected Readings,* edited by H. J. Parad, p. 101. New York: Family Service Association of America, 1965.

Blaker, Karen. "Systems Theory and Self-Destructive Behavior." *Perspectives in Psychiatric Care* 10 (1972): 168-172.

Bloom, B. L. "Definitional Aspects of the Crisis Concept." In *Crisis Intervention: Selected Readings,* edited by H. J. Parad, pp. 303-311. New York: Family Service Association of America, 1965.

Bluebond, Myra H. "I Know, Do You?: A Survey of Awareness, Communication and Coping in Terminally Ill Children." Conference on the Foundation of Thanatology, New York, April 14, 1972.

Braceland, F. "Psychological Concepts of Aging." In *Problems of the Aged,* edited by C. Vedder and A. Lefkowitz. Springfield, Ill.: Charles C. Thomas, 1965.

Brown, Esther Lucille. *Newer Dimensions of Patient Care: Improving Staff Motivation and Competence in the General Hospital.* New York: Russell Sage Foundation, 1962.

———. *Newer Dimensions of Patient Care: Patients as People.* New York: Russell Sage Foundation, 1964.

Bryan-Logan, Barbara N., and Dancy, Barbara L. "Unwed Pregnant Adolescents: Their Mothers' Dilemma." *The Nursing Clinics of North America* 9, no. 1 (March 1974): 57-68.

Caplan, Gerald. *An Approach to Community Mental Health.* New York: Grune & Stratton, 1961.

———. *Principles of Preventive Psychiatry.* New York: Basic Books, 1964.

Cath, Sidney. "Some Dynamics of Middle and Later Years." In *Crisis Intervention: Selected Readings,* edited by H. J. Parad, p. 187. New York: Family Service Association of America, 1965.

Coleman, John. "Life Stresses and Maladaptive Behavior." *Nursing Digest* 1 (Dec. 1973): 4-15.

Dancy, Barbara L. "The Unwed Pregnant Adolescent's View of the Label Illegitimate." Unpublished master's thesis, University of Illinois College of Nursing, Chicago, 1972.

Davidites, Rose Marie. "The Extended Roles of the Prepared Professional Psychiatric Mental Health Nurse in the General Hospital Setting." In *The Roles of Psychiatric Nurses in Community Mental Health Practice: A Giant Step,* edited by Gertrude Stokes, pp. 80-87. New York: Faculty Press, 1969.

———. "A Social Systems Approach to Deviant Behavior." *American Journal of Nursing* 71 (Aug. 1971): 1588-1589.

DiFalbio, Susan. "Crisis: A Complex Process." *The Nursing Clinics of North America* 9, no. 1 (March 1974): 47-56.

Donner, Gail. "Parenthood as a Crisis: A Role for the Psychiatric Nurse." *Perspectives in Psychiatric Care* 10, no. 2 (1972): 84-87.

Erikson, E. H. *Identity and the Life Cycle.* New York: International University Press, 1959.

Futterman, F. H.; Hoffman, I.; and Sabshin, M. "Parental Anticipatory Mourning." In *Psychosocial Aspects of Terminal Care,* edited by B. Schoenberg, et al. New York: Columbia University Press, 1972.

Goldstein, Kurt. "Methodological Approach to the Study of Schizophrenic Thought Disorder." In *Language and Thought in Schizophrenia,* edited by J. S. Kasanin. New York: W. W. Norton and Co., 1961.

Halstead, Louis. "The Use of Crisis Intervention in Obstetrical Nursing."
    The Nursing Clinics of North America 9, no. 1 (March 1974): 69-76.
Harrison, Mary. "Lindemann's Crisis Theory and Dabrowski's Positive
    Disintegration Theory." *Perspectives in Psychiatric Care* 3, no. 6 (1965): 8-13.
Herman, Sonya. "Divorce: A Grief Process." *Perspectives in Psychiatric
    Care* 12, no. 3 (1974): 108-111.
Hill, Rubin. "Genetic Features of Families Under Stress." In *Crisis
    Intervention:Selected Readings,* edited by H. J. Parad, p. 36. New York:
    Family Service Association of America, 1965.
Hirschowitz, R. "Crisis—A Crossroads." Presented at the 5th Annual
    Clinical Nursing Symposium, University of Illinois at the Medical Center,
    Chicago, April 1971.
Hitchens, Emily. "Denial: An Identified Theme in Marital Relationships of
    Sex Offenders." *Perspectives in Psychiatric Care* 10, no. 4 (1972): 152-159.
Hoffman, Irwin. "Parental Adaptation to Fatal Illness in a Child."
    Unpublished doctoral dissertation, University of Chicago, December 1972.
Jacobson, G. F. "Some Psychoanalytical Considerations Regarding Crisis
    Therapy." Presented at American Psychoanalytic Association,
    New York, April 1965.
Janken, Janice K. "The Nurse in Crisis." *The Nursing Clinics of North
    America* 9, no. 1 (March 1974): 17-26.
Johnson, M., and Martin, H. "A Sociological Analysis of the Nurse Role."
    American Journal of Nursing 58 (1958): 373-377.
Jourard, S. *The Transparent Self: Self-Disclosure and Well-Being.* 2d ed.
    New York: Van Nostrand Reinhold Co., 1971.
Kaplan, D. M., and Mason, F. A. "Maternal Reactions to Premature Birth
    Viewed as an Acute Emotional Disorder." In *Crisis Intervention: Selected
    Readings,* edited by H. J. Parad, pp. 118-128. New York: Family Service
    Association of America, 1965.
King, Joan. "Denial." *American Journal of Nursing* 66 (May 1966): 1010-1013.
Klein, D. C., and Ross, A. "Kindergarten Entry: A Study of Role Transition."
    In *Crisis Intervention: Selected Readings,* edited by H. J. Parad, pp. 140-148.
    New York: Family Service Association of America, 1965.
Klopf, Joan K. "Please Don't Go Away. A Crisis When Nobody Intervened."
    The Nursing Clinics of North America 9, no. 1 (March 1974): 77-80.
Logan, Barbara. "Negotiating the Mothering Role." Unpublished master's
    thesis, University of Illinois College of Nursing, Chicago, 1972.
Lorenze, E., ed. *Physical and Mental Health: Background and Issues.*
    White House Conference on Aging. Washington, D.C.: U.S. Government
    Printing Office, 1971.
McClellan, Muriel. "Crisis Groups in Special Care Areas." *Nursing Clinics
    of North America* 7 (June 1972): 363-371.
Maloney, Elizabeth. "The Subjective and Objective Definitions of Crisis."
    Perspectives in Psychiatric Care 9 (Nov.-Dec. 1971): 257-268.
Mann, Sylvia A. "Coping Patterns of Parents Living With the Fatally Ill
    Child." Unpublished master's thesis, University of Illinois College
    of Nursing, Chicago, June 1973.

Maslow, A. *Motivation and Personality.* New York: Harper and Row, 1970.

Menzies, I. "A Case Study in the Functioning of Social Systems as a Defence Against Anxiety: A Report on a Study of the Nursing Service of a General Hospital." *Human Relations* 13 (May 1960): 95-121.

Morley, W. E.; Messick, Janice M.; and Aguilera, Donna C. "Crisis: Paradigms of Intervention." *Journal of Psychiatric Nursing* 5 (Nov.-Dec. 1967): 538-540.

Moses, Dorothy V. "Reality Orientation in the Aging Person." In *Behavioral Concepts and Nursing Intervention,* edited by C. Carlson. Philadelphia: J. B. Lippincott Co., 1970.

Murray, R., ed. *Income: Background and Issues.* White House Conference on Aging. Washington, D.C.: U.S. Government Printing Office, 1971.

Parad, H. J., ed. *Crisis Intervention: Selected Readings,* pp. 1-4. New York: Family Service Association of America, 1965.

———. "Preventive Casework: Problems and Implications." In *Crisis Intervention: Selected Readings,* edited by H. J. Parad, pp. 284-298. New York: Family Service Association of America, 1965.

Perlin, S., and Butler, R. "Psychiatric Aspects of Adaptation to the Aging Experience." In *Human Aging: A Biological and Behavioral Study,* edited by J. Birren et al. Bethesda, Md.: U.S. Department of Health, Education, and Welfare, 1963.

Peterson, Margaret. "Understanding Defense Mechanisms—Programmed Instruction." *American Journal of Nursing* 72 (September 1972): 1651-1674.

Plutchik, R. et al. "Reliability and Validity of a Scale for Assessing the Functioning of Geriatric Patients." *Journal of American Geriatric Soc.* 18 (1970): 491-500.

Rapoport, I. "The State of Crisis: Some Theoretical Considerations." In *Crisis Intervention: Selected Readings,* edited by H. J. Parad, pp. 22-34. New York: Family Service Association of America, 1965.

Robinson, Kathy D. "Therapeutic Interaction: A Means of Crisis Intervention With Newly Institutionalized Elderly Persons." *The Nursing Clinics of North America* 9, no. 1 (March 1974): 89-96.

Rudd, T. *The Nursing Management of Elderly Sick: A Practical Handbook of Geriatric Nursing.* Philadelphia: J. B. Lippincott Co., 1954.

Satir, Virginia. *Conjoint Family Therapy.* Palo Alto: Science and Behavior Books, 1967.

Schneidman, E. "Crisis Intervention: Some Thoughts and Perspectives." In *Crisis Intervention,* edited by G. A. Specter and W. L. Claiborn, pp. 9-15. New York: Behavioral Publications, 1973.

Searles, Howard. *Collected Papers on Schizophrenia and Other Related Subjects.* New York: International University Press, 1965.

Solomon, P., and Patch, V. D., eds. *Handbook of Psychiatry.* 2nd ed. Los Altos, Calif.: Lange Medical Publications, 1969.

Spiegel, John. "The Resolution of Role Conflict Within the Family." In *A Modern Introduction to the Family,* edited by Norman Bell and Ezra Vogel, p. 363. Glencoe, Ill.: The Free Press of Glencoe, 1963.

Stein, L. "The Doctor-Nurse Game." *Archives of General Psychiatry* 16 (1967): 699-703.

Strauss, A.; Schatzman, I.; Ehrlich, D.; Bucher, R.; and Salishin, M. "The Hospital and Its Negotiated Order." In *The Hospital in Modern Society,* edited by E. Friedson. London: Collier-Macmillan, Ltd., 1963.

Sullivan, H. S. *The Interpersonal Theory of Psychiatry.* New York: W. W. Norton, 1953.

Verwoerdt, A. "Clinical Geropsychiatry." In *Working With Older People— Clinical Aspects of Aging.* Bethesda, Md.: U.S. Department of Health, Education, and Welfare, 1971.

Williams, Florence. "Intervention in Maturational Crises." *Perspectives in Psychiatric Care* 9 (Nov.-Dec. 1971): 240-246.

———. "The Crisis of Hospitalization. *The Nursing Clinics of North America* 9, no. 1 (March 1974): 37-46.

Zind, Roberta K. "Deterrents to Crisis Intervention in the Hospital Unit." *The Nursing Clinics of North America* 9, no. 1 (March 1974): 27-36.

CHAPTER FOUR: # PSYCHOSOMATIC AND NEUROTIC COPING STYLES

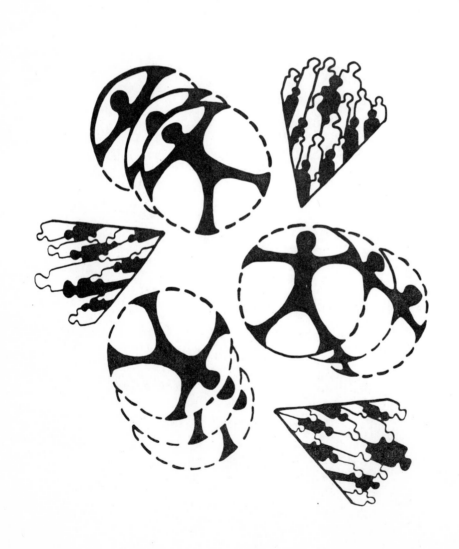

While the connection between "mind" and "body" has been a part of both medical lore and knowledge for centuries, it has come into its own in more recent times. Traditionally, emphasis has been placed on the physical treatment of disease, while a psychological component may or may not have been recognized. Further, when it was recognized, it was not so easily dealt with as the physical aspects of the disease. For example, it has always been far easier to provide antacids to coat the stomach and protect it from the ravages of gastric juices than to figure out what psychological factors are implicated in the development of an ulcer—and then to eliminate those psychological factors. In addition, people have always been more amenable to taking antacids as a reasonable remedy for their malady than to accepting the suggestion that the problems might be in their style of dealing with situations. Doctors, faced with having to please patients and to provide a service that they can accept, have been doubly encouraged to focus on the physical aspects of disease, first, because of the reciprocal nature of their relationships with patients, and second, because of the ease of dispensing medications without having to go into problematic areas of the patient's life aside from his or her physical condition. There have always been situations in which doctors and patients are unable to reach a reasonable détente about the patient's symptoms, In such instances, patients may wander from doctor to doctor in search of a solution, while doctors, recognizing this type of patient, cringe when they see them enter their office. In these kinds of situations, solutions other than the usual physical remedies are somtimes tried, one of them being to send the patient for some other type of help.

Historically, it was just this kind of situation that led to the development of psychoanalysis as a branch of medicine. These maladies, not surprisingly, reflect certain aspects of the culture of the time. One of the coping styles open to women in Victorian times was to have "the vapors," weeping, fainting, and other "nervous" symptoms. It was perfectly acceptable to be physically ill and be concerned about it, whereas many other areas of behavior were considered unseemly and not to be acknowledged, discussed, or treated. In his practice with many such patients, Sigmund Freud was led to discover a host of psychological factors, the presence of which was both unknown to people and very displeasing to them. But it was Freud's conviction that another layer of meaning did indeed exist which led to his formulations of psychoanalytic theory.

PSYCHOSOMATIC COPING STYLES

Since Freud's time, the theory that underlying conflict or stress is associated with physical symptoms has gone through valleys and peaks of popularity with medical practitioners, surfacing always in wartime, when combat exacted a physical toll of disability of one sort or another for which doctors could find no organic basis. In this century, research such as that pioneered by Cannon's[1] studies in the 1920s of the defensive functions of the adrenal medulla demonstrated beyond doubt that, to the body, stress is stress, no matter what its origins. Psychological stressors, such as anger or fear, brought about the same physiological responses as organic stressors. Two basic themes underlie further research in this area: one relates to the general effects of stress in the development of physiological disorder, the other to the identification of specific sets of conflicts or coping styles that underlie the development of specific types of disorders, such as peptic ulcers or asthma.[2]

The theme of stress as a factor in the development of physiological disorders has come to the fore since the 1950s as a result of studies demonstrating that numerous physical diseases not generally associated with psychological causality do occur within a short time after some experience of stress. Loss of a loved one is a frequently acknowledged stress. In studies of immediate survivors, it has been demonstrated that the rates of both

1. W. B. Cannon, *The Wisdom of the Body* (New York: W. W. Norton, 1939).
2. Theodore Lidz, "General Concepts of Psychosomatic Medicine," in *American Handbook of Pyschiatry,* ed. Silvano Arieti, vol. 1 (New York: Basic Books, 1959), pp. 647-657.

disease and death are much higher than would be predicted by chance. In studies of patients admitted to the hospital for various conditions, it has been shown that a much higher number than could be expected by chance have suffered some easily identifiable stress during the preceding six months. Many of these stresses could be identified as following losses or changes of the kind that we have discussed as contributing to crises, such as relocating, change of employment, change in marital status, and changes in social roles.

Exactly how such illnesses occur is not understood at the present time. Explanations usually focus on the thesis that the body is rendered either less capable of defense or more susceptible to attacks than under normal circumstances. Whether these situations in fact represent previously unknown mechanisms at work or are simply extensions of previously established theories about the effects of stress remains to be seen.

One widely accepted theory of physiological stress follows from the early work of Selye[3] and focuses on the fact that stress is mediated through the autonomic nervous system. The autonomic nervous system has two functions: to prepare the organism to fight and to maintain homeostasis through its control of autonomic body functions such as respiration and digestion. These two functions can be antagonistic. "The stomach, while responding to fear or anger, will not meet digestive needs properly."[4] One function can be activated or reinforced at the expense of the other; in the individual's response to an overload of stress, the homeostatic mechanisms are often sacrificed so that the body may be in a state of preparation for fight. Considerable current research is exploring the relationships between the autonomic nervous system and other body systems, such as the endocrine, muscular, cardiovascular, and reticular systems. These relationships have interesting implications for psychosomatic disorders.

Learning theorists hypothesize that psychosomatic illnesses are learned in much the same way as any other behavior is learned, that is, by conditioned response. The person associates his or her physiological reaction to stress with the stimulus causing the stress and so comes to overgeneralize it. As an example of the learning theory view, let us consider the mother of a toddler who bangs on pots and pans incessantly. When the mother

---

3. Hans Selye, *The Stress of Life* (New York: McGraw Hill, 1956).
4. Ibid., p. 649.

hears this noise, her blood vessels constrict and her blood pressure starts to rise. Soon this physiological response occurs whenever she hears any noise at all. As she feels this occurring, she feels angry, confused, and frustrated. If it continues, she may feel irritated by the slightest noise her child makes.

Other hypotheses also come within the theme of the general effects of stress as contributing to the development of psychosomatic coping styles. In one such approach, differences are noted between coping styles developed by people who will become neurotic and by those who develop psychosomatic disorders. The person who is neurotic has used defense mechanisms, such as those described earlier, in such a way as to deceive himself or herself about the real nature of situations that provoke anxiety, while the person who is prey to psychosomatic illness is someone who has suffered serious insecurity but has not erected adequate mechanisms to protect against the danger. Lidz summarizes this theoretical view: "... he avoids the reoccurrence of the insecurity or trauma by patterning his life so that he will never be exposed again."[5] The little boy whose mother does not fulfill his dependency needs, for instance, becomes very self-sufficient so he does not have to ask people for help. This maneuver succeeds in encapsulating the problem area, but it is still there unresolved. On the surface, this person seems to be in good shape, but when his defensive pattern of living collapses, he is exposed to the same intentsity of feeling he originally experienced, since he has never developed adequate defenses. Lidz describes as an example a peptic ulcer patint:

> The patient with the peptic ulcer who has defended himself against loss of dependency by insistent self-sufficiency, may be overwhelmed by any business setback even though he is already wealthy.[6]

He is still as overwhelmed as he was in childhood. For such people the "illness" seems to start when the defensive pattern crumbles. The wealthy businessman Lidz describes will suffer an ulcer attack at the time of a business setback even though it makes no long-term difference in his situation from the point of view of reality.

One could examine the development of this same situation from a

---

5. Lidz, "General Concepts of Psychosomatic Medicine," p. 652.
6. Ibid., p. 652.

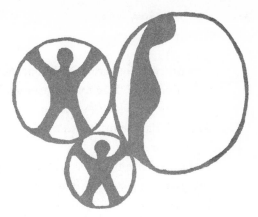

Reciprocity of roles

sociological view, rather than from this solely psychological perspective, and come out with some modifications that make the development of the disorder seem quite reasonable. One could examine this businessman from the viewpoint of the roles he has learned throughout life and note that roles are always reciprocal. When he was the little boy whose mother, for whatever reason, did not meet his dependency needs, he was learning something about her expectations of how he should perform the role of "boy" in the family. Probably this expectation was that he should not look for anyone to meet his dependency needs. One could expect that self-sufficient behavior was encouraged in this family setting. Therefore, any shift in subsequent roles relating to his self-sufficiency results in the feeling that he is violating the requirements of the people who play reciprocal roles to him. One could also assume that his wife, business associates, and other important people in his adult life have roles structured around a perception of him as a self-sufficient and competent person. Therefore, from a sociological point of view, one would not say that he is responding simply to the reality from his childhood, but also to the reality of his current situation. The two views are not necessarily antagonistic, but it means that in treating this man one could consider him to be responding to the stress in his current situation, not simply to historical life events.

Let us turn now to the second general theme that appears in research and theory related to psychosomatic disorders: that there are specific sets of conflicts that underlie the development of specific types of disorders. This theoretical view implies that certain body organs are susceptible to certain types of stress, and that certain people have body organs that will be vulnerable. For example, it is felt that certain people are able to develop ulcers while others, no matter what stress they experience, cannot. Mirsky[7] has demonstrated that certain people have pepsinogen and uropepsin levels higher than those of the general population and that, under certain situations, these persons develop ulcers. Other examples of theories involving organ specificity attempt to identify genetic or physiologic factors that may predispose a person to certain organic problems, or to identify psychological states—specific conflicts or types of personalities—that predispose the individual to specific diseases. For instance, the hypertensive mother with the pan-banging toddler may be described as having a conflict over expressing anger. A mother without that particular conflict would not develop hypertension, though she might have some other conflict leading to a different disorder. Another example of an organ-specificity theory is that asthmatics have a conflict centered around dependency needs; their wheezing is seen as a "cry" that elicits a response of someone caring for them. Migraine headaches are another common example. Here the victim is presumed to be an overconscientious and ambitious person, who reacts to genuine enjoyment with guilt and is unable to express or acknowledge anger or resentment.

In summary, there appear to be connections between a wide range of organic illnesses and psychological stress. The exact nature of these connections remains unclear, although many promising research studies are now attempting to explicate them. As these connections become clearer it may be possible to develop direct approaches, such as those available through the use of biofeedback, in which people may be trained to modify their physiological responses to stress. But even though a person may be trained to control physiological responses to stress, the issue of the underlying psychological underpinnings of the illness response still remains, as well as the meaning of this particular illness within the context of his or her social network. Even though the mother of the noisy toddler may be deconditioned so that her blood pressure does not rise, what has she learned about dealing more effectively with anger or altering the role-reciprocity between herself and her child? And if this symptomatic re-

---

7. I. A. Mirsky, "Psychoanalysis and the Biological Sciences," in *Twenty Years of Psychoanalysis,* ed. F. Alexander and H. Ross (New York: W. W. Norton, 1953).

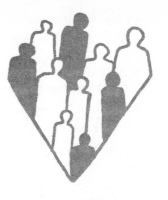

Neurotic coping styles

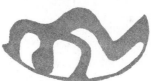

sponse is taken away from her without dealing with these other issues, will something else replace it?

NEUROTIC COPING STYLES

The hallmark of a neurotic coping style is the way anxiety is managed. There are always several steps in the development of a neurotic style. Initially the person is faced with a conflict so serious and anxiety-laden that he or she cannot go through the usual problem-solving steps, and so comes out with neither an accurate assessment of the nature of the problem nor an effective plan of action to eliminate the source of the anxiety. Because of overwhelming anxiety and lack of ability to take any action to solve the conflict, the person retreats from it, a measure that, although it eliminates the anxiety, prevents him or her from having certain types of experience that would have resulted in learning. Retreating from this conflict requires that the person block out the original experience and avoid future situations that would serve to reactivate the original conflict, but the attempt is never successful because of the nature of the conflict. These two factors—that one cannot recall the original conflict and that one must avoid all situations that would reawaken it—lead to behavior that is commonly labeled neurotic. This person experiences anxiety whenever he or she is stimulated by anything associated with the original conflict. If the original stimulus was something the person can successfully avoid, he or she may not experience subsequent problems. For example, if the source of anxiety were an experience with funny green critters from Mars, one could probably avoid this stimulus. But more commonly, the original source of anxiety relates to highly charged interpersonal situations that are not easily avoided. Thus, the anxiety experienced tends to pervade the person's life and to recur with regularity. He or she is unable to identify the true source of the anxiety and so cannot achieve reasonable conflict resolutions; such persons usually redefine a situation for themselves focusing only on the felt anxiety and the mechanisms that succeed in eliminating it for them. The particular form of neurosis is labeled according to the mechanisms people employ in dealing with the anxiety. Thus, some persons develop phobias, others are consumed with obsessive thoughts, some become preoccupied with physical symptoms, while others convert their anxiety into some form of hysterical behavior.

It is important to note that although this behavior originates out of some crucially important unresolvable conflict, it comes to contaminate every facet of one's life. One develops a neurotic life style in which he or she has a propensity to handle many situations using, for instance, the same phobic mechanisms that he or she initially learned in handling the original conflict. As this life style develops, persons in reciprocal relationship to the person tend to respond to him or her in terms of these particular neurotic patterns.

Let us take as an example a young woman nursing student who has a basically obsessive coping style. She probably developed this style very early in her life, under circumstances that she does not now recall, although they probably conflicted with her parents over highly charged issues, possibly power struggles over toilet-training. Now at this point in her life, even though she is in no way involved with conflicts about the original issue, she tends to keep herself free of anxiety by using the same obsessive mechanisms that have been successful in the past. For example, as exams approach, she may find herself checking five times rather than her usual twice to see if she has locked her dorm door. If she is on a first date with a new man, she may be convinced that her make-up is not on right

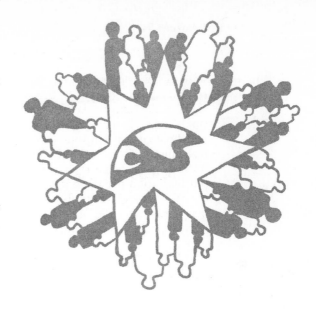

The neurotic life style

and keep checking her appearance in the mirror. She may have a hard time feeling convinced that she is wearing the right clothes for the occasion, and she spends a great deal of time worrying about whether she is properly attired. Actually she spends a good bit of time on this date consumed with questions of this sort, which save her from the anxiety of relating to this new man in her life.

All persons experience anxiety as a normal condition of living. Neurotic anxiety differs from that common to most people in that the nature of what threatens the individual is not clear, nor is it apparent what is endangered. One cannot readily discern the cause of the anxiety nor the probable hazardous outcome to oneself. A third factor that differentiates neurotic anxiety from that experienced as a common part of life is the degree of involvement in attempting to defend oneself in the face of the threats perceived. One's whole life becomes organized around a legion of unidentified fears and anxieties. The life style developed in an attempt to cope with these unnamed anxieties is described by Angyal:

> The basic situation in neurosis is that of life lived in isolation; it is the state of being "narrowed in," working one's course within narrow confines, not daring to move out into the wider areas that could be encompassed by personal life . . . . Anxiety is the emotional expression of the

state of being narrowed in, but the presence of the state can be objectively determined, even in the absence of anxiety, through the observations of the person's behavior and the general pattern of his life. You can see, e.g., how he sits on the edge of the chair, or hides in a corner, how he shrinks when you try to talk to him; you know that although he feels miserable in his job he has kept it for thirty years; or that he always stays at home even though he professes to love company. The self-limitation need not always be as obvious as this; it can take a variety of form and be subtly disguised. However, by closely examining a person's total mode of living one can determine whether he treads a narrow path or is genuinely expansive.[8]

The key factor underlying neurotic behavior is that the person becomes a captive of these unnamed anxieties and fears. His or her total life becomes organized tightly as a means of controlling and managing anxiety, usually in relative isolation from warm, meaningful interpersonal relationships.

The person feels and functions as if he were not really a part of the world; he does not feel that the world is his home. As a result of his isolation, both his capacity to exercise mastery, to determine his own fate, and his capacity to live are impaired; one cannot reach out to others and share in their lives without coming out of one's shell.[9]

Neurotic behavior is characterized by a set of general features. First is the *overemphasis on safety* as a response to any type of fear.

For the neurotic, almost his entire life is devoted to the pursuit of safety, to protecting himself against danger. When he is making decisions his considerations are overwhelmingly centered on the dangers to be avoided rather than on the objectives to be achieved.[10]

One's attempts to ward off the dangers are reflected in behavior that tends to be compulsive. A person finds that some type of behavior works in controlling his or her anxiety in a certain situation, and he or she tends to call repeatedly on the same mechanisms in response to any anxiety-provoking situation. As the cycle becomes repetitive, the person's range of behavioral responses to situations becomes increasingly limited, to the degree that he or she feels that he or she *must* do certain things or something

---

8. Andras Angyal, *Neurosis and Treatment: A Holistic Theory* (New York: John Wiley & Sons, Inc., 1965), pp. 76-77.
9. Ibid, pp. 80-81.
10. Ibid., p. 81.

dangerous will ensue. Thus, one's entire life becomes patterned around warding off the unidentified impending dangers that surround one, rather than being free to engage in activities that bring gratification and fulfillment.[11]

Neurotic behavior may take several different forms. The A.P.A. specifies a classification based on (1) anxiety reaction, (2) phobic reaction, (3) dissociative reaction and conversion reaction, (4) obsessive-compulsive reaction, and (5) depressive reaction.[12]

ANXIETY NEUROSIS

In *anxiety neurosis,* the primary symptom is a free-floating anxiety experienced in varying degrees at unpredictable intervals. The person frequently suffers acute episodes of anxiety which are very distressing and can progress to the point of panic. The person cannot tell what the anxiety is about, but only knows that he or she is anxious. The attacks of anxiety are episodic, and between them the level of anxiety is greatly diminished. The course of this particular neurosis is unpredictable; its onset may be either insidious or acute, and the duration of any one episode may range from a relatively few minutes to hours or days. Sometimes it is possible to discern what precipitates an anxiety attack, while at other times there is no discernible precipitating event. A person might typically describe an anxiety attack in the following manner: "I don't know what's happening to me. My heart is pounding and I can't seem to sit down. I just pace back and forth. I don't know what's wrong; I've never been so nervous in my life. The children are out playing, my husband is on a fishing trip, but I just feel that something dreadful is going to happen. I feel that if I sit here any longer, I'm just going to start screaming; maybe I'll flip my lid like my mother did. My stepmother always said I would some day. I just don't know what is happening to me."

The individual who is experiencing an anxiety attack has a sense of impending doom, a feeling that "something dreadful is going to happen." He or she may be able to state specifically what terrible thing might happen or may just have a pervasive sense of doom, more or less nameless.

---

11. Ibid., pp. 80-88.
12. George A. Ulett, *A Synopsis of Contemporary Psychiatry* (St. Louis: C. V. Mosby, 1972), p. 162.

Some common expressions would be "Something terrible is going to happen to me," "I'm going insane," "I am going to die," or "I have a terrible disease." In addition to these feelings, the person has the usual physiological responses, which contribute to his or her distress. Tense muscles may result in pains in the head and back as well as tremors. Respiration is rapid and shallow, and other manifestations of shock may be present. If this is the person's first attack, both he or she and family members may be alarmed to the point of seeking emergency medical assistance.

Frequently people with this type of anxiety problem will complain of other symptoms as well, some of which are directly caused by a constant degree of more than the usual amount of anxiety in their lives. Such symptoms as fatigue, insomnia, gastrointestinal complaints, headaches, and various muscle aches are common. All of these symptoms may be the direct result of a physical reaction to stress. The chronically anxious person goes through life with his or her body in a constant state of readiness to ward off a host of unnamed dangers. The bodily toll of anxiety is manifested in the list of symptoms commonly reported by increasingly large numbers of people. Instead of responding by giving a pill to stop the headache, aid the digestive process, or relax the back muscles, the nurse might view these complaints as symptomatic of an underlying state of chronic anxiety and direct his or her therapeutic work with patients accordingly.

PHOBIC NEUROSIS

In contrast to anxiety neurosis, in which there is relatively free-floating anxiety not attached to specific ideas or objects, *phobic neurosis* is characterized by persistent fear of a specific place or thing which is impossible to banish from one's mind. All the anxiety is bound in one object that has particular significance in terms of the originating conflict. A key factor here is the use of the mechanism of displacement, which allows the person to function without undue anxiety in areas not connected with the phobic object. Another hallmark of a phobia is the irrational nature of fear, which persists even though the person recognizes it. While most people have fears, sometimes irrational ones, the mere presence of such fears is not sufficient to constitute a neurosis. What does constitute a neurosis is the serious and pervasive nature of the conflict, which encompasses a larger dimension of the person's life than is usual.

Some common objects that are the focus for phobic reactions include closed places, open spaces, high places, crowds, germs, school (the most common phobic object for children), sharp objects, and vehicles. Note the restrictive qualities inherent in the development of the phobic life style. The person progressively becomes walled off; the development of a phobia is basically an avoidance maneuver in which one progressively retreats from whatever it is that causes the anxiety. Again, the conflict leading to the neurosis is so great that one cannot simply wall it off by avoiding it; thus anxiety is constantly generated, and the person will have to spend increasing amounts of time and attention on phobic maneuvers attempting to avoid it. It is therefore fairly common to have multiple phobias rather than just one. The person who has a phobic reaction comes to rely on the phobia as a tool in satisfying other significant areas of living.

As an example of how a phobia can contain the original anxiety and then come to serve other purposes for the individual, let us consider the situation of a middle-aged suburban housewife with teen-aged children. During the past two years, this woman, Anne Johnson, has become increasingly fearful about going out of the house. Initially her fear was centered on the supermarket so that she soon became unable to do the family shopping, a task which then had to be taken care of by either her husband or two middle-teen daughters. Her fears then became more generalized, so that she experienced difficulties in almost any shopping transaction, including dry cleaners, beauty parlors, and restaurants; as a result, her daughters had to take care of her hair for her, and she could no longer be a part of the usual dinners with her husband's business friends. As time progresses, one can see the pattern of her essentially removing herself from outside activities and having to remain home. Mrs. Johnson's stated fears center on germs, contamination, and "dirt" kinds of issues, although if one were to talk with her eldest daughter she would recount numerous incidents in which Mrs. Johnson has had difficulties relating to clerks and other salespeople. As a matter of fact, three months before the onset of her fear of the supermarket, she had changed supermarkets because she had trouble with the store manager over weevils she had found in flour products. A more recent development is that she now fears being in the house alone and will not stay there unless at least one of her family is with her. She is especially afraid of going into the kitchen because she has begun to have obsessive thoughts about serving garbage for dinner. She is relying increasingly upon her daughters to prepare meals and do other kitchen activities.

Now although we have defined the basic mechanism of a phobia as the displacement of anxiety from the originating conflict to some other object or idea about which the person comes to have a morbid fear, it is easy to see that the situation of the phobic person is vastly more complicated. As in the case of all other neuroses, the person comes to have a very constricted coping style; in this case she has to rely more and more on phobic mechanisms to negotiate much of her daily business and relationships with other people. In looking at the activities of Mrs. Johnson, one can readily see that a feeling of insecurity and threat pervades her life. Her coping style is such that she relies on avoidance mechanisms to diminish anxiety rather than taking any measures to understand the underlying source of the anxiety; in a sense she is always "on the run."

We mentioned that the conflicts underlying neurosis must involve a central portion of the individual's life as opposed to some easily isolated, one-shot stress. Mrs. Johnson's situation epitomizes this fact. Notice how most of her interactions and concerns center on the issue of control. She is both being controlled and controlling others; by removing herself from the fulfillment of various role requirements, she is forcing other members of her family to pick up these unfulfilled tasks; others also are required to pick up the slack when she can no longer meet her obligations because of the fears connected with them. The phobia becomes a vehicle for conducting her life; thus she has a feeling of being cared for and loved by her daughters because they must attend to her phobia, not her. People with this style of coping are afraid to ask for anything directly; they can ask for certain considerations because of the phobia, not because of anything that they might personally want for themselves.

The central conflict in this instance may well have to do with issues of control generated back in the second stage of development. One can only speculate about this, since Mrs. Johnson would have no recall of the circumstances, but one could assume that she does indeed have difficulty with asserting herself with others in either a positive or a negative way. thus it is easier to change supermarkets than to go into a scene that provokes anger. One might say that the conflict here relates to the early anger she experienced toward her parents, which was thoroughly unacceptable in her family. The phobia then becomes the vehicle for expressing her anger when she is, in a sense, punishing people. She punishes herself as well, as she is genuinely distressed by these symptoms and very disappointed in having to endure them. People with phobias generally have a very limited capacity for recognizing their own feelings, either positive or negative, but one can assume such feelings from symptoms such as her terrible fear of serving her family "garbage" and in her maneuvering to receiving a "caring" response from her family.

OBSESSIVE-COMPULSIVE NEUROSIS

An *obsessive-compulsive neurosis* has many features in common with the phobic behavior described above, particularly in relationship to the element of control and the pervasiveness of defense mechanisms which come to constitute the person's entire life style. The obsessive-compulsive person conducts most of his or her negotiations around obsessions or compulsions. He or she cannot be very direct in expressing feelings, either positive or negative, and has an avoidance approach to mitigating anxiety. Specifically, obsessions are the presence of thoughts, usually distressful and somewhat strange; these thoughts, which are never perceived by the person as reasonable, always precipitate anxiety, yet cannot be banished from consciousness. A compulsion is an uncontrollable, persistent urge to perform a certain behavior. As with obsessions, the behavior is never perceived by the person to be either reasonable or worth performing. The compulsion causes anxiety both before and after the behavior; before, because one has the urge, and after, because one has given in to it. It is also thought that the particular behavior itself symbolizes the committing of some prohibited action and the restitution for this "sin of commission." Typical forms of compulsive behavior include handwashing, checking doors to see if they are locked, checking the stove to be sure it is out, and always performing a given task in a particular order.

One might reasonably think that structuring the situation to prevent the person from performing a particular compulsive act would short-circuit the anxiety and therefore be useful. Unfortunately, compulsive behavior does not follow such reasoning, and the person prevented from performing a compulsive act suffers an increased urge toward it, and so any prohibition causes greater amounts of anxiety. Some think that the reason for such urgency to perform a compulsive act lies once again in the symbolic nature of the behavior; that compulsive behavior not only involves handling anxiety generated from some earlier conflict, but also symbolically represents acting out the initial wish. The obsessions and compulsions are thought to involve the mechanisms of reaction-formation and undoing. In other words, the original conflict involved some impulse to act that was unacceptable, and for protection against this impulse and its attendant anxiety, the person adopts the opposite response; for instance, instead of insisting on smearing feces, he is concerned with cleanliness. The cleanliness is both a reaction-formation against the wish to soil and an undoing of the act of dirtying. That is, a particular symptom expresses both the wish and the undoing of it. Handwashing may express the reaction-formation to a wish to be dirty; in suffering sore hands from excessive washing, the person also enacts a form of atonement for the unacceptable wish.

In addition to understanding the significance of obsessional thoughts or compulsive acts for an individual, it is important to notice the function they serve in the person's interpersonal relationships. It is common for a person to become so involved with obsessions and compulsions that they take the place of relating to people and thus protect him or her from the stress of getting close to others and experiencing feelings, either positive or negative. These maneuvers play a predominant part in how one structures his or her social roles; one seeks to involve people who play reciprocal or complementary roles.

In some instances, it may be difficult to discern that the roles being enacted are indeed reciprocal, because of the seeming distress that at least one of the role partners shows. For example, take the compulsive husband who constantly complains about his wife, who cannot keep the house orderly. First, they center most of their communications around the dirty house and whose fault it is, thus maintaining a certain degree of distance from one another. Second, the husband can act out his wish to be dirty through his wife's dirtiness, while never having to feel guilty, because it is her fault, not his; in this way he avoids some of the anxiety he would experience if he were the one creating the "mess." Third, he can spend a great deal of time straightening up the house, undoing the impulse to mess. As it turns out, this kind of wife is the perfect complementary foil for a man with such a compulsive coping style, and he probably would have difficulty establishing a safe relationship with some other kind of woman. The husband in this situation generally regards his wife as inferior because of her obvious difficulties in managing, and thus maintains his own shaky self-esteem. In essence, if he had nothing to complain about, he might well fall apart. If the wife "shaped up" by becoming a more competent housekeeper, the husband would probably suffer more severe symptoms because he would no longer have her to carry out these meaningful behavior patterns for him. Also, she would be likely to demand a more mature, meaningful interpersonal relationship with him, thereby increasing his anxiety and the accompanying need to maintain control through the rigidity of his compulsive behavior.

HYSTERIA

Hysteria was one of the earliest neuroses to be described; it was common in earlier times such as the Victorian era. Possibly the prevalence of this form of coping style was due to predominant social conditions at that point in history, particularly the role of women, which necessitated that they play a passive, dependent role. The classical form of conversion hysteria described at an earlier period is rarely seen today, though textbooks still describe the characteristic symptoms.

The basic mechanism involved in the development of this coping style is conversion, in which anxiety from the original conflict is converted into specific physical manifestations. The reader will remember that the mechanism of conversion is also implicated in the development of psychosomatic disorders, but it is important to bear in mind that psychosomatic disorders altered body physiology, while in classic hysteria there is no such physiologic involvement. The most common forms of conversion hysteria interfere with the person's motor or sensory capacities. Classic conversion symptoms include weakness of a body part, paralysis or anesthesia (loss of a sensation) of a limb, lessening of vision, and seizures. Therapists have frequently noted that in the face of such severe symptoms as paralysis or anesthesia, the person expresses remarkably little concern. Therapists think that these persons have no anxiety; that the symptoms have served both to bind their anxiety and to produce other advantages, commonly referred to as secondary gains.

As in the other neurotic coping styles, the form that a particular conversion hysteria takes symbolizes the underlying conflict; for example, a boy wishing to strike his father may develop paralysis of his arm. This serves two purposes; in a primary way it protects him from his impulses, and in a secondary manner he gains other benefits, such as sympathy and attention. Note the cultural determination of how people handle anxiety. There are not too many boys today who would choose this route of handling conflict with their fathers, since our current culture dictates other means for expressing aggression. Boys today would probably be far more likely to get into difficulty at school, shoplift, take drugs, or simply go ahead and hit the father. In the Victorian era, by contrast, people did not have as many alternative forms of behavior available to them, and they were much more restricted in terms of a network of social relationships. It is interesting to note that it is now people in very restricted networks, such as the armed services during war, who are the most likely candidates for such conversion reactions.

An equally unsophisticated neurotic coping style, uncommon today probably because of the availability of other alternatives, is *dissociative hysteria.* Here there is a gross disturbance of awareness and memory. Several terms are used for the different manipulations of one's state of consciousness with regard to behavior carried out. In a *fugue,* the person usually acts out certain impulses without any awareness of his or her current behavior. For example, a man may travel many miles and not remember how he got there or what he did along the way. A fugue is a temporary state and commonly develops in conjunction with the use of alcohol or with other factors that serve to loosen the usual defensive personality structure. In *amnesia,* the person completely walls off all of his or her prior experience. Amnesiacs cannot remember who they are nor any of the prior circumstances of their lives. Usually dissociative reactions develop in response to intensely stressful emotional experiences. A third form of conversion reaction is represented in the development of multiple personalities. Sybil[13] is a classic example of such a phenomenon. While multiple personalities are classic and colorful forms of hysterical coping styles, they are rarely seen in such a pure form today.

More commonly, a number of persons cope with anxiety by renouncing their true selves and going through life putting on a role performance that will elicit certain favorable responses from others; they go through

13. Flora R. Schreiber, *Sybil* (New York: Warner Paperback Library, 1974).

life playing a part rather than being or expressing themselves. As Angyal has pointed out, there are two basic hallmarks of neurotic behavior: the prevalence of *fear* and the determining role of fantasy.[14] The person's life is built around avoiding anxiety-provoking experiences. Angyal feels that the hysteric has early experiences that lead him or her to feel unlovable and unworthy, leading in turn to a massive denial of the personality that is spontaneously his or her own. The person then maneuvers to avoid the anxiety over these unacceptable feelings by playing the role of someone other than his or her true self. He or she is thus forced into a position of adopting a facade, giving an "as if" quality to all of life. The problem becomes compounded when significant others begin to respond favorably to the "false" self.

As Angyal describes the situation:

> Even more powerful are the effects on the child of being explicitly cast into a false role by the parents, and being faced with expectations he cannot fulfill without totally disregarding himself. The parent may, e.g., praise him as a diligent student, a scholar who has no interest in childish pranks and play, and thus give him a powerful motive to suppress his genuine wishes and to cultivate a false front. This bribing is the counterpart and the complement of the influences that result in repression; the parents ascribe to the child not just "purity from evil" but positive merits which are equally untrue. He pockets them, but he knows deep down that his self-image is false, that he is a fake. In measuring himself against the excessive parental expectations he secretly begins to feel utterly worthless.[15]

The most frequently censured behaviors on the part of children in our society concern some expression of sexual impulses. Common examples are the parental responses to children exploring their genitals in any manner that might relate to masturbation, or examining one another's bodies in playing "doctor," or going through the Oedipal stage and getting locked into a struggle with the parents that is interpreted as "bad" because of its sexual overtones. Such sexual endeavors, in whatever way they are experienced by the child, become a prominent part of what must be repressed, and they are acted upon only symbolically by whatever form the neurosis takes.

---

14. Angyal, *Neurosis and Treatment,* pp. 139-148.
15. Ibid., p. 141.

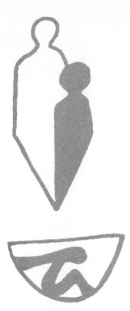

Development of a negative self-image

An example of this is the adolescent girl who acts out her sexual feelings toward men by creating a very sexy appearance and displaying behavior that may be perceived only as a "come-on." When the adolescent boy accepts the sexual invitation at its face value, the response is a slap in the face and a vehement protestation of outrage by the girl, who never intended to become involved in such an intimate manner as an expression of her "real" self. She may even deny that her behavior is sexually stimulating and insist on perceiving it as part of being a well-mannered, friendly approach to people that other people can admire. Instead of viewing her manner of dress as provocative, she identifies it as appropriate for a girl of her status. As with other forms of neurosis, the major part of her life becomes entangled in a series of negotiations with others that relate to this cycle of repression and "as if" living; whenever she is threatened by having to be herself, she seeks release by engaging in behavior that again is representative of a "false" self.

The same type of hysterical pattern is evidenced in the lives of women who attach themselves to strong men, usually those who have either wealth or prestige (and frequently both), and then forevermore live in their shadow. Again these women are not faced with having to be their true selves, but are preoccupied with the role of wife of the important man. These women are at a great loss if something happens to interrupt the relationship, even for a time, because they have no idea of what to do as independent, free-standing people.

TREATMENT ISSUES

As can be seen from our discussion of psychosomatic and neurotic coping styles, many people with these types of symptoms never appear for psychiatric treatment. In fact, many of them appear to be faring tolerably well. The compulsive businessman is making a profit, even though he may suffer from ulcers and other forms of psychosomatic problems. That he has an ulcer is perceived by himself and others as the price he has had to pay for being successful; it is not necessarily viewed as problematic, other than for the discomfort it causes him. Most persons with such life styles would be insulted at the suggestion that they might be in need of treatment. Some appear for treatment not because of the personal pain they are experiencing, but because they are causing troubles for others. The husband of the phobic wife may insist, when he has had to take over all her responsibilities, that she needs some kind of help. Still others present themselves as wishing relief from certain symptoms such as obsessive thoughts, compulsive rituals, panic attacks, or misunderstanding by others. Rarely do such persons present themselves as wishing an improved life for themselves; they are unable to formulate any goals for therapy other than getting rid of the problematic symptom.

In treating neurotic behavior, then, one is faced with a number of problematic issues. First, persons coming for help are focusing to a great extent on the symptoms that are causing them difficulties. They wish relief from these symptoms. The therapist knows, even though the patient may not, that treatment of the symptom is going to precipitate changes in a person's overall life style. Furthermore, it is important to bear in mind that even though patients may complain about their symptoms, their particular patterns of behavior form the basis of their relationships with significant others. Their roles in social groups are built around their particular styles of coping. Removal of the symptoms frequently creates problems for those in reciprocal roles, for they must also alter their manner of relating. Again taking the example of the husband of the phobic woman; should her phobias be removed, she may become much more independent and self-directed, and he may feel abandoned and no longer needed, suffering a loss of self-esteem that may culminate in the accentuation of his neurotic patterns. A central issue in treatment, then, is whether to treat only the person as an individual or to relate to that person as a member of a social network, such as a family or other significant reference groups.

A further issue about which there are differing views relates to the goals of treatment. Some hold that the central goal should be to alleviate the particular problematic symptom, while others argue that the total life style of the person is in need of alteration and that this should be the central treatment goal. Some argue that alleviation of the symptom in itself will precipitate massive changes in the person's total life style; while others say it is not necessary to pay attention to the symptom, for the person treated as a whole will gain insight into himself or herself, and the symptoms will disappear. A related treatment issue is whether it is necessary for the person with a psychosomatic or neurotic coping style to gain a cognitive understanding of the nature of his or her problems, past or current, or whether a behavioral change without concomitant understanding is sufficient. Take, for example, a girl who has many conflicts with her mother, while in fact the real problem may be that the mother is working out remaining Oedipal conflicts by trying to steal the daughter's boyfriend. Some would argue that the daughter may not be cured of her neurotic symptoms until she cognitively understands the Oedipal situation with her mother, while others would maintain that simply helping the girl to win the struggle with her mother would eliminate the issue.

While these issues are particularly pertinent in considering treatment of psychosomatic and neurotic problems, they also are representative of more general issues of intervention, and in this light they will be discussed in much greater detail in Section II.

SUMMARY

The nature of psychosomatic disorders is still a matter of controversy, with many people believing that stress of a psychological nature is implicated in one way or another with the development of the physical pathology. Two basic theoretical views are advanced regarding the relationships between psychological and physiological processes: (1) that stress generally is a contributor to a wide range of physiological disorders and (2) that specific sets of conflicts contribute to specific types of disorders, such as ulcers or asthma. Significant losses are most frequently associated with the development of psychosomatic problems.

Neurotic coping styles develop out of particular maneuvers used to manage anxiety. One's whole style of living shows the restrictions and difficulties in relating that are an outgrowth of his or her persistent and persuasive attempts to manage anxiety. Common to all of them is their crippling effects on the person's total outlook and style of living. Neurotic people tend to become captives of their anxieties and fears, develop tightly organized lives as a means of control, and live in relative isolation from warm relationships.

The particular categorizations are based on the most prominent symptomatology. The current A.P.A. classifications include (1) anxiety reaction, (2) phobic reaction, (3) obsessive-compulsive reaction, (4) dissociative reaction and conversion reaction, and (5) depressive reaction (discussed in Chapter 7). In an anxiety reaction, the primary symptom is free-floating anxiety experienced in varying degrees at unpredictable intervals. In a phobic reaction, the person's anxiety is attached to specific places or things. Displacement is the chief defense mechanism. The avoidance of objects featured in the phobic reaction pervades all aspects of the person's life and significantly influences his or her interpersonal relationships. A person who has an obsessive-compulsive reaction likewise conducts most of his or her interpersonal negotiations around particular obsessions or compulsions. Anxiety is contained by obsessive thinking or compulsive action. Dissociative or conversion reactions are forms of hysteria. In these reactions the original conflict is handled either through amnesia (dissociative reaction) or through converting the conflict into a specific physical manifestation.

Treatment controversies center on whether the symptoms or the originating conflict is to be the central focus.

FURTHER READINGS

"Anxiety—Recognition and Intervention." *American Journal of Nursing* 65 (Sept. 1965): 120-152.

Burkhardt, Marti. "Response to Anxiety." *American Journal of Nursing* 69 (Oct. 1969): 2153-2154.

Drage, Elaine. "Recall of Panic Episodes." *American Journal of Nursing* 68 (June 1968): 1254-1257.

May, Rollo. *The Meaning of Anxiety,* pp. 190-234. New York: The Ronald Press, 1950.

Melton, Janet. "A Boy With Anorexia Nervosa." *American Journal of Nursing* 74 (Sept. 1974): 1649-1651.

Neylan, Margaret. "Anxiety." *American Journal of Nursing* 62 (May 1962): 110-111.

Parks, Suzanne. "Allowing Physical Distance as a Nursing Approach." *Perspectives in Psychiatric Care* 4, no. 6 (1969): 31-35.

Peplau, Hildegard. "Interpersonal Techniques: The Crux of Psychiatric Nursing." *American Journal of Nursing* 62 (June 1962): 50-54.

Peplau, Hildegard. "A Working Definition of Anxiety." In *Some Clinical Approaches to Psychiatric Nursing,* edited by Shirley Burd and Margaret Marshall. New York: The Macmillan Company, 1963.

Roncoli, Marianne. "Bantering: A Therapeutic Strategy With Obsessional Patients." *Perspectives in Psychiatric Care* 12, no. 4 (1974): 171-175.

Schmidt, Mary, and Duncan, Beverly. "Modifying Eating Behavior in Anorexia Nervosa." *American Journal of Nursing* 74 (September 1974): 1646-1648.

Schwartz, Morris, and Shockley, Emmy. *The Nurse and the Mental Patient,* pp. 182-198, 277-280. New York: John Wiley & Sons, Inc., 1954.

CHAPTER FIVE

DRUG
DEPENDENCE

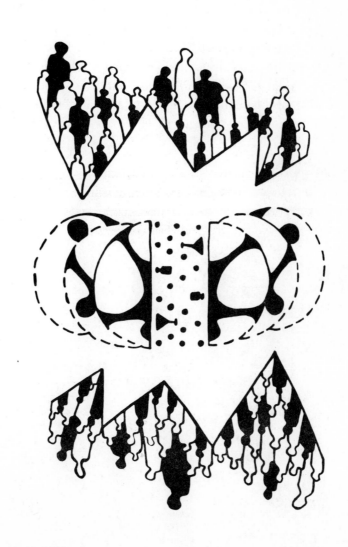

We have described several means of coping with problems, some productive and others less so. The wish to eliminate the anxiety engendered by problems is a universal phenomenon. People usually take anxiety as a signal that something is amiss and in need of problem-solving attention. However, some people develop styles in which anxiety is considered the central problem rather than the signal. They attempt to short-circuit the process by eliminating the anxiety without going through the usual problem-solving steps. A side effect of this technique is that they never learn much detail about what triggered the anxiety, nor do they develop skills related to eliminating its cause. These persons automatically engage in behavior to dull the discomfort experienced when they are anxious, much the way Linus (in "Peanuts") clings to his security blanket.

The use of objects to ameliorate anxiety is familiar to us all to some degree. This use of objects is not, in itself, of paramount significance. But a distinction can be made between using objects as a help in attacking the original problem, and using them as a substitute for action to deal with the problem. It is the latter case that gets incorporated into a style that substitutes maneuvers to eliminate anxiety for an aggressive attack on

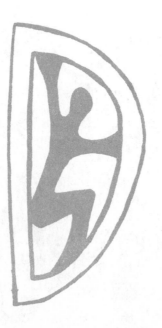

Use of objects to ameliorate anxiety

problems to reach a resolution. In either case, the outcome of the technique depends on many factors; important among these is the choice of objects. Relying on a good luck charm produces a much different response from "shooting up" on heroin.

In considering the whole problem of addictions, it is important to keep constantly in mind the meaning of the individual's choice of objects within the framework of the culture. For instance, in the 19th century women were big consumers of highly alcoholic "tonics," which were supposed to strengthen them. Although taking tonics was thought proper and ladylike, consuming the same amount of alcohol at a bar would have resulted in social ostracism. Thus, it is important to keep in mind not only the effects of the object upon the individual, but the meaning associated with the use of a particular object within a particular social setting.

A further point to note is that while a person may rely initially on a particular object as a way to short-circuit anxiety, a secondary effect may result from the social context. For example, a highly anxious student who fears taking an exam may try marijuana for the first time to reduce her anxiety, but she does this within the context of a group who are also smoking marijuana. Not only does the drug work to reduce the anxiety, but the social group provides support for her which helps to block out the anxiety-producing stimulus. Another student might gravitate toward a marijuana-smoking group to relieve his feelings of loneliness and isolation from other students. He seeks out the group and, as a condition of membership, participates in smoking pot. He relies on his ability to engage in the primary activity of the group—marijuana smoking—as easier than developing skill in interpersonal relationships that might be required in other groups. The fact that he allies himself with a marijuana-smoking group may or may not have major consequences, depending on how this activity is defined, both within this group and within the larger social setting. If the group's activities are not brought to the attention of anyone who is concerned about the dangers of smoking marijuana or the fact that they are engaging in illegal activity, the consequences might be positive, in that the student finds his place as a member of a social group. Perhaps, as the group develops over time, the quality of relationships within the group will form the basis for membership rather than solely the use of marijuana.

In some instances, the group will remain as a haven for lonely, isolated people who either never develop any interpersonal ties or develop ties on the basis of antisocial themes. In these cases, the group does little to help the individual develop an improved coping style. Negative outcomes of being a participant in a marijuana-smoking group may result from the responses of other significant groups. For example, if the university police raid the group and take them off to the police station, it is likely that this group will become publicly labeled as "drug users." In some instances, legal action will be taken and the student will begin developing a police record. Frequently parents become involved at this time and further push the student into a deviant role. One can imagine the irate father appearing at the police station delivering a lecture on how much his son's college education is costing him, and how the son is "ungrateful and no good"—when *he* went to school he had to work his way through and had no time for such foolishness. A frequent additional response is for the group to become solidified on another dimension, that of developing further their anti-establishment views. Pot smoking becomes a symbol that identifies "us," the pot smokers, in contrast to "them," those who do not smoke pot. If this student visited another city, he would identify pot smokers as kindred to him, and this commonality would serve as a unifying element in his life style.

Some people who start out using an object to help in attacking problems find themselves in a different situation, in which, instead of using the object as a means, they begin to use it as an end in itself. An example of this is the suburban housewife who has a cocktail by herself so she will not notice that her husband is late coming home again. She may find herself drinking cocktails in other situations; then gradually look forward to the cocktail itself, even when her husband is not late, and start having one earlier so she can have a second when her husband arrives home.

In our culture, drugs are frequently the object of choice for the relief of anxiety or discomfort. We are conditioned to view drugs as a way of relieving a wide variety of discomforts—tension, anxiety, sleeplessness, and fatigue. Looking into the medicine cabinet of the average American home or viewing television commercials for an evening will attest to this. The use of prescription and nonprescription drugs is encouraged and condoned. "Take Sominex tonight and sleep" echoes through the minds of a large number of Americans.

Many common substances not usually thought of as drugs also are used for their emotional effect, and sometimes they are habit-forming—such as caffeine in coffee, tea, and cola drinks, and nicotine in cigarettes. America has become a drug-taking culture.

The particular types of drugs Americans take are closely tied to predominant values of the overall culture. As Ray points out, most of the drugs used in Western culture "are those primarily affecting arousal levels"[1] rather than those that distort information processing. Drugs that either stimulate or depress the individual, causing a loss of some inhibitions, are "compatible with our aggressively achieving but tightly moral society. Whether speeded up or slowed down, the user is still focused on the outside 'real world.' "[2] In the late 1960s, when a predominant theme among young people was the rejection of achievement-oriented values of society, there was a rise in the taking of mind-altering drugs such as LSD and mescaline. In the early 1970s, as this theme dissipated to some extent, the drugs of choice tended more to be stimulants or depressants ("uppers" and "downers"). The choice of using drugs, and of what drugs to use, is closely tied both to larger cultural values and the norms and values of one's own social groups.

DEFINITION OF TERMS

Before proceeding to discuss types of drugs and their effects, let us first clarify the meaning of some terms commonly used when discussing drug use. Drug *use* refers to ingesting, in any manner, a chemical substance that has an effect on the body. Drug *abuse* is a value-laden term in our society, and the definition of what constitutes abuse varies from person to person and from special interest group to special interest group. For example, a brochure called "Drugs and You" circulated to public school students gives this definition of drug abuse: "Drug abuse occurs whenever a person takes a drug without a prescription in an attempt to *influence* his mind or body to escape from reality. Drug abuse can cause *legal, social,* and *medical* problems. It can 'unbalance' a healthy body and cause physical or mental illness or even death!"[3] According to this definition, the crucial

---

1. Oakley S. Ray, *Drugs, Society, and Human Behavior* (St. Louis: C. V. Mosby, 1972), p. 271.
2. Ibid.
3. "Drugs and You" (Greenfield, Mass.: Channing L. Bete Co., 1969).

variable is whether the drug was obtained from a doctor on prescription. And so a woman who receives amphetamine "diet pills" from her doctor and takes them with increasing regularity would not be considered to be abusing drugs. On the other hand, there are physicians who hold the view that prescribing amphetamines for weight reduction in any case is an example of drug abuse. Further, the above definition emphasizes the physical or mental illness that might develop from taking drugs. These examples illustrate the clouding and relativity of the drug issue.

Another way of attempting to clarify the definition of drug abuse is to distinguish drugs taken for medicinal purposes from those taken for recreational purposes. Again the issue is cloudy, since there can easily be disagreement about what constitutes a medicinal purpose. Is taking sleeping pills because one is too anxious to go to sleep medicinal or an escape? Taking a glass of wine before bedtime may be interpreted as a form of relaxation by some and as medicinal by others. A further complicating example is the practice in England of regularly prescribing heroin for addicts. Because of the lack of clarity of the term, "drug abuse" is frequently a term of choice.

Addiction is still a commonly used term, though it too has dropped out of favor because of problems of clarity and specificity like those described for the term "drug abuse."

Drug dependence is currently more frequently used and has a more precise definition. There are two types of drug dependence: physical and psychological. *Physical dependence* means that the body has accommodated to the presence of the drug so that it is required to maintain normal functioning. If the drug is stopped, withdrawal symptoms occur. Tolerance develops as the body accommodates to the drug and requires increasing doses to maintain the desired effect. Both tolerance and physical dependence are variables; either one may depend on the drug and on individual factors that have not been clearly identified. The term "addiction," used properly, refers only to physical dependence. *Psychological dependence* refers to the reliance on drugs solely for nonphysical reasons; the psychologically dependent person feels that he or she cannot get along without the drug.

While the definitions given above seem rather clear-cut, there are a number of problematic questions related to the nature of dependence. The exact physiological and psychological mechanisms underlying addiction are not really understood. For example, it is possible to break physical dependence upon a particular drug, but the "craving" or desire for drugs still lingers on. As Brecher describes it:

> Most addicts who mainline heroin, when asked what happens when they 'kick the habit' describe the classic withdrawal symptoms—nausea, vomiting, aches, and pains, yawning, sneezing, and so on. When asked what happens after withdrawal, they describe an equally specific 'post-addiction syndrome'—a wavering unstable composite of anxiety, depression and craving for the drug. The craving is not continuous but seems to come and go in waves of varying intensity, for months, even years after withdrawal. It is particularly likely to return in moments of emotional stress.[4]

A contrasting example is provided by reports of the Vietnam veterans. It was feared that large numbers of soldiers returning from Vietnam would be permanently addicted, according to the established views concerning physical dependence. However, Lee Robins of Washington University School of Medicine (St. Louis) studied 1,000 1971 returnees and found that during the eight to ten months after their return, 53 percent of them drank heavily and 45 percent used marijuana. The use of other drugs reverted to pre-service levels. Only 14 percent of those who had been seriously addicted to narcotics in Vietnam became re-addicted..[5]

In the instance of Vietnam veterans it is important to note that although addiction to heroin was not evident, a large percentage of returned veterans substituted heavy drinking. This evidence points to the incomplete state of knowledge; contradictions abound and there are more questions than answers. One of the biggest areas of questions concerns the physical factors involved in dependence, the psychological and social questions, and the way in which they are inextricably interrelated.

TYPES OF DRUGS

Drugs are commonly divided into central nervous system depressants, central nervous system stimulants, hallucinogens, marijuana and hashish

---

4. Edward M. Brecher, *Licit and Illicit Drugs* (Mount Vernon, N.Y.: Consumers Union, 1972), pp. 13-14.
5. *Science News* 106, no. 1 (13 July 1974), p. 26.

(which do not fit into the usual categorization system), and inhalants. Table 5-1 lists the major drugs in each of these categories.

DEPRESSANTS

The use of depressants, particularly opium derivatives and alcohol, has a long history, and the taking of these drugs has taken on different meanings at different times. All cultures have, through the years, developed mind-altering potions, sometimes as a relaxant to be used on festive occasions, sometimes as a part of religious ceremonies, and sometimes as a pacifier to numb the minds of those in deprived circumstances so they will be less aware of their plight and will exert no pressure to change their condition. An example of the last is the tot of rum provided for seamen by the British navy. This was regarded as a right of the men and was withheld only as a form of punishment. If the ship ran out of rum, a crisis would occur and mutiny would be imminent. In contrast, if a seaman was harshly treated for a minor offense, there would be little complaining about this treatment. The use of depressants follows a cultural pattern. Where they have been used, it is always possible to trace how their use has been consistent with some overall social norms.

OPIATES

Although heroin is today the most frequently abused opiate, such was not always the case. In the nineteenth century, the sale of opium was legal. It could be purchased with or without prescription and was available in drug stores, in grocery and general stores, and even through the mail. It was also contained in many patent medicines, some of which were given to babies and children. In about 1890, approximately two-thirds of the opium addicts were middle-aged women of the upper and middle classes. According to prevalent social norms, the taking of tonics laced with opium was permissible, and in fact advocated, as a means of handling a number of physical complaints. Opiates were not viewed as any type of menace to society. In fact, they were perceived to have the effect of "calming the person," a characteristic important in the Victorian era, and therefore they were not restricted. The fact that women were the prime users is perhaps related to another social norm of this era, that cultured women did not

Table 5-1   Major Drugs by Category

DEPRESSANTS	STIMULANTS	HALLUCINOGENS	*MARIJUANA AND HASHISH	INHALANTS
Opium and its derivatives	Cocaine	LSD		Airplane glue
Morphine	Amphetamines	Mescaline		Plastic cement
Heroin	Dextroamphetamine	Psilocybin		Hair spray
Codeine	Dexedrine	DMT		Toluene
Synthetic narcotics	Methamphetamine			A wide
Meperidine (Demerol)	Methedrine			variety of
Methadone (Dolophine)	Desoxyn			substances
	Caffeine			whose vapors
Alcohol	Nicotine			may be inhaled
				(paint thinner,
Barbiturates				gasoline, etc.)
Phenobarbital				
Pentobarbital (Nembutal)				
Secobarbital (Seconal)				
Nonbarbiturates				
Hypnotics				
Glutethimide (Doriden)				
Ethchlorvynol (Placidyl)				
Diazepam (Valium)				
Chlordiazepoxide (Librium)				
Meprobamate (Miltown, Equanil)				
Nicotine				

*Difficult to categorize since its chemical and physiological effects are unique, and its properties do not adequately fit in any of the other categories.

frequent places where alcoholic beverages were sold; only women defined as "loose" or lower class and otherwise uncultured would drink alcoholic beverages. As the addicting characteristics of opium became recognized, the major objection to their use surrounded their damage to "moral character"; opium users were not socially ostracized or labeled deviant. Many addicts led useful and productive lives, since opiates do not, in themselves, interfere with an addicted person's functioning.[6]

With the increasing awareness of the addicting qualities of opium, laws were developed to control its use. A first step toward the development of laws regulating opium use was embodied in the Pure Food and Drug Act of 1906. For the first time, labeling of medicines containing opiates was required, to be followed by a requirement that the quantity of each drug be specified and that it meet standards of identity and purity.[7]

The Harrison Act of 1914, an outgrowth of the international agreement resulting from the opium war between Britain and China, was the first attempt to license drug dealers and was aimed primarily at the regulation of drug traffic through taxing distributors. Legal sources of drugs, such as doctors, were licensed to dispense drugs only in the course of their professional practice. Others were licensed to dispense drugs under specified conditions; the act was an attempt to provide for an orderly flow of drugs. The long-range effect of this bill, however, was the reverse; immediately many physicians were arrested under the provisions of the law. Very rigid controls specifying the use of opiates only for medicinal purposes became, in effect, a prohibition measure. Some physicians were prosecuted for making opiates available to addicts; as many physicians refused to treat them, addicts were forced to obtain their drugs from illegal sources.

In the past fifty years, the reaction of federal and state legislators to this illegal traffic has been to pass more and stricter laws to control narcotics and to punish offenders. The effect of such laws has been to create a thriving black market where heroin is readily available if one can pay the price; thus a whole deviant counter-culture has been created in which the predominant group goal is to obtain sufficient money to support the habit, with little regard to how the money is obtained.

Through the years since the passage of the Harrison Act, addiction

6. Brecher, *Licit and Illicit Drugs,* pp. 3-19.
7. Ibid., p. 17.

patterns have changed drastically. In contrast to the middle-class Victorian women with their opium-laced tonics, addicts in the 1950s and early 1960s were primarily young, lower-class black males. Heroin became the drug of choice. The late 1960s and early 1970s saw an increase in heroin addiction among young, middle-class white suburban dwellers. The number of addicts has increased since 1900, but not proportionately to the population. In 1971, there were an estimated 250,000 to 315,000 heroin addicts.[8] Because of the laws governing drug use, and the accompanying inflated prices of illegally obtained drugs, many addicts pursue lives of crime to support their habit, and their existence centers on procuring enough money to buy their daily supply. The heroin black market has developed into a well-organized system of suppliers and pushers, and addicts exist in their own subculture apart from the mainstream of society.

Let us examine some of the facets of addiction through considering an episode in the life of Larry, a hypothetical 19-year-old, white middle-class addict who started pill popping while in high school. During the past year he has left his high school group and gravitated toward a group of hard-core drug users. When Larry first started on heroin, he was invited to a party where all the slightly older, "cool guys" congregated. He had looked up to the guys in this group during high school, and while he recognized that two of them were kind of "messed up," he felt that the rest of the group were "capable of handling it." The "messed up" guys were ones whose drug habit was out of control and whose personal lives were deteriorating. They were regarded as weak by the others. As the party progressed and a number of the guys started shooting up, they asked Larry if he wanted to try it. Larry agreed out of curiosity and a wish to gain status with the others. Of course, he was not going to be like those other guys—he just wanted to see how it compared with the other stuff he had been taking. Since Larry was given his dose intravenously, he experienced what is usually described as a sudden "rush" of warmth in the pit of his stomach. In contrast to other drugs, it really did not give him the kick he had expected. As the initial phase passed, he felt slightly nauseous and removed from what was going on around him. It made him feel pleased with himself, that he was grown-up and important. Thus, for Larry, one of the important factors in initially taking heroin was the meaning of the

8. Ibid., pp. 49-58.

group experience for him. The initial drug-taking of other people may be associated with the reduction of discomfort, not with pleasure.

Larry continued to join the weekly party on Saturday night. As he returned to work each Monday, he was pleased with himself that he could take heroin and have no desire for it other than on weekends—he could take it or leave it like all the other drugs he had experimented with. However, on Wednesday he had a disagreement with his boss, who he thought was too critical of his performance, and he walked out. On his way out of the plant, he met his friend Sam, who was part of the Saturday night group. Sam invited him to his pad, and during the evening Larry had a shot of heroin. He spent the next couple of days there, and in the course of those few days had a couple more shots of heroin in the company of the group. The next week he went back to his parents' house, went job-hunting, and kept on meeting turndowns. He thought back to the previous week and remembered that when he had had a shot he did not really worry so much about not having a job. So on Wednesday he again went to his friend's house and had a shot. During this period of time, he felt that his drug use was definitely under control, but he had shortened the intervals; the jobs that he was able to find were not particularly satisfying, and he increasingly looked forward to the times spent with the group as a time of relaxation when he did not feel as hassled as he did the rest of the time, when he was either looking for a job, being criticized by his parents, or working in an unsatisfactory line of work.

This pattern of Larry's is fairly typical. He was at the age when most people are introduced to drugs on occasion, as they progress; the intervals become shorter to a point at which they become "hooked." The drug occupies an increasingly larger place in their lives. People who are very wealthy and do not have money problems in securing the drug can often be addicted without gaining much attention. But people like Larry, who have limited resources, eventually structure more and more of their lives around the problems and activities involved in securing a supply of the drug.

At some point after Larry became a daily user, he noticed that if he did not take the drug daily he experienced unpleasant symptoms—withdrawal symptoms. Some people describe withdrawal symptoms as similar to the flu, with the severity of the symptoms related to the extent of the habit. The only way to relieve these symptoms was to have a fix; then

The addicted life style

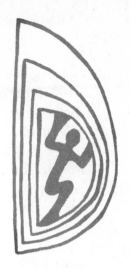

Larry began to notice that the same amount of drug no longer resulted in the same good feelings, and he began to increase the dose.

From this point on, the life of the addict varies considerably, depending on his or her circumstances and on the responses of people to him or her. Some addicts must take to the "street life," which is generally a rather regimented, antisocial, all-engrossing life style that revolves around the various kinds of hustling necessary to get enough drug to, at best, produce a high, but at any rate to avoid withdrawal symptoms. Since Larry was still living at home, he had his parents' resources to run through. The usual pattern for Larry was that, although he had many disagreements with his parents about many of his activities, he could always rely on them for money whenever he was in a tight spot. As his habit increased and he was working less frequently, his requests for money from his parents increased, and they became more upset with him and critical of his behavior; they did not understand why he spent so much time just lying around. Larry reached the point where he stole money from his parents when he could, and the family increasingly became involved in a series of confrontations that culminated in Larry's leaving home and living with his friends. Larry now adopts a hand-to-mouth existence of jobs when he can get them, pilfering and petty stealing, concern about always having a pusher available and hoping that he will not be cheated, and constant fear of being apprehended. The "fix" has become the central organizing point to his life.

Larry is caught and arrested, and since it is his first offense, he is sent to the local drug treatment center. The initial stage of treatment, withdrawal from drugs, goes rather easily for Larry. He has, in fact, a successful career in all phases of the treatment program. He fulfills his responsibilities as a member of the live-in group, participates actively in the "rap" sessions designed to help him get to know himself and his weaknesses, and lands a job which he holds for a month before graduating from the treatment program. Larry stays clean three months but then finds himself gradually back on the "stuff." When asked about how he got back on drugs, Larry can give no adequate explanation; he can just report that he felt an intense craving at various times and that he gradually succumbed. Larry's experience with "kicking the habit" is fairly typical. It is a relatively simple matter for addicts to have their physical dependence on drugs eliminated, but to have the craving persist, which ultimately leads to their re-addiction.

■ *Theories About the Cause of Addiction.* A number of theoretical views as to why people become addicted to heroin are presented in the literature. These theories fall into three major categories: psychological, sociological, and biochemical. Most psychological theories revolve around the theme that persons become addicted because of an "addictive personality"; the focus of these theories is on understanding the psyche of the addict.[9] Jaffe, for example, points out that while chance, curiosity, and availability may lead an individual to experiment with a drug, they do not explain why he or she continues to use it. Those who become dependent on drugs do so because of some personality or emotional disturbance that they attempt to relieve through drugs. Narcotics relieve anxiety in a passive way by suppressing the source of the conflict, while alcohol and barbiturates release inhibitions and promote aggressive behavior.[10]

Research following this theoretical point of view seeks to discern the personality traits of drug users. Cohen et al., in a study comparing multidrug users seeking therapeutic help with a control group of nonusers also seeking help, discovered certain personality traits and family relationship patterns in the drug-using group that were not present in the control

9. Ibid., p. 67.
10. Jerome Jaffe, "Drug Addiction and Drug Abuse," in *The Pharmacological Basis of Therapeutics,* ed. Louis Goodman and Alfred Gilman, 4th ed. (New York: The MacMillan Co., 1970).

group. They found that the drug users behaved in a dominating and critical manner, although underneath this behavior they had self doubts and preferred to be passive. They described their parents as being self-reliant and efficient, but not emotionally warm, with a minimum of affection displayed in their homes.[11] In considering research of this nature, it is important to note its ex post facto nature, addicts are studied, and the personality traits discerned are then attributed to them without any data about their pre-addictive personality patterns, or how they compare to a nonaddicted population. Further, it is difficult to differentiate between psychological and sociological factors. As Abrams et al. noted in their study of black ghetto residents addicted to heroin, both psychological and sociological factors are implicated in addition. They argue that while it is true that drugs are used to relieve anxiety, much of the anxiety comes from the individual's environment, that is, the economic and social deprivation of the ghetto. Heroin is readily available, and experimentation with it is common. It is not unusual for a ghetto resident to use heroin in an attempt to block out the harsh realities of his or her life.[12]

Sociological theorists generally hold that the social context is the key factor in understanding drug use. Brecher summarizes this point of view:

> These views hold in general that society creates addicts and causes ex-addicts to relapse into addiction again. The sense of hopelessness and defeat among the dwellers in our city slums, the sense, among young people today, of impotence to affect change, the needs of young people to belong to a group and their consequent drift into groups of heroin users—countless sociological factors such as these are cited to explain both addiction and relapse following "cure."[13]

Disenchanted with both psychological and sociological theories, a number of researchers are investigating biochemical factors that might be related to drug use. Regarding physiological causes of drug dependence, the primary consideration is the fact that certain drugs, namely central nervous system depressants, produce physical dependence or addiction. This fact is not related to why individuals begin to use drugs, but it is

---

11. Charles Cohen et al., "Interpersonal Factors of Personality for Drug-Abusing Patients and Their Therapeutic Implications," *Archives of General Psychiatry* 24 (April 1971): 355-358.
12. Arnold Abrams et al., "Psychosocial Aspects of Addiction," *American Journal of Public Health* 58 (Nov. 1968): 2142-2155.
13. Brecher, *Licit and Illicit Drugs,* p. 67.

definitely related to why, once addicted, they continue to use them. Biochemical research is directed toward identifying changes in the structure of the chemical molecule during withdrawal and the effect of these changes upon the cells of the nervous system.[41] Current physiological research has not been able to identify factors that account for re-addiction. With heroin, a post-addictive syndrome has been described: the anxiety, depression, and craving experienced by former addicts, even after prolonged abstinence. This syndrome occurs most often during stressful periods and is the cause of many relapses.[15] Even though the exact factors have not been identified, proponents of biochemical theories hold that the propensity for re-addiction is attributable to the effects of the opiate molecule on the nervous system.[16]

ALCOHOL

> An alcoholic is someone who drinks too much, and you don't like anyway. Anonymous.[17]

Alcohol (ethyl alcohol or ethanol), though not often thought of as a drug, is a mind- and mood-altering chemical and is classified as a central nervous depressant. Although officially classified as a depressant, alcohol produces a number of contradictory effects. At low levels it may have no apparent effect upon the drinker, at moderate levels it may make one euphoric, while at other levels it acts as a sedative and puts one to sleep. The World Health Organization classifies alcohol as "a drug intermediate in kind and degree between habit-forming and addicting drugs."[18]

Definitions of what constitute "normal" drinking as contrasted with alcoholism are numerous and contradictory. As with other types of drug use, the definitions are closely tied to the point of view of the definer. The National Institute of Alcoholism and Alcohol Abuse (NIAAA) defines excessive use as taking two forms: (1) *alcohol abuse,* which is defined as "repeated episodes of intoxication or heavy drinking which impairs health, or consistent use of alcohol as a coping mechanism in dealing with the problems of life to a degree of serious interference with the individual's

---

14. Ibid., p. 68.
15. Ibid., pp. 13-14.
16. Ibid., p. 68.
17. Ray, *Drugs, Society, and Human Behavior,* p. 78.
18. Ibid., p. 79.

effectiveness. . . ."[19] and (2) *alcoholism,* which, in addition to the above, infers that the individual is physically dependent or addicted and has developed tolerance. Based on these definitions, it is estimated that while alcohol is used by about two-thirds of the adult population, it is used excessively by about 7 per cent.

The World Health Organization incorporates a consideration of the general norms of the community in their definition of "alcoholism as a chronic behavioral disorder manifested by repeated drinking of alcoholic beverages in excess of the dietary and social uses of the community and to an extent that interferes with the drinker's health or his social and economic function."[20] Using this definition, a person may not be defined as having a drinking problem so long as he or she stays within a particular cultural context, but in another setting where drinking patterns are very different, the same person may suddenly find himself or herself labeled as alcoholic. In France, where the quantity of wine drunk regularly far exceeds the usual limits set in other cultures, a person who consumes large quantities of alcohol would rarely be defined or define himself as having a drinking problem. Yet, should a Frenchman come to America and ask to be served wine for breakfast, he might be perceived differently.

Most definitions include as part of their criteria some statement related to whether the use of alcohol interferes with one's social and occupational behavior.[21] Using this definition, a person who drinks heavily but is able to maintain himself or herself in occupational and social roles may be able to avoid being labeled an alcoholic. For example, the business executive who has an efficient secretary to do much of his work for him and who has a considerable amount of freedom in setting the parameters of his work may be able to avoid being labeled an alcoholic even though he consumes three double martinis at lunch every day and continues to drink steadily throughout the remainder of the day. Many such persons who finally join AA (Alcoholics Anonymous) look back retrospectively and define themselves as having been alcoholic, although at the time they did not so define themselves. In contrast, the assembly-line worker who must be precise and speedy in doing his or her task may get into trouble by

---

19. Department of Health, Education, and Welfare, *Alcohol and Health* (Washington, D.C.: U. S. Government Printing Office, 1971), p. 1.
20. George A. Ulett, *A Synopsis of Contemporary Psychiatry* (St. Louis: C. V. Mosby, 1972), p. 184.
21. Ray, *Drugs, Society, and Human Behavior,* p. 92.

drinking even a minimal quantity while on the job, particularly if he or she has an accident or cannot keep up the pace.

Still other definitions are closely tied to the precise amounts that someone drinks. An example of this is given by Ulett, who defines *episodic excessive drinking* in terms of becoming intoxicated as frequently as four times a year; while "persons who become intoxicated more than twelve times a year or are recognizably under the influence of alcohol more than once a week, even though not intoxicated, are classified as *habitual excessive drinkers.*"[22] "Alcohol addiction" is used to describe persons who are dependent on alcohol and suffer withdrawal symptoms should they abstain. Although these definitions are an attempt to be precise, it is important to note the relativity of their criteria.

Estimates of the seriousness of the problem of alcoholism are closely tied to the definitions one uses in determining who is an alcoholic. Most authors stress the magnitude of the problem. The NIAAA estimates that there are five million persons in this country who suffer from alcoholism and another four million who are alcohol abusers. One person in five reports that someone close to him or her, usually a family member, abuses alcohol.

Mulford, taking a different perspective, reports that 8 per cent of the adult population may be classified as heavy drinkers, and only a part of that number might be considered to be alcoholic. Based on this report he concludes: "The major portion of the nation's adults are either abstainers or have such a low consumption level that they can hardly contribute to the 'alcoholism problem.' "[23]

In any event, there are a number of persons who do use alcohol to excess. Contrary to popular belief, however, most alcoholics are not derelicts. That we should hold this stereotype is perhaps a reflection of how vulnerable the poor person with few role options is to being labeled as in some deviant category. In fact, Mulford reports:

> . . . heavy drinkers tend to be concentrated in the following social segments: males, the college educated, the cities, the above $5,000 income group, the next-to-highest and the third from lowest status occupations,

---

22. Ulett, *A Synopsis of Contemporary Psychiatry*, pp. 183-184.
23. Harold Mulford, "Drinking and Deviant Drinking, U.S.A. 1963," *Quarterly Journal of Studies on Alcohol* 25 (1964): 649.

and the unmarried. Among the religious categories the Protestants who did not specify a denomination have the highest rates of heavy drinkers while the Methodists, Baptists and Jews stand out with low rates. . . . Jews had the highest rates of drinkers of any religion, but next to the Methodists, the lowest rates of heavy drinkers.[24]

These findings would appear to support the view that the use of alcohol is closely related to one's involvement or lack of involvement in social groupings that have developed social norms governing drinking patterns. Involvement in certain groups, such as religious or ethnic groups, position in certain socioeconomic categories, and marital and family status seem clearly related to the incidence of both alcohol use and alcoholism.

Note also that certain categories of persons who have a high incidence of alcoholism may be under higher levels of stress than those with lower incidence rates. The upwardly mobile male living in the city and striving to "make it" may rely on the use of alcohol as a means of coping with his anxieties and on excessive amounts of alcohol to dull the realization that he has not as yet "made it." Because of the pronounced effect of alcohol in producing euphoria, reducing inhibitions, and in general making the world appear rosier, it is very easy for people to incorporate its use into their repertoire of coping styles, and particularly to use it as a means of avoiding a problem, rather than as a help in tackling it. As the effect of the alcohol wears off, the problem that was avoided once again surfaces, thus setting off another round of anxiety that may again trigger the use of alcohol as a means of coping.

As this pattern begins to develop, it receives considerable encouragement within our societal structure, where the before-dinner cocktail reigns supreme. At some point, however, this coping style may interfere with the way a person carries out his or her social role obligations, and people in complementary roles may put pressure on the person to modify his or her drinking behavior. For some people the cycle may stop at this point, but for others this pressure becomes an additional source of stress which induces further drinking. The continuation of drinking behavior results ultimately in the person's becoming socially defined as an alcoholic, and as he or she moves on this path it becomes inceasingly difficult to break out of the drinking pattern. For other people, defining the person as an alco-

---

24. Ibid., p. 647.

holic provides a handy explanation for why he or she cannot cooperate in fulfilling certain role obligations.

Alcoholics, unlike addicts using opiates, do usually suffer from varying degrees of physical impairment. Some of these difficulties may be a direct result of alcohol on the biochemical structure of the body, while others are probably more related to the life patterns that accompany alcoholism. Prominent among these is wretched nutrition; alcoholics usually do not eat. Vitamin-B deficiencies leave the nervous system in a poor state to withstand the effects of alcohol, and peripheral nerve damage is frequently noted. Lack of sleep and neglect of other health habits render them more susceptible to illness than they might normally be. Since alcohol is metabolized by the liver, excessive use frequently leads to cirrhosis of the liver. Because of these complications, the life span of alcoholic individuals is shortened by an average of ten to twelve years. Since the person under the influence of alcohol suffers from lack of judgment as well as slowed reaction time, he or she is frequently involved in accidents of various kinds. At least 50 percent of all traffic accidents, for instance, are thought to be associated with the use of alcohol.

Prolonged use of alcohol does result in physical dependence, and abrupt withdrawal results in a number of pronounced physiological changes that may be life-threatening. Unlike opiate use, in which withdrawal symptoms are noted immediately after a certain time interval, symptoms do not appear immediately when alcoholics are withdrawn. Symptoms are noted progressively. The initial signs of tremors and anxiety may appear in a few hours, but the person remains rational. Over the next day or two, he or she may begin hallucinating and becomes increasingly terrified. If no medication is given, delirium tremens frequently develops, occasionally accompanied by convulsions; some individuals die at this stage. The most frequent causes of death are heart failure and pneumonia.

■ *Theories About the Cause of Alcoholism.* As with drug dependence, there are a number of psychological, physiological, and sociological theories advanced to explain alcoholism. Psychological theories usually involve descriptions of the "alcoholic personality." As with similar theories related to drug-taking, it is difficult to ascertain whether these characteristics are typical of the person before he or she becomes an alcoholic or are, instead, a reflection of the psychological effects of drinking. The alcoholic personality is usually characterized by dependency, feelings of inferiority, low frustration tolerance, and inability to profit from experience. It should be noted that the shortcoming of most research in this area is that there is no comparative data that would provide evidence that these traits are not also characteristic of a similar proportion of the population who are not alcoholic.

Learning theorists, instead of asking the question "What type of personality leads to alcoholism?", focus their explanations on alcoholism as learned behavior resulting from either positive or negative reinforcement (reward or punishment).[25]

Physiological research is primarily concentrated on attempting to identify differences in enzymes or in other biochemical factors that distinguish the metabolism of alcohol in the addict and in the similarly exposed nonaddict. Geneticists have attempted to identify an inherited vitamin or enzyme deficiency that creates a craving for alcohol. To date, the studies on vitamin deficiencies have been inconclusive.[26] There is evidence, however, that enzyme variations do exist in individuals; the enzyme in question is alcohol dehydrogenase, which is developed in the metabolism of alcohol in the liver. It is believed that these metabolic variations may explain why some persons become alcoholic while others do not. Genetic studies of twins and of the children of alcoholics do not indicate a genetic inheritance of alcoholism. Other researchers are exploring endocrine disorders as they relate to alcoholism; the studies in general are inconclusive but seem to suggest that endocrine disorders are a result of alcoholism rather than a cause.

Sociological theories relate primarily to cultural differences regarding alcohol use, for rates of alcoholism are noticeably higher in some cultures than in others. Studies of drinking behavior in varying primitive tribes seem to indicate that tribes with heavy drinking patterns have a much looser social structure—for example, hunting groups—while some sober tribes live in settled communities with a structured social system. As has been noted, France is a country with one of the biggest drinking problems. Ray attributes this to a number of factors: "This high level of consumption (32 quarts of pure alcohol per year) is maintained by a variety of factors including nationalism, the relating of wine drinking to virility by the

---

25. Department of Health, Education, and Welfare, *Alcohol and Health,* pp. 64-66.
26. Ibid., p. 63.

French, and a very strong wine lobby that places ads in the subway such as 'Water is for frogs.' "[27] Certainly the use of alcoholic beverages is strongly influenced by the cultural norms surrounding drinking.

Recent sociological studies indicate that an even better predictor of whether or not a person will drink is the type of family background he or she comes from. Forty percent of all alcoholics come from broken homes, and 40 percent report drinking as a problem of one or both of their parents. Studies of juvenile drinkers indicate that they come from families where one or both parents drink heavily.[28] Studies such as these would indicate that children in families where drinking is an integral part of the parents' coping styles learn to resort to the use of alcoholic beverages as their way of coping.

SEDATIVES AND BARBITURATES

Although barbiturates were first synthesized in 1862, they did not gain popularity as a drug of choice with drug users until the 1940s. Until that time they had been used therapeutically for insomnia, anesthesia, and epilepsy.[29] In the early 1940s several articles appeared as part of an informational campaign designed to warn people of the danger of barbiturates. A number of states passed laws limiting the sale of barbiturates to prescription use only. These articles seemingly backfired; instead of preventing people from taking "barbs," they introduced the possibility of their use to a large number of people who normally would not have been familiar with them. The barbiturates became known as "thrill pills," and instead of being used for their sedating effects they were used increasingly to produce a state of intoxication similar to that produced by alcohol.

Barbiturates have many of the same effects as alcohol, as well as the same dangers. Some people go so far as to consider "barbs" alcohol in solid form; but while it would be difficult to consume a fatal dose of alcohol at one sitting, it is only too easy to swallow enough "barbs" to accomplish this end (as indicated by the number of people who choose barbiturates as a way of committing suicide). Another difference to note is that of social acceptability. Barbiturates are not generally used at social gatherings to

27. Ray, *Drugs, Society, and Human Behavior,* p. 92.
28. Ibid.
29. Ibid., pp. 173-175.

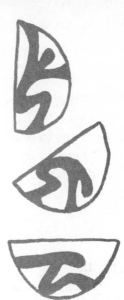

Becoming hooked

promote the camaraderie of the group; they still retain the aura of a medication taken for health purposes, such as calming nerves or controlling anxiety. Although numerous religious groups frown on the consumption of any alcoholic beverages, they usually condone the taking of medication such as a barbiturate. Many alcoholics become so under an initial cover of socially approved activity; barbiturate addicts, likewise, sometimes ease themselves through the first stages of becoming addicted by considering themselves to be taking a medication, and then find themselves "hooked."

One of the dangers encountered by those who take barbiturates is the tendency to take other drugs at the same time. Many barbiturates have a synergistic action with other drugs, and cross-tolerance develops. Many people take alcohol and barbiturates interchangeably or together. One of the problems of taking these drugs together is the narrow margin between the maximum dose an addict can manage and a lethal dose. Mixing the two often results in death, as, for instance, when someone takes his or her "usual" dose of barbs following an evening of heavy drinking.

In general, the stages leading to the development of barbiturate addiction are similar to those leading to alcoholism, as are the symptoms that accompany withdrawal. Many of the commonly used minor tranquilizers also have been discovered to have addicting qualities like the barbiturates.

The one difference is that people do not become as sleepy on tranquilizers. Because they have not generally been assumed to be addicting, tranquilizers have been grossly misused by doctors. The pattern is for the family doctor to prescribe mild tranquilizers indiscriminately for a wide variety of nonspecific ills, and in this way some persons with a propensity to abuse drugs have become addicted.

NICOTINE

Nicotine is a unique drug in that it acts as both a stimulant and a depressant. Tobacco has been used in some form since the 1500s, and at different times it has been viewed as an herb to be used in the treatment of a number of ailments and as a poison to be avoided. Perhaps one of the most detailed accounts of nicotine addiction is provided in the private letters and biographies of Sigmund Freud. His struggle with nicotine addiction in the form of cigar smoking (up to twenty-five cigars per day) extended over forty-five years, during which time he made repeated attempts to stop and was fully aware that his cigar smoking was exacerbating his serious mouth cancer.

Nicotine is one of the most toxic drugs known; 60 milligrams is a lethal dose.[30] Although a cigar contains double this amount, it is not directly absorbed into the body. While nicotine has been demonstrated to be an addicting drug, is it commonly identified in the folklore as merely habit-forming. Many people feel that if smokers really wanted to stop, they could break themselves of this habit, not recognizing the physiological dependence of some people upon nicotine. The case that nicotine is, in fact, an addicting drug rests on the evidence that persons who begin smoking on a regular basis continue and are noticeably bothered by a lack of the drug. Furthermore, persons who are heavy smokers have noticeable withdrawal symptoms. With nicotine, as other drugs, it is not the addictive quality of the drug itself that is so damaging but the dangerous effects of constant drug use upon the body. Nicotine has been demonstrated to be related to lung cancer, coronary artery disease, and emphysema.

In the light of these dangers, why do people continue smoking? A common psychological explanation relates to smoking as a way of meeting

---

30. Ibid., p. 103.

the "oral" needs of the person. Physiological research suggests that one of the effects of smoking is cortical arousal. Other studies indicate that heavy smokers naturally have a higher cortical level and that smoking serves to depress this activity. This latter explanation fits the commonly voiced reason that smoking is a means of relaxing. In any case, more persons are addicted to nicotine than to any other drug.

STIMULANTS

The use of stimulants is not new. Perhaps the oldest stimulant known to man is coca, whose leaves were chewed by the ancient Incas. In 1844, the chief active ingredient in coca leaves, the alkaloid cocaine, was isolated in pure form. In the late 1800s, cocaine was issued to Bavarian soldiers during maneuvers to counter fatigue. Freud, reading this account, took cocaine to relieve himself of depression, chronic fatigue, and other neurotic symptoms. Brecher, quoting Ernest Jones's biography of Freud, reports that he "tried the effect of a gram and found it turned the bad mood he was in into cheerfulness, giving him the feeling of having dined well 'so that there is nothing at all one need bother about' but without robbing him of any energy for exercise or work."[31] This account of Freud's use of cocaine shows the characteristic way stimulants have been used. In contrast to depressants, which are used to numb one's awareness of anxiety, stimulants work to produce euphoria. Freud, for instance, took cocaine at a time when he was experiencing many self-doubts. Again, in considering the effects of taking stimulants, it is important to note what the user does with the euphoria that accompanies the taking of the drug. In Freud's case, it allowed him to become suddenly very productive in his writing, which then brought him many accolades. These positive appraisals of his work in turn helped to relieve some of his self-doubts and perhaps propelled him to a resolution of some of his underlying problems. But in the usual case, the use of a stimulant mainly brings a misleading sense of euphoria so that one temporarily feels that all is well with the world and does nothing about working actively toward problem resolutions.

Amphetamines, the most commonly used stimulants today, were first synthesized in 1887, but medical uses were not noted until 1927, when the

---

31. Brecher, *Licit and Illicit Drugs,* p. 272.

effects of raising blood pressure, enlarging the nasal and bronchial passages, and stimulating the central nervous system were considered in formulating Benzedrine.[32] By 1971, at least thirty-one amphetamine preparations had been developed. The effects of the amphetamines are similar to those of cocaine:

> The main results of an oral dose . . . are as follows: wakefulness, alertness, and a decreased sense of fatigue; elevation of mood, with increased initiative, confidence and the ability to concentrate; often elation and euphoria; increase in motor and speech activity. Performance of only simple mental tasks is improved; and, although more work may be accomplished, the number of errors is not necessarily decreased. Physical performance, for example, in athletics, is improved. These effects are not invariable, and may be reversed by overdosage or repeated usage.[33]

Amphetamines, unlike cocaine, have been readily available to a large number of people. These drugs have been prescribed by doctors for weight reduction, depression, and fatigue; they have been given to athletes to improve their performance. As with cocaine, users experience depression when they discontinue the use of amphetamines, and it is frequently the attempt to avoid this letdown that propels users to take another dose. While these stimulants are not considered to be physically addicting, psychologically they are the most reinforcing of drugs.[34] Individuals who abuse these drugs sometimes develop a tolerance to them, although this is not as clear-cut a process as with other drugs. Children who have been placed on amphetamines for the treatment of hyperkinesis are maintained on the same dose over a prolonged period of time, while those who take amphetamines for mood elevation or appetite suppression sometimes find they need increasingly higher doses to accomplish the same effect.

Cocaine, by and large, has a shorter duration of action, and a person taking cocaine to maintain a "rush" must take intravenous injections every 5 to 15 minutes to maintain the exhilaration,[35] while a person taking methamphetamine will need to take a dose every two to four hours. Amphetamines taken intravenously to achieve this effect are commonly re-

---

32. Ibid., p. 278.
33. Ibid., p. 278.
34. M. H. Seevers, "Characteristics of Dependence on and Abuse of Psychoactive Drugs," in *Chemical and Biological Aspects of Drug Dependence,* ed. S. J. Mulé and Henry Brill (Cleveland: CRC Press, 1972), p. 16.
35. Ray, *Drugs, Society, and Human Behavior,* p. 161.

ferred to as "speed." Such intravenous use of methamphetamines was popularized in the late 1960s in a small segment of the anti-establishment adolescent drug culture. Such use of stimulants is particularly damaging in that it produces loss of appetite and sleeplessness, which are then accompanied by weight loss and malnutrition, when the user stops taking the drug, extreme fatigue and depression follow.

Heavy use of cocaine and amphetamines, both central nervous system stimulants, is frequently identified with the development of a particular type of paranoid state.[36] It is important to note that this state is believed to be a direct result of the drug and not related to the pre-psychotic personality. There are distinctive differences between a drug-induced psychosis and other forms of psychotic behavior. The person in a drug-induced state experiences visual and auditory hallucinations, but maintains a state of clear consciousness. Generally visual hallucinations predominate and there is no thought disorder.[37] A particular type of hallucination common to the drug-induced psychosis is the appearance of "cocaine bugs" (technically called formication), in which the person feels that bugs are crawling under his or her skin. The effects may be so pronounced that the person will try to cut them out with a knife. A further characteristic of drug-induced behavior is compulsive and repetitive action which may or may not be bizarre.[38]

The use of "speed" reached its peak in the late sixties in the well-known Haight-Ashbury section of San Francisco, the unofficial "hippie" center of the time. "Speed" users characteristically were white, middle-class adolescents who suffered disaffection from the world of their parents, had noticeably lowered self-esteem, and were attracted to the use of these drugs as an instant "cure" for these feelings.[39] It is important to note that, under the effects of "speed," one can get into a number of problematic situations. As is pointed out, the average user of "speed," unlike the heroin addict, is not acquainted with "street life" and therefore may be a ready prey for others more familiar with the scene. Further, "the paranoid behavior of the speed freak may at times look superficially like murderous

---

36. Brecher, *Licit and Illicit Drugs,* pp. 285-287.
37. D. S. Bell, "Comparison of Amphetamine Psychosis and Schizophrenia," *British Journal of Psychiatry* 3 (1965): 706.
38. Ray, *Drugs, Society, and Human Behavior,* p. 172.
39. Brecher, *Licit and Illicit Drugs,* p. 284.

aggression."[40] Even more hazardous is the taking of barbiturates with speed. Barbiturates have the effect of reducing inhibitions, while speed provides a burst of energy that may mobilize the user to all types of anti-social acts. Speed seems to have been primarily a creature of the late 60's, a fad that appears to be on the wane.

HALLUCINOGENS

The hallucinogens also have a long history. Various peoples have incorporated substances that produce hallucinations into their religious rites. An example of this type of use is the peyote used ritually by some Indians of the Southwest. In considering hallucinogens, it is important to note that their use as part of the ceremonial life of a culture did not pose problems; it is only as the use of hallucinogens became popular outside a ceremonial context that they have become problematic to society.

LSD, mescaline (a peyote derivative), and psilocybin are called "hallucinogens" because of their capacity to distort perceptions. LSD ("acid") was synthesized in 1938; its hallucinogenic properties were discovered in 1943. During the ensuing years it was widely used for experimental purposes in various types of psychotherapy. From this early beginning, wideranging research projects were initiated. In these studies, a number of students were incorporated as research subjects and thus were "turned on" to the use of LSD.

As with the other drugs we have discussed, it is important to consider the context in which the hallucinogens became popular. For youths disillusioned with the world of their parents, where the primary emphasis was on competitive striving and "making it" and where the Vietnam war was an ever-present reality, the availability of hallucinogens provided a ready escape. The average user of hallucinogens is characterized as

> . . . predominantly middle class in economics and beliefs. Usually they are non-athletic, above average in intelligence, and poor in competitive situations. They are frustrated with life and angry with their parents, but their response is one of passivity. They deny their hate in the easiest way possible, by turning it to love.[41]

---

40. Ibid., p. 286.
41. Ray, *Drugs, Society, and Human Behavior*, p. 237.

A characteristic pattern for those who become users of hallucinogens is a growing preoccupation with the supernatural and metaphysical world. Again, this is a convenient way of escaping the anxieties of the present world; instead of confronting problems, one seeks to avoid them, and this approach does little to develop a more adept coping style.

Although the hazards of taking LSD were widely proclaimed, there is little evidence to support the claims. Usually these drugs are taken within the context of a group, and norms are established for managing the one real danger, the "bad trip." A "bad trip" occurs unpredictably and for no apparent reason; the user has very frightening, unpleasant distortions of perception, instead of the desired pleasant, uplifting, "insightful" experience. The person on a "bad trip" has a frightening time and may go into a panic. It is at this point that medical attention is frequently sought to short-circuit the process. Intramuscular injections of chlorpromazine are most commonly given. A further adverse reaction to LSD may be the "flashback," which is the recurrence of symptoms weeks or months after taking LSD.

The evidence so far suggests that the use of hallucinogens as part of one's coping style is a passing phase, unlike the use of alcohol or barbiturates, which tends to escalate. LSD is not addicting. Tolerance develops rapidly but there are no withdrawal symptoms.

MARIJUANA AND HASHISH

Marijuana and hashish (the dried resin of marijuana, five to eight times more potent) are derived from the leaves and flowering tops of the plant *cannabis sativa,* or hemp. The use of these drugs is recorded since ancient times, and the popularity of marijuana in the United States was widespread by the late 1970s. The number of persons estimated to have used it varies from 15 to 24 million, with over half using it at least monthly. The users tend to be young people, a fact that may be due to the period over which marijuana smoking has achieved widespread popularity. The generation that embraced marijuana smoking so enthusiastically has not yet advanced to old age.

Marijuana and hashish do not produce physical dependence, and the evidence about whether tolerance develops is inconclusive, though tending toward the negative. As with other drugs, cold, hard facts are difficult to establish because of the paucity of research and the highly charged emotional climate surrounding the drug. Proponents of marijuana use argue that there are no negative effects and point to the dangers of alcohol and cigarettes to build their case for "pot" smoking. Opponents argue just as strenuously that there are many negative effects yet to be identified, that "pot" smoking may lead to genetic defects in offspring, that it is associated with sterility in the male, and that it leads to the use of other drugs.

The use of marijuana parallels that of alcohol in that both are generally used in a social situation, although there may be isolated pot smokers, just as there are isolated drinkers. The effects a person experiences as a result of smoking pot are closely tied to the social situation. However, most users report that they have a pleasant feeling of increased well-being and become introspective and tranquil. Short-term memory is impaired, and the sense of time is altered. The question of whether marijuana produces physical damage is unresolved.[42] The repeated user of marijuana may be equated with the alcoholic and differs from the occasional smoker as does the social drinker from the alcoholic. As Ray notes: "Once heavy use is started, of either alcohol or marijuana, the cycle continues, with the use of the drug reducing discomfort, but setting things up to cause more discomfort so that more drug is needed."[43] However, the physical effects of marijuana are apparently not nearly so damaging as those of alcohol.

INHALANTS

In recent years inhalants have been gaining public attention as a further source of "kicks," largely within the school age population who have ready access to a number of substances that might be inhaled and less chance to obtain other drugs. The inhalants, of which airplane glue has been most publicized, can produce a state similar to alcohol intoxication and sometimes a hallucinogenic-like experience.[44] Although warnings about the dire consequences of "glue sniffing" have been widespread in the news media, the actual physical damage caused by the practice has

---

42. *Marijuana and Health: Second Annual Report to Congress* (Washington, D.C.: U. S. Government Printing Office, 1972), pp. 19-23.
43. Ray, *Drugs, Society, and Human Behavior,* p. 265.
44. Brecher, *Licit and Illicit Drugs,* p. 309.

Functions of drug use

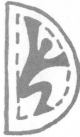

been limited. The ill effects so publicized are due primarily to long-term industrial exposure rather than recreational use. Deaths are sometimes attributed to use of inhalants, but many reports are unsubstantiated and attributable to related causes, such as suffocation because of the plastic bag used in the inhalation process.

In summary, a large variety of substances are taken to alter experience. In any discussion of drug use, it is important to note that the use of drugs throughout history is embedded in an overall cultural milieu. At certain periods, the inclination is toward drugs that will dull awareness, while at other times the push is toward mind expansion. Some drugs are taken primarily within social groups, and drug-taking is governed by the norms of the group. Other drugs are taken in solitude, usually in attempt to hide the fact that the person is taking an excessive amount of drugs or alcohol. The explanations of why people take drugs are numerous, including psychological explanations related to certain personality structures that predispose one to drug-taking; sociological explanations that relate to the overall cultural milieu; and physiological explanations that seek to identify predisposing biochemical factors. In any event, it is our view that the use of drugs serves recreational purposes as well as altering one's perceptions of the problems of living that surround him or her. Anxiety is temporarily quelled, but once the impact of the drug wears off, the problems facing the person remain and the use of drugs has not assisted him or her in becoming a more adept problem solver.

TREATMENT ISSUES

OPIATES

Attempts at treating opiate addiction through the years have not been notably successful. At the turn of the century, sanitariums were established for the treatment of addicts and extensive efforts made to get people off drugs, but permanent cures were not the rule. People would remain off the drug while in the sanitarium, only to become re-addicted once they were home. Such failures were commonly ascribed to a lack of motivation or "weak will" on the part of the addict. Some were hospitalized in mental institutions, but again little other than withdrawal from drugs was accomplished. A predominating view was that addicts could not be successfully treated. It was only in the 1960s that a number of approaches to the treatment of opiate addiction were developed.

There are two major approaches to the treatment of opiate addiction: (1) psychosocial, which emphasize relearning patterns of living; and (2) pharmacological, which are based on the substitution of other drugs for the opiates.[45] A number of treatment programs provide some combination of these approaches.

■ *Psychosocial Approaches.* In recent years a number of therapeutic communities have been established in an attempt at a psychosocial approach to the treatment of addiction. Perhaps the best known of these is Synanon, established in 1958 in California. Synanon, modeled after Alcoholics Anonymous, is based on the premises that "once an addict, always an addict," and that a person must truly want to be helped if he or she is to stop using drugs. Individuals wishing this form of treatment must be highly motivated and able to invest their full time for one to two years. Life at Synanon is highly structured around a number of activities:

---

45. Ray, *Drugs, Society, and Human Behavior,* pp. 204-205.

Several things do make living at Synanon, and thus staying off drugs, effective. One is work: the ex-addict is kept busy. Another is faith, a religious-like belief of any sort. A third practice is to relate the type of work, the freedom, and the responsibility the individual has to the degree of his acceptance of a non-drug life style, and thus, in their terms, to his emotional maturity. Last is the assumption that an addict has difficulty in expressing his emotions and in identifying his own and others' emotions. The formal group encounters which occur three to five times a week are often psychologically violent, but are the arena in which the ex-addict learns to stop using destructive guards to protect himself and above all learns to see himself and others as they really are.[46]

The addict is completely involved with the community, and all his or her outside contacts are subject to group scrutiny. The therapeutic process is essentially one of resocialization. Initially, the addict is treated as one who is a child emotionally and who must prove an ability to be independent and trusted. Initiation rites are designed to test the person's motivation to change. House rules are strictly maintained, infractions are severely punished, and the person who breaks the rules is publicly degraded. Each member of the community shares in the work. The therapeutic community is structured in such a way that there are definite progressive steps; the first is the initiation phase, and at later stages the person is moved into positions of increasing responsibility.

Inherent in the philosophical underpinnings of many therapeutic communities like Synanon is a view that "it takes an addict to treat an addict." Thus the highest grade in the therapeutic community is usually that of being part of the "treatment" staff. Ex-addicts in this way find a role for themselves within the therapeutic community, but never make it beyond this to a legitimate role in society outside the drug community. Although some persons who have been treated in Synanon programs do make it into jobs within the community, they live nearby and remain integrally involved in the activities of the therapeutic community. Other therapeutic communities being established, primarily by ex-addicts, are attempting to bridge the gap so that addicts may move out into socially accepted roles in the larger community. The cure rate of therapeutic communities is questionable. Synanon no longer makes claims of curing ad-

---

46. Ibid., pp. 205-206.

dicts but offers itself as a way of life for those who wish to pursue it.[47]

In any event, therapeutic communities are built upon a recognition that the world of the drug user represents a total way of life for the person who is addicted. The mere withdrawal of the individual from drugs does not constitute treatment, but an alternate world of meaningful relationships needs to be structured if the treatment is to be successful.

■ *Pharmacological Approaches.*   Methadone maintenance, first used experimentally in 1963, has been the most commonly used form of pharmacological treatment. Other chemical treatment methods have limited but potentially useful applicability; for example, cyclazocine, a drug that does not relieve the craving, but does make the addict sick if he or she takes heroin.

Methadone is a synthetic narcotic that does produce addiction, but an addiction that, in the opinion of its proponents, has fewer deleterious effects on the social functioning of its subjects. People maintained on methadone experience none of the sedation or euphoria associated with heroin, and so they can turn their attention to other social obligations rather than struggling for an existence on heroin. That methadone is provided legally, instead of being secured surreptitiously by the addict, is a variable that has not been evaluated. A notable characteristic of methadone is that it blocks the effect of heroin. If the addict is being maintained on a high enough dose of methadone, he or she will not experience any pleasurable effects from taking heroin. Addicts report that knowing this makes them feel safer from temptation.

Other factors that make methadone an appealing treatment approach are, first, that it may be taken orally, and second, that it has, as far as is currently known, no untoward side effects. In any form of drug treatment, the first step is detoxification, which basically involves freeing the individual of physical dependence on drugs. In actual practice, the term is used for treatment in which the dosage of the drug is gradually lowered, not limited to the process of eliminating the drug altogether. Methadone is frequently used in detoxification; the technique is to provide enough methadone to eliminate withdrawal symptoms, the dose being gradually lowered. Detoxification may be done on an in-patient or out-patient basis

---

47. Brecher, *Licit and Illicit Drugs,* pp. 81–82.

and usually takes about two weeks, although it frequently takes considerably longer for out-patients. During this initial phase, it is important to be aware of accompanying problems, such as infections and hepatitis, which may be a result of contaminated equipment, malnourishment, and other physical problems associated with the addict's street life.

The main usefulness of methadone as a maintenance drug is that the addicted person may take it indefinitely, if necessary, as treatment for his or her addiction. Without the need for all the activities associated with heroin addiction, the person has considerably more time and energy to devote to more socially accepted activities, such as work and involvement with significant others. In many cases, psychosocial treatment approaches are coupled with methadone maintenance to assist the person to move into these more socially accepted roles. Legal, vocational, and social service counseling are usually available as part of the overall treatment program, with social rehabilitation the goal. Although the person is still addicted, now to methadone, the methadone plays a relatively small, but enabling, place in his or her life, in contrast to the all-encompassing, disabling effects of heroin addiction.

Urine testing to detect the presence of narcotics and certain other drugs is an important feature of methadone treatment programs. Methadone must be taken daily, which means that persons on such programs either must have a supply of methadone themselves or report daily to a treatment center to get their dosage. There is now a newer drug, methadol, which lasts two to three days; its use could eliminate the need for daily reporting without risking black-market trafficking in methadone by addicts supplied with more of the drug than they need at one time.

Another use of methadone is in programs intended to withdraw the person totally from drugs. Here methadone is given during withdrawal, with a steady decrease in the dosage. To accomplish this goal requires four to eight months. Although this is the stated goal of a number of programs, it is rarely achieved; methadone maintenance is the more usual approach.

Cyclazocine, a narcotic antagonist with low abuse potential, has been mentioned as having a limited current use in the treatment of narcotic addiction. This drug blocks the effect of heroin and makes the person sick, much as does Antabuse with the use of alcohol. Cyclazocine does not block the craving and has unpleasant side effects. In one study involving thirty-five patients, after three years, seven were off both cyclazocine and opiates, and another seven were still on cyclazocine but opiate-free. It is believed that this method of treatment may be useful for those who have been addicts only a short time and for whom methadone maintenance is contra-indicated, but more studies on this drug are needed, as well as on other drugs now being investigated for possible use in the treatment of opiate addictions.[48]

A common feature of most drug treatment programs is that they are staffed primarily by ex-addicts. The reasons given are that these people have an inside knowledge of the problems addicts face and therefore can be more helpful. It is further argued that those who have been in a similar plight are not so likely to be manipulated as some other well-meaning drug counselors might be. This type of arrangement serves numerous purposes other than those advanced for "therapeutic" reasons. First, the management of the drug problem remains in the hands of those who have used the drug, and they therefore maintain control rather than relinquishing it to the psychiatric establishment. Second, this arrangement serves as an employment route for ex-addicts so that they do not really risk going out into the larger community to establish a place for themselves. Third, it is not necessarily true that it takes an addict to treat an addict; while it is true that drug counselors who have not used drugs may readily be "conned," it is also possible that those who have used drugs can also be conned, perhaps in a slightly different way. In any event, maintaining such a staffing pattern creates a social unit in which one is either an addict or ex-addict, a rather homogeneous grouping. Two-thirds of the persons on methadone maintenance programs remain in the treatment program.[49]

As is readily apparent from this discussion, there are no easy solutions to the problems of opiate addiction. The problems associated with heroin addiction are deeply embedded within an overall societal context. Any solution will arise only out of some broader social changes and cannot be confined solely to the medical or psychological aspects of the treatment of addicts.

---

48. David Lackowitz et al., "Cyclazocine Intervention in the Treatment of Narcotics Addiction: Another Look," in *Major Modalities in the Treatment of Drug Abuse*, ed. Leon Brill and Louis Lieberman (New York: Behavioral Publications, 1972), pp. 85-105.
49. Edward Senay and Pierce Renault, "Treatment Methods for Heroin Addicts: A Review," *Journal of Psychedelic Drugs* 3, no. 2 (Spring 1971): 48-49.

ALCOHOL

Like the question of narcotics addiction, the treatment of alcoholism in this country is complicated in that we are in conflict as to whether the problem is moral, legal, medical, or social. This grows out of our tendency to problem-solve, as we must categorize in order to make judgments and arrive at courses of action. The judgments that twentieth-century American society fosters are definitive, black-and-white contrasts. Questionable, less settled, grey areas pose problems. Many people prefer to be definite, though "black," than to be indefinite.

For instance, a moralistic view of alcoholism immediately implies that it is wrong and sinful, and the efforts then are directed toward converting the sinner. Legalistic views are similarly straightforward: a person either breaks the law or does not. The tendency, in our country, has been to view alcoholism in the framework of the legal system. The moral or abolitionist movement against alcohol was powerful enough in this century to secure the enactment in 1919 of the Eighteenth Amendment to the Constitution, imposing national prohibition. Although ultimately it was repealed, prohibition remained law for thirteen years until passage of the Twenty-first Amendment. In the legal realm, public intoxication was considered a criminal offense in all states until as recently as 1966 when, through test cases, some of the laws prohibiting public drunkenness were declared invalid. Since that time, a number of states have changed their laws, and alcoholism increasingly is being viewed as a medical problem rather than as a crime.

Although there has been considerable interest in transforming alcoholism into a medical problem, it is again important to consider the long-range implications. It is considered more humanistic to view the alcoholic as "sick," in that this implies it is not the person's fault; he or she now is viewed as a victim of a disease that has some cause and presumably some treatment. In our view, taking the legal or moral view paints a "black" picture of the alcoholic as either a sinner or a criminal. The alternate medical approach tends to place the alcoholic in the position of a victim and therefore "white." In contrast, the social view is quite "grey," with no clear-cut simplistic view of causality and related treatment, but rather a tangle of factors all interacting to produce a situation that is not well understood and not easy to deal with.

Since alcohol is one of the most physically damaging drugs, the treatment of the alcoholic person is of prime importance and takes place on several levels. The alcoholic usually denies his or her problems until they become of great magnitude, influencing physical well-being as well as relationships within a number of social networks. For this reason, treatment programs frequently include physical, emotional, and social aspects.

The first step in treatment usually is detoxification, or treatment of withdrawal symptoms. At this stage the concern is to prevent seizures and delirium tremens (as is also true in withdrawal from barbiturates). Withdrawal symptoms occur when the individual abruptly stops drinking, usually beginning within twelve to forty-eight hours afterward; they include tremors, anxiety, profuse sweating, and nausea. The person may also experience the severe and potentially lethal condition of delirium tremens, which is characterized by severe agitation, confusion, disorientation, hallucinations, and autonomic and metabolic dysfunction. Anti-convulsant and sedative drugs are used in this phase of treatment, generally accompanied by other drugs, such as high-potency vitamins, to treat accompanying physical conditions. This phase of treatment lasts for one to two weeks, during which the person should be thoroughly examined for other physical illnesses, since disorders of the liver, heart, central nervous system, and gastrointestinal system occur as a result of prolonged excessive ingestion of alcohol. Alcoholics frequently have problems in eating because they have no appetite. Usually hospitalization is required in the detoxification phase because of the multiple problems involved.

The role of chemotherapy in the treatment of alcoholism is usually limited to the use of tranquilizers, anticonvulsants, and sedatives during the withdrawal phase. In fact, these drugs are contraindicated after withdrawal because of the danger of substituting one addiction for another and the cross-tolerance effects. One drug sometimes used is disulfiram (Antabuse), a chemical that has no effect on the body except when alcohol is present. If a person has had Antabuse and takes alcohol, the Antabuse interferes with the metabolism of the alcohol, creating extremely unpleasant symptoms. The blood pressure decreases, while pulse and respiration rates increase. The person experiences dyspnea, coughing, pounding of the heart, tingling and numbness of the hands, and sometimes dizziness, blurred vision, and headaches. The usefulness of disulfiram is that these bad side effects reduce the temptation to drink. It may be especially help-

Group treatment for alcoholism

ful early in treatment but should be used discriminately with persons who have medical complications. Another undesired effect is that sometimes persons are completely "turned off" treatment by the negative side effects of disulfiram.

Many alcoholics discontinue treatment after they are detoxified, resolving never to resume drinking. This rarely works, and they probably again re-establish the alcoholic pattern. For this reason, forms of treatment directed toward social and psychological problems usually accompany detoxification programs. The most successful organization in treating alcoholics is Alcoholics Anonymous (AA), but unfortunately a large number of alcoholics are not ready to make the necessary commitment of acknowledging that they have a problem beyond their conrtol. The basic philosophy of AA is to acknowledge that one has a drinking problem and needs help, both spiritual and social. Members of AA are encouraged to put themselves in God's hands and ask for help. They are helped to feel worthwhile, a feeling most members do not have about themselves as they enter. AA also allows the person both to accept any kind of help he or she needs and to provide help to others; people in AA know absolutely that they can depend on one another. Also, if they slip they know that they can return, even if they have another episode of uncontrolled drinking. The focus is on living one day at a time without alcohol. Alcoholics are not encouraged to plan, so far as their drinking is concerned, for the rest of their lives, or even for tomorrow, but only for one day at a time, and in this way their problem is cut down to manageable dimension.

Members of Alcoholics Anonymous tend to give their lives a service orientation and become heavily involved in providing help to other people through a variety of civic, church, and related types of activities. It is worthwhile to note that when alcoholics do maintain a role within their own nuclear families, the whole family network is likely to need professional attention, since the process of having an alcoholic member has created role shifts and a warping of everyone's roles. It is not uncommon to find the family functioning more effectively with someone in the alcoholic role and to resist efforts on the alcoholic's part to move out of this role; for example, the woman who needs an inadequate husband so that she can take over and thereby feel adequate. AA, recognizing these types of family problems, provides subgroup organizations for family members: Al-Anon for spouses, Al-Ateen for teenage children, and Al-Atots for younger children.

A number of persons in the process of becoming alcoholic become isolated from their family and friends, a factor that frequently interferes with their motivations to stop drinking. AA is particularly helpful in this regard by providing a fellowship of persons who have experienced similar problems. New members are accepted as equals and given the warmth and support they so desperately need.

In the total treatment of alcoholism, early discovery and prevention are as necessary as treatment and rehabilitation. Frequently the person with a drinking problem is ignored until his or her drinking reaches an advanced stage. Of particular importance in this aspect is the potential role of employers. Absenteeism and poor job performance often are indications that a person is drinking excessively. Instead of ignoring the problem or firing the individual for inadequate performance, it would be preferable if employers encouraged him or her to receive treatment for the problem as a condition of keeping the job. In this way a person would necessarily become involved in treatment, but would also remain within a supportive social structure. Community education in the schools and through the media is a further important aspect of prevention and early case finding.

OTHER DRUGS

In the treatment of persons addicted to barbiturates, nonbarbiturate hypnotics, and minor tranquilizers, gradual withdrawal or detoxification is essential; abrupt withdrawal can be fatal. Withdrawal takes from two to three weeks and is usually carried out in an in-patient setting, since these persons are prone to some of the same complications that beset alcoholics. As with all drugs, detoxification is one phase, but attention must be paid to how drugs are used as part of the person's coping style. Unless the person makes some shift in his or her way of coping with problems, he or she is likely to revert to drug-taking behavior. Treatment, therefore, consists of trying to help drug users develop alternate coping mechanisms.[50]

Although amphetamine and cocaine users suffer no physical withdrawal symptoms, they do suffer from fatigue and depression that usually last several weeks. Persons hospitalized for treatment of amphetamine addiction are usually "speed freaks" who come into the hospital at the end of a "run," often in a paranoid state. For this reason they are usually hospitalized when they are taken off drugs. Phenothiazines are often used as an adjunct to treatment. Attention should be paid to any accompanying medical problems, such as abscesses at the site of injection, hepatitis, malnutrition, skin problems, and respiratory and gastrointestinal distress. The more florid symptoms of paranoia fade within a couple of weeks, but these people typically remain confused and have some memory loss for six to twelve months; these symptoms, too, gradually fade. Most commonly, ex-users report slightly greater difficulties in remembering. Ex-speed freaks generally report that they feel their personalities have undergone a favorable change. We referred earlier to the low self-esteem reported by speed freaks; evidently during the drug experience or recovery a good many of these young people manage to come to more favorable terms with themselves.

Persons seeking treatment while on hallucinogens do so because they are having a "bad trip." As the effects of hallucinogens are greatly influenced by the environment, reassurance or "talking down" is effective in dealing with most reactions. The person is given emotional support, encouraged to ventilate, and oriented to reality; all actions are directed to reducing anxiety and dealing with the panic state that the person is in. Someone should remain constantly with a person on a "bad trip" until he or she is over the effects of the drug. For extreme agitation or psychotic

---

50. Carl Chambers and Leon Brill, "The Treatment of Non-Narcotic Abusers," in Brill and Lieberman, *Treatment of Drug Abuse*, pp. 257-265.

symptoms, Thorazine or a sedative may be prescribed. The same type of treatment is indicated for the person suffering from "flashbacks."

THE NURSE'S ROLE IN TREATMENT OF DRUG DEPENDENCE

Given the problematic facets of drug dependence that have been outlined, the nurse's role in the treatment of addicts is equally problematic. Perhaps the most characteristic term describing work with drug users and alcoholics is "frustrating." Not only are nurses constantly confronted by people making bad decisions, but they are also caught up in some of the ambivalences about the use of drugs in our society. One tendency is either to perceive drug users as having no "will power," equating them with criminals because of the legal connotations of drug-taking; or to see them as "sick" and therefore helpless and dependent. The nurse's role, by and large, is reciprocal to his or her view of the person's problem. For example, if the nurses sees drug abuse as an example of weakness of will, it is likely that his or her orientation toward the drug user will be moralistic or legalistic. This nurse will probably find herself or himself involved in a whole series of negotiations with the person to "shape up," use "will power," and "repent from such wicked ways." One may assume that the person has already gone through a set of these same types of admonitions to himself or herself and has not been able, by strength of will, to refrain from the use of drugs or alcohol. Therefore, the effects of such negotiations will frequently be further alienation from people who might give help.

Nurses are perhaps most comfortable in adopting a view of alcoholics as "sick" because it fits their image of "curing the sick." In studies of nurses' attitudes toward alcoholics, nurses have shown most positive attitudes towards alcoholics who are being detoxified—the stage of the process in which they are most able to treat the person as one who is "sick" rather than as a rational person who has made some bad choices in life. This is probably a reflection of the fact that when the alcoholic is at the stage of being "sick," the nurse can feel that he or she is doing something tangible to make the person feel better; while after detoxification, he or she tends to resist the help the nurse might try to offer.

It is particularly important that the nurse enlarge his or her view of this role so that it becomes more than merely providing things that the patient can take from the nurse. If the nurse sees drug dependence and alcoholism as a reflection of the person's attempt to cope with stressful situations, it is likely that she or he can reconceptualize the nurse's role as that of an active listener in encouraging the person to explore alternative means of coping, identifying the types of stressful situation that lead to taking drugs, and in other ways more rationally appraising the nature of the drug user's dilemma.

It is particularly important that nurses generally be aware of the symptoms of drug use and drug withdrawal. Frequently on medical and surgical units, patients are admitted for reasons other than manifest symptoms related to drug withdrawal, for example, for fractures and other accidental injuries. Withdrawal symptoms and delirium tremens are a particular danger in such patients if they are not appropriately treated. Because of the cross-dependence of drugs, the identification of withdrawal symptoms is sometimes clouded. For example, the addict who comes in for surgery often does not experience withdrawal symptoms until a period after surgery, primarily because of the drugs given pre- and post-operatively. Similarly, sedatives may preclude withdrawal symptoms in the alcoholic for a period of time. In any event, the nurse should be aware of this possibility so that the appropriate therapeutic measures might be taken.

A nurse is frequently one of the few nonaddicts who is allowed to participate in drug treatment programs. It is therefore doubly important that she or he be aware of some of the particular pitfalls of treating addicts. The nurse needs to understand a great deal about how the system of that particular program works and to discover her or his particular position in the network. Nurses frequently are employed to administer methadone and supervise the medical procedures, such as seeing that the urine samples are properly collected and processed. In many instances, there is a wish to confine the nurse solely to this role, leaving all the counseling aspects to others. It is possible for the nurse to become caught in all types of conflicts between counselors, clients, and other medical authorities about such things, for example, as dosages of methadone. The exact procedures should, for these reasons, be clearly spelled out and agreed on by everyone involved. In fact, channels of communication in all instances, not just in matters relating to methadone, should be examined. All too easily the nurse may become enmeshed in "conflict of interest" arguments that do nothing to enhance the quality of the treatment program. Remember the addict's propensity to "con" others. If staff members are not clear about their relationships to one another and the rules by which they will operate, the system is open for the conning operations of the addicts, which in turn contribute to their problem.

The nurse working in drug treatment programs or with alcoholics needs to guard against a tendency toward gullibility and believing the addict's protestations that he or she wishes to remain "clean"; the nurse can be of greatest help by being a firm, consistent person who listens as the person tries to sort things out for himself or herself. The nurse should resist a tendency to provide care and nurturance, for this may contribute to the addict's maintenance of the habit.

SUMMARY

In summary, the addictive pattern of coping is a multifaceted problem deeply rooted within a cultural matrix. The use of varying forms of substances in dealing with anxiety-fraught situations has been a common pattern throughout history and in different cultures. The popularity of certain substances is closely correlated with dominant social themes. In considering drugs, it is particularly important to distinguish drugs used to reduce anxiety to a level where people might actively attack their problems as distinct from drugs used to avoid problems totally. People with addictive patterns have chosen the latter course.

Depressants of one form or another have been particularly popular. Opium derivatives, alcohol, and a wide range of sedatives and barbiturates all have a depressive effect. While the problem of addiction related to opium derivatives has generated the greatest amount of public concern, alcohol and barbiturates are more physically damaging. Definitions of alcoholism vary depending on their source, but there is general agreement that alcoholism is a prominent public health problem.

Other large numbers of people rely on stimulants to produce a sense of well-being that they otherwise do not feel. Cocaine and amphetamines are well-known stimulants. Excessive use of stimulants may sometimes produce a paranoid state.

The use of caffeine and tobacco generally escape being labeled as forms of addiction, although they also produce damaging effects. The hallucinogens have recently been popular in the younger segment of the population. The use of marijuana seems to be more enduring than other forms of drug use, and it will be interesting to follow the attendant legal processes.

The nursing role in the treatment of addictions has not been settled and so is problematic. A theme that frequently arises among drug users is that other drug users can help them more effectively than professionals. Treatment efforts generally range from multi-faceted attempts to change basic living styles to replacement with a less damaging form of addiction.

FURTHER READINGS

Abrams, Arnold, et al. "Psychosocial Aspects of Addiction." *American Journal of Public Health* 58 (Nov. 1968): 2142-2155.

B., Elaine (pseud.), et al. "Helping the Nurse Who Misuses Drugs." *American Journal of Nursing* 74 (Sept. 1974): 1665-1671.

Barbee, Evelyn. "Marijuana: A Social Problem." *Perspectives in Psychiatric Care* 9, no. 5 (1971): 194-199.

Brecher, Edward, and the Editors of Consumer Reports. *Licit and Illicit Drugs.* Boston: Little, Brown and Company, 1972.

Byrne, Marcella. "Resocialization of the Chronic Alcoholic." *American Journal of Nursing* 68 (Jan. 1968): 99-100.

Canning, Mary. "Care of Alcoholic Patients." *American Journal of Nursing* 65 (Nov. 1965): 113-114.

Caskey, Kathryn. "The School Nurse and Drug Abuse." *Nursing Outlook* 18 (Dec. 1970): 27-30.

Dambacher, Betty, and Hellwig, Karen. "Nursing Strategies for Young Drug Users." *Perspectives in Psychiatric Care* 9, no. 5 (1971): 200-205.

Department of Health, Education, and Welfare. *Alcohol and Health.* Washington, D.C.: U.S. Government Printing Office, 1971.

Department of Health, Education, and Welfare. *Second Special Report to the U.S. Congress on Alcohol and Health.* Preprint ed. Washington, D.C.: U.S. Government Printing Office, (June) 1974.

Distasio, Carol, and Nawrot, Marcia. "Methaqualone." *American Journal of Nursing* 73 (Nov. 1973): 1922-1925.

Estes, Nada. "Counseling the Wife of an Alcoholic Spouse." *American Journal of Nursing* 74 (July 1974): 1251-1255.

Finnegan, Loretta, and Macnew, Bonnie. "Care of the Addicted Infant." *American Journal of Nursing* 74 (April 1974): 685-693.

Fitzig, Charmaine. "Nursing in an Alcohol Program." *American Journal of Nursing* 66 (Oct. 1966): 2218-2222.

Foreman, Nancy Jo, and Zerwekh, Joyce. "Drug Crisis Intervention." *American Journal of Nursing* 71 (Sept. 1971): 1736-1739.

Freed, Earl. "The Crucial Factor in Alcoholism." *American Journal of Nursing* 68 (Dec. 1968): 2615-2616.

Garb, Solomon. "Narcotic Addiction in Nurses and Doctors." *Nursing Outlook* 13 (Nov. 1965): 30-34.

Gillespie, Cecilia. "Nurses Help Combat Alcoholism." *American Journal of Nursing* 69 (Sept. 1969): 1938-1941.

Harris, T. George. "As Far as Heroin is Concerned, the Worst is Over: A Conversation About the Drug Epidemic With Jerome Jaffe." *Psychology Today* 7 (Aug. 1973): 68-79.

Hecht, Murray. "Children of Alcoholics Are Children at Risk." *American Journal of Nursing* 73 (Oct. 1973): 1764-1767.

Huey, Florence. "In a Therapeutic Community." *American Journal of Nursing* 71 (May 1971): 926-933.

Jones, Ann. "My Birthday Is Not the Day I Was Born." *American Journal of Nursing* 67 (July 1967): 1434-1438.

Kimmel, Mary. "Antabuse in a Clinic Program." *American Journal of Nursing* 71 (June 1971): 1173-1175.

Levine, David, et al. "A Special Program for Nurse Addicts." *American Journal of Nursing* 74 (Sept. 1974): 1672-1675.

Morgan, Arthur, "Minor Tranquilizers, Hypnotics, and Sedatives." *American Journal of Nursing* 73 (July 1973): 1220-1222.

Morgan, Arthur, and Moreno, Judith. "Attitudes Toward Addiction." *American Journal of Nursing* 73 (March 1973): 497-501.

Morton, Elvera. "Nursing Care in an Alcoholic Unit." *Nursing Outlook* 14 (Oct. 1966): 45-47.

Mueller, John. "Treatment for the Alcoholic: Cursing or Nursing." *American Journal of Nursing* 74 (Feb. 1974): 245-247.

Muhlenkamp, Ann. "Personality Characteristics of Drug Addicts." *Perspectives in Psychiatric Care* 6, no. 5 (1968): 213-219.

Nelson, Karin. "The Nurse in a Methadone Maintenance Program." *American Journal of Nursing* 73 (May 1973): 870-874.

Pillari, George, and Narus, June. "Physical Effects of Heroin Addiction." *American Journal of Nursing* 73 (Dec. 1973): 2105-2108.

Price, Gladys. "Alcoholism: A Family, Community, and Nursing Problem." *American Journal of Nursing* 67 (May 1967): 1022-1025.

Randall, Brooke Patterson. "Short-Term Group Therapy With the Adolescent Drug Offender." *Perspectives in Psychiatric Care* 9, no. 3 (1971): 123-128.

Rodewald, Rosemary Roth. "Speed Kills: The Adolescent Methedrine Addict." *Perspectives in Psychiatric Care* 8, no. 4 (1970): 160-167.

Russaw, Ethel. "Nursing in a Narcotic Detoxification Unit." *American Journal of Nursing* 70 (Aug. 1970): 1720-1723.

Senay, Edward, and Renault, Pierce. "Treatment Methods for Heroin Addicts: A Review." *Journal of Psychedelic Drugs* 3, no. 2 (Spring 1971): 47-54.

Singer, Ann. "Mothering Practices—Heroin Addiction." *American Journal of Nursing* 74 (Jan. 1974): 77-82.

Walker, Lynna. "Crises of Change: A Case Study of a Heroin-Dependent Patient." *Perspectives in Psychiatric Care* 12, no. 1 (1974): 20-25.

Yolles, Stanley. "The Drug Scene." *Nursing Outlook* 18 (July 1970): 24-26.

CHAPTER SIX

DEPRESSIVE COPING STYLES

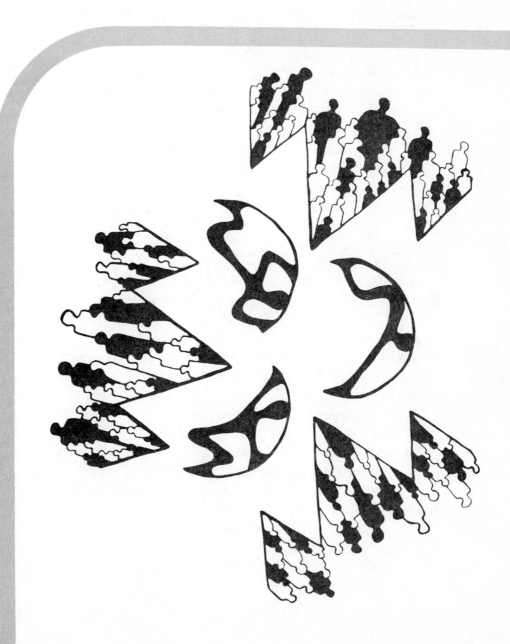

The phenomenon of depression, with the attendant risk of suicide, may be viewed in many different ways. The term "depression" has wormed its way into common usage and may be used to describe anything from one's response to a bad day at the office to a severe, long-term, stuporous state requiring intervention in order to avoid tragic results such as suicide. Thus "depression" represents anything from a transient lowering of one's mood to a well-defined "disease" entity.

Although depression is a fact of life for everyone under certain situations, some persons are particularly vulnerable to depression in relation to any number of real life situations. These are people who, in their early relationships, became convinced that their continued security and status of being loved and cared for were entirely dependent on "shaping up" and fitting the requirements set for them by significant others. Persons who develop a depressive coping style feel that deviations from these requirements rupture relationships and render them worthless and helpless. They also feel that they alone are responsible for these disruptions.

Such a pattern may develop in a number of ways at a very early period of life. For example, a young toddler who is always compared negatively with an older sibling can be made to feel that the only way for her to achieve status and worth in the family is to deny her own self and become a mirror image, if not better, of the older sibling. The child's existence then becomes an "as if" one. All her efforts are invested in being like her sibling, which is what she perceives others require if she is to be held in the same esteem as the sibling. An important concomitant of this process is that the child becomes out of touch with her real self, except to feel that it is quite unlovable and in need of change.

Another typical situation occurs when parenting figures have very high, unrealistic expectations about a child's behavior. The child is usually envisioned as fulfilling some type of family-saving or elevating role. The child comes to feel that just being himself is not sufficient to be accepted and loved in that family, and thus finds himself in a position like that of

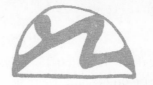

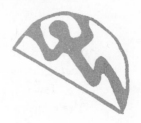

The depressive life position

the child in the first example. He generally adopts the same solution as the "as if" child does and spends all his efforts in playing out the role required by his parents. Failure to play the required role results in messages from the parents, either overt or covert, that he is inferior, that he is not measuring up, that he is more or less unloved, and that it is his fault.

Looking at this basis for a depressive style, it is clear that our culture is rampant with this form of reality construction. Take, for example, the very common occurrence of a child spilling milk. Adults are likely to focus on the child's carelessness, lack of attention, and similar elements instead of acknowledging that the child has to have such experiences in learning manual dexterity. The child is, in a sense, demoted to baby status and given utensils that will not spill. Usually, accompanying chastisements about the spilled milk involve some aspect of being "bad" which, instead of being attached to the act itself, somehow become directly related to the child. Situations like this are inevitable, human nature being what it is. The critical factor that determined how great a problem is thus created for the future adult is whether such occurrences are infrequent or a pervasive pattern of interaction between parent and child.

In all these instances, the child suffers a loss—of love, of status, of self-esteem—and directs his or her activities toward reducing these losses. People who have developed this central style of coping are those who have experienced this loss to a point where their feelings of security are conditional; they are secure only so long as they have direct signs from important people around them that they are approved and loved. Securing these signals of approval and love becomes a central motivational factor governing their activities. Their energies are directed toward discerning what will please others, and their behavior toward fulfilling others' expectations.

While all depressions have certain mechanisms in common, they differ in several aspects such as degree, duration, and etiology. As can be imagined, there is lack of agreement as to whether depression is one distinct entity, varying in duration and intensity, or a wastebasket category, similar to a "fever" in general medicine. Seligman has characterized depression as "the common cold of psychopathology."[1]

Despite ambiguities of terminology, there is some agreement on a set of attributes commonly associated with a depressive syndrome. Beck summarizes these attributes:

1. A specific alteration in mood; sadness, loneliness, apathy.
2. A negative self-concept associated with self-reproaches and self-blame.
3. Regressive and self-punitive wishes; desires to escape, hide, or die.
4. Vegetative changes; anorexia, insomnia, loss of libido.
5. Change in activity level: retardation or agitation.[2]

THE CONCEPTS OF GRIEF AND LOSS

Some mechanisms common to all depressive syndromes may be understood through an examination of the concept of grief. Grief is a typical response to situations of loss—no matter what the source of the loss may be. In fact, the best definition of a loss may well be anything at all that an individual values, that one perceives he or she once had or had aspirations for, and now has no possibilities for acquiring. One experiences this loss as losing a piece of oneself and, in a sense, has to repair the damage. This "damaged" condition leads to a diminished self-esteem, to anger, and to feelings of helplessness. Depending on his or her past experiences with the object of loss, the person has more or less ambivalent feelings about the object. It would be rare indeed for a relationship not to involve some measure of ambivalence. When these ambivalent feelings have been either unacknowledged or not integrated comfortably, the old conflicts involving them come to the fore when the loss occurs.

---

1. Martin E. P. Seligman, "Fall Into Helplessness," *Psychology Today,* June 1973, p. 43.
2. Aaron T. Beck, *The Diagnosis and Management of Depression* (Philadelphia: University of Pennsylvania Press, 1973), p. 6.

Freudians[3] talk about some of these responses being due to the psychic energy that the individual has invested in a highly ambivalent way in the object. When a loss occurs, the person is faced with the necessity of taking that energy back from the lost object and reinvesting it in something new. It is common for people during this phase to feel "down." They typically have no energy and feel somewhat withdrawn and self-contained; they may either sleep a lot or have insomnia; and they find it harder to concentrate and attend to their usual interests. Self-critical, derogating thoughts are common, as are somatic complaints such as difficulty with digestion. Angry thoughts about the loss are frequent, and these are troublesome to people who cannot understand why they feel angry.

If persons undergoing the grief reaction do not have too much unresolved conflict surrounding the particular loss in question, they generally will be able to "work through" their grief in a fairly reasonable, time-limited fashion. They will begin to reinvest their energies, will succeed in severing their ties with the lost object, and will start mobilizing themselves to replace the lost object.

As an example, consider Debbie, a twenty-year-old college sophomore, who just last week discovered that her boyfriend, whom she had planned to marry, has found a new girlfriend during the summer vacation; he has asked to terminate their relationship, even though he expressed a wish that they would "still be friends." Debbie is now, and probably will be for some time to come, engaged in "working through" what may be called the grief process. She is feeling very sad, "down," having a lot of angry feelings about the untrustworthiness of men in general and this man in particular, wondering if she is lacking some quality that the other girl has, and feeling very self-depreciatory. She probably even looks different, down in the dumps and certainly not as perky as her usual self. People may notice from her appearance and general sad demeanor that something is wrong in her life. She may well be irritable, have trouble sleeping or getting up in the morning, and have difficulty in concentrating on her school work. It may be anticipated that these symptoms will diminish in time, according to the common folk statement that "time heals." Debbie will go through a number of steps that will end up with her being able to put this man on a "back

---

3. For example, see Edith Jacobson, *Depression: Comparative Studies of Normal, Neurotic, and Psychotic Conditions* (New York: International Universities Press, 1971).

burner," so to speak, and she will once again be able to view other men as attractive and to consider developing new relationships. She will similarly be able to invest energies in activities that engage her interest and give new meaning to life. The process just described may be considered a rather normal "depressive" reaction.

To contrast with Debbie's story, let us assume a similar situation for another student, Mary. Let us also assume that Mary's relationship with this man was fraught with unrecognized and unresolved issues, which really carried out some old problems with her parents that had never been settled during her early years of development. Her relationship, then, was an ambivalent one, with many facets being double-edged, since they belonged as much to earlier relationships as to the reality of the current situation. Mary thought that the relationship was rather ideal in that her man had seemed content; she had done everything possible to please him. After they started dating, she had acquiesced in all his decisions, developed a new set of friends, and even learned how to play chess and eat with chopsticks. Mary could not imagine what fault her boyfriend could find with her.

In the aftermath of his leaving, even though she reassured herself that she had done everything for him, the nagging doubt persisted that maybe she was not good enough. Early conflicts that Mary experienced have resulted in a fear of rejection; her patterns of behavior are fairly submissive and compliant, all designed to prevent rejection from occurring. Part of the reason that she loves this young man relates to the fact that she could apparently get him to love her, could behave in a way that gained his approval. This approval confirmed her as a person of worth, not the inferior person she really perceives herself to be. Any argument between them was very significant to Mary and got blown up out of proportion. She responded with both fear and anger, although she overtly expressed neither one to him. Her usual behavior was to be somewhat sulky and aggrieved for a few days, and then to do more and more to try to please him.

For Mary, this final break becomes tied to her earlier feelings about not really being able to please anyone; not only is she faced with a current loss, but with her earlier, poorly resolved, losses as well. Her situation is much more complicated than Debbie's, and Mary can be expected to have much more difficulty in working toward a resolution. She is more likely to have sufficient trouble to be categorized as being "depressed."

A person suffering a loss of this type is expected to go through a grieving process. Lindemann describes the typical steps of this process as including (1) somatic distress, (2) preoccupation with the image of the loss—be that a person, condition, or thing, (3) guilt, (4) hostile reactions, and (5) loss of usual patterns of conduct.[4] In comparison with Debbie, Mary is likely to have much more pronounced symptoms in all these areas. She may be more troubled with somatic complaints, be unable to sleep or eat well. Mary will probably spend long hours thinking of her lost man, going over every detail of the relationship to see how she might have managed something differently that would have led to a different outcome. She will be preoccupied with feelings that she really is not a very attractive or brilliant person and that it was a wonder he was interested in her in the first place. At some points, she will spend a great deal of time thinking about how undependable people are, will flare out in sudden sarcastic statements, and in general will seem markedly different from the compliant, generally pleasant person others have assumed her to be. With Mary's pattern, it is most likely that she will feel that the termination of the relationship was her fault and that continuing to live as she has is really problematic. She may even entertain thoughts of suicide as a way out of her hopeless situation.

TYPES OF DEPRESSION

Although there are commonalities in all depressive reactions, there are different point of views about how depressions can be categorized and what, in truth, they represent. Some argue that differences in types of depression are merely differences in degree, while others maintain that they are separate entities: that the person who will become neurotically depressed is a different kind of person from the one who will become psychotically depressed. Probably the most common viewpoint is that there are two different types of depression: organic, or endogenous; and psychogenic, sometimes called exogenous.[5] In this view, the endogenous (organic)

---

4. Erick Lindemann, "Symptomatology and Management of Acute Grief," in *Crisis Intervention: Selected Readings,* ed. Howard J. Parad (New York: Family Service Association of America, 1965) p. 8.
5. Beck, *Diagnosis and Management,* pp. 59-62.

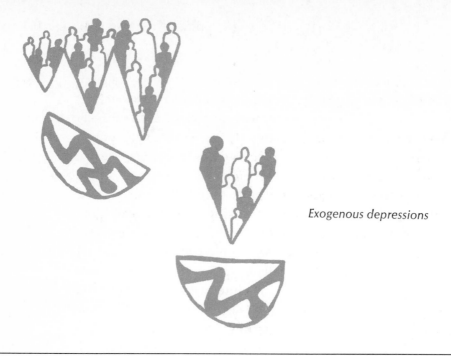

Exogenous depressions

type is regarded as being very much the product of biological factors and relatively uninfluenced by environmental or psychological factors. Psychotic depressions, including manic-depressive and involutional states, are frequently considered in this way. Exogenous (psychogenic) depressions are frequently called reactive. These depressions are seen as being the product of environmental or psychological factors and include the less severe neuroses.

Theoretical questions aside, the matter of how a person's depression will be regarded depends very much on a few accompanying circumstances. Generally speaking, differentiation between psychotic and neurotic depression is based on four specific variables: (1) intensity, (2) severity of ego impairment, (3) degree of regression, and (4) precipitating factors.

If there is an easily identifiable factor, such as a loss, that serves as a precipitant, the person is likely to be considered neurotic rather than psychotic. The more prominent the other three factors appear, the more likely it is that the person will be considered psychotic. In the case of regression, if the person merely becomes whiny and self-pitying and perhaps sleeps through some engagements, he or she will most likely be considered neurotic; but if the person cannot get out of bed at all for weeks, and cannot eat unless fed by someone, he or she would most likely be considered psychotic. In the area of ego impairment, if the person has difficulty concentrating on studies, is absent-minded and unable to follow directions well, and keeps ruminating over the past, he or she may be neurotic. However, if the individual's thinking patterns are fragmented or show changes such as delusions (e.g., "I have committed the unpardonable crime"), which show an inability to perceive reality with accuracy; and if he or she demonstrates poor judgment, it is most likely that this person will be considered psychotic. As for intensity, the person is "down" but can marginally manage commitments and meet role obligations, he or she will be considered neurotic; whereas if he or she is devastated, totally engrossed in bad feelings, markedly retarded (slowed down) or agitated, both mentally and physically, he or she will most likely be considered psychotic.

Bear in mind that the subjective element of this schema of labeling lends itself to ambiguity and problems in application. There are no discernible objective demarcations between categories, and in any type of labeling situation such as this, a number of other variables enter into the decision-making process. For example, a middle class person who seeks private psychiatric help is more likely to be labeled neurotically depressed, since this classification is generally regarded as less stigmatizing than the psychotic one. This classification sometimes remains until the person, still functioning poorly but unable to continue in private care because of finances, is sent for other types of psychiatric care. At that time it is likely that the classification will be changed from neurotic to psychotic, for only under those conditions is the person's state likely to gain him or her access to other forms of psychiatric treatment. (The poor person by and large falls on the mercies of prevalent public attitudes about mental care, since the treatment available in the public sector is determined and paid for by the public through government channels.) Currently, that sector requires the more serious diagnostic labels before treatment is available.

A further compounding factor arises from circumstances surrounding the person. A poor person probably does not come to the attention of anyone until he or she has done something quite weird as judged by the usual social norms, such as sitting on a park bench after midnight, wringing the hands, and crying in despair. In this instance, the police are probably the key persons in making a judgment that the person is psychotically depressed, and they act accordingly by bringing him or her to the closest psychiatric hospital.

Another variable is the sex of the person. Women are especially vulnerable to being classified as depressed, particularly as psychotically depressed. In this society, a whole set of circumstances that surround the roles traditionally provided for women would warrant a pained reaction, a lack of mastery, and a subsequent syndrome that might well be classified as a reactive depression. Past tendencies have been to discount factors in reality that could be seen as losses, and to focus instead on more endogenous (biological or organic) factors that might contribute to the depression. This is particularly true for women at a menopausal stage of life or women in any phase of the childbirth process (while pregnant, at delivery, immediately following delivery, and sometimes for a couple of years following the birth of a child). Instead of saying a woman is depressed because she has no way to retain her self-respect or to influence the world since her children have left, it is far easier to consider her depression as a result of hormonal imbalances from menopause. This is not to say that hormonal imbalances may not play a part; but it should be noted that they are frequently considered as the entire cause.

With these considerations in mind, classifying depressions according to exogenous or endogenous causes does not seem as useful as considering them to represent an interplay between physiological and psychological factors, each of these components having a different weight in varying types of depressions. Formerly, depressions that could not be accounted for by some external event in a person's life, and that had certain regularities or familial patterning, were considered endogenous. Examples of this are manic-depressive psychosis, involutional melancholia, and post-partum depression. Persons manifesting these forms of depression go through cyclic stages that appear unattached to any external factors. However, appearances are frequently deceptive, and it is difficult to be sure there are no external factors.

One example of mistaken classification can be seen in our past predilection for judging minorities according to the majority cultural position. Majority cultural views have clouded some very realistic problems of minority members, i.e., women, the aged, and those of minority ethnic backgrounds. When the predominant cultural view begins to change, the relationship of depressive responses to external reality factors becomes much clearer, and previous classifications no longer seem accurate. Thus, the powerless position of minority group members in our culture now is viewed as an explanatory factor for a depressive reaction. Our prior concepts of causality are in the process of being changed. Depressions experienced by women, minority cultural groups, and the aged are being recast in this perspective of powerlessness.

On the other hand, numbers of studies have amply demonstrated that some altered physiology does play a contributory part in the depressive process. Just what the balance is between external and internal factors may vary from case to case and is difficult to ascertain with any certainty. With these areas of ambiguity in mind, let us consider the various physiological factors believed to be related to the development of depressive reactions.

PHYSIOLOGICAL FACTORS

Genetic factors have long been studied, particularly in relation to manic-depressive disorders. These studies indicate a higher incidence of manic-depressive psychosis in relatives of patients suffering from this disorder than in the general population.[6] It should be noted that to generalize from this type of finding to a conclusion that there is a genetic base for manic-depressive psychosis is controversial. It is difficult to determine whether the greater incidence is due to genetic factors or is a result of a cyclic process in which the psychological environment set up by persons with this type of coping behavior tends to produce the same kind of coping behavior in this next generation.

Another common avenue of study concerns the neurohormonal balance of persons suffering from depressions. Most of these studies have focused upon hormonal levels, particularly those in women. The prevalence of studies of women is perhaps due to the more demarcated cyclic patterns associated with menstruation, although there is some evidence that men similarly have cycles in which their hormonal levels are altered. These studies have pointed to the increase in depression and irritability prior to, and accompanying, the menstrual period. As Bardwick summarizes the findings of these studies,

> . . . testosterone seems to be clearly related to levels of hostility or assertiveness or dominance . . . . It seems to me possible that characteristic

---

6. Frederich Redlich and Daniel Freedman, *The Theory and Practice of Psychiatry* (New York: Basic Books, 1966), p. 539.

affect differences between midcycle and premenstruation could reflect not only levels of testosterone in women but also the interactive effect of a high level of testosterone and low levels of both estrogen and progesterone premenstrually. A high midcycle testosterone level in addition to high estrogen might add to the probability of increased assertiveness or competitiveness along with feelings of self-esteem. In contrast, the premenstrual testosterone effect might increase the probability of aggression experienced as hostility.[7]

It is readily apparent from these findings that women's hormonal balances are closely tied to their emotions, though these findings do not support the conclusion that a woman's emotions are entirely determined by her hormonal state.

Further research along this line has been directed toward identifying the sequence of synapse activity and the transmission of nervous impulses. This research has focused primarily on the biochemical activities of monoamine oxidase (MAO) and the catecholamines. As Bardwick describes the process:

> When the neuron is activated and the catecholamine is released so that an impulse crosses the synapse, then that amount of the catecholamine must be deactivated. It must be metabolized so that the neuron can go back to its original resting capacity in preparation for refiring. Monoamine oxidase is an agent that causes the catecholamines to metabolize back to their initial state. Therefore, the presence of a high level of MAO means a low level of the catecholamine at the synapse. This is a condition associated with depression.[8]

It has been found that the MAO level is high in certain conditions: premenstrually and at menopause women have high levels of MAO, and depression is common also at these times.

Bardwick, summarizing findings in this general area, states: "The data thus support the general hypothesis that there are neural changes associated with steroid levels, and sensory, preceptual, cognitive, emotional, and activity level measures may alter significantly as endocrine levels or combinations alter."[9] Physiological studies definitely indicate the

---

7. Judith Bardwick, "System Hormones, Nervous System and Affect Irritability," in *Women in Therapy,* ed. Violet Franks and Vasanti Burtle (New York: Brunner/Mazel Publishers, 1974), pp. 34-35.
8. Ibid., p. 42.
9. Ibid.

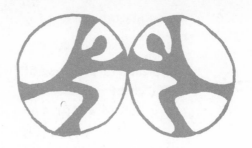

Dependency

interaction between hormones, nervous system, and affective state, but the precise nature of their interaction is not known at this time. It seems fair to say that the most reasonable view to adopt in considering depression would be one that combines physiological and environmental factors rather than looking solely at one or the other.

PSYCHOLOGICAL FACTORS

Constructs most frequently identified as being involved in depressive syndromes are dependency, with an associated diminished self-esteem, and powerlessness. Another related constellation consists of anger, a severe superego, guilt, and ambivalence. As can be seen, some of these difficulties originate in early relationships that one has experienced.

In discussing general coping style, we referred to some typical themes common in relationships at an early developmental level. A child feels that he or she has been a disappointment and in turn feels disappointed by parents because the child is never able to get what he or she hopes for. Thus, it is hard for the child to accomplish the developmental tasks of this period, and he or she never fully learns to trust and to become an effective, autonomous person. Instead he or she, as an adult, is left with specific vulnerabilities about needing people to lean on and is beset by fears that they will not be available or will reject him or her as unworthy. Because of this dependency, the person strives to do what other people require in an effort to be favored. Relationships are always fraught with ambivalences, usually unrecognized by the person, but due to the extreme positive and negative feelings attached to a significant other and also to the contradictory demands the dependent person places on significant others. The person both wants others to allow him or her to remain dependent and blames them for not allowing him or her to become autonomous and self-sufficient.

It is reasoned that a good bit of this ambivalence stems from the rage during a very early developmental period when the child was not unconditionally loved and accepted for what he or she was. The person always retains the hope of securing approval and becomes enraged when it is not forthcoming. The pattern of wanting acceptance very much and being angry when it is not received continues to be the way the susceptible person constructs his or her relationships with others. Depression is viewed as a turning inward of angry impulses originally directed toward significant others.

During early years when the child was acquiring this general coping style, he or she was unable to deal with conflicts inherent in relationships with important people. If he or she expressed anger toward significant others, they might vanish, or be destroyed, or destroy the child, and thus he or she would have nothing. This configuration is not only a product of primary process thinking but also a result, usually, of the parents' style of responding to negative feelings and messages directed toward them by their children.

Parents frequently do make comments that legitimate children's fears, such as the mother who is "going to have to go away" or "is made sick" by the child's behavior. Frequent threats of abandonment if the child "is bad" affirm children's worst fears of what their anger might do. Blocked in expressing anger toward others and being made to feel that somehow they are to blame for the trouble, children set up the pattern of feeling that they are unable to achieve what it is they want, unable to "bring off" a loving relationship because they are unlovable. This pattern becomes the base for feelings of helplessness and lowered self-esteem. It is also the base for a continual source of aggression that cannot be directly expressed and therefore must be managed in devious ways. People in this situation become so involved in protecting their own wounded selves that they do not have enough energy to invest outside themselves. Such self-involvement, called narcissism, can be discerned in many adults who would be shocked at hearing themselves so described.

A mother "giving her all" to her family, the PTA, and various other charities or civic enterprises may be genuinely altruistic. On the other hand, she may be doing these things to maintain her own security with others, to enhance her sense primarily of being loved. A person so involved never has had the opportunity to become truly autonomous because he or she is so involved in providing performances that will foster positive feedback. This pattern is established in childhood when parents become involved in turning the child into what they wish him or her to be rather than relating to the child he or she really is. It is possible that there are some children who automatically are what their parents wish them to be and so are spared from the development of the problems we are now describing.

Some theorists emphasize a set of problems relating the superego in their discussions of depressed people. Parents of children who later develop a depressive coping style are likely to have rigid standards that their children are expected to attain. These standards are incorporated as unreasoned, automatic givens that remain unaltered as the person matures. One characteristic of such children's very early lives is that they cannot reason and tie together in a logical fashion their ideas or interpretations of what they experience. Because of the primitive, magical nature of children's early thinking processes, standards that they incorporate are likely to be primitive and harsh. They lack the ability to apply reason and logic to experiences and view things in a black-or-white, all-or-none, magical fashion. The impact of this pattern is that, in some sense, the child's mental image of what he or she ought to be will be made up of a number of unrealistic standards that he or she cannot achieve. Although the ego ideal is formed in this way by all children, the particular child who will be prone to depression is in a worse position in that he or she has never been able to satisfy the parents, while the standards of those parents, to begin with, were more unrealistic than most.

This constellation of factors is usually very apparent, to one degree or another, if one examines the behavior patterns of someone in a depressive episode.

COGNITIVE VIEW

More recently, attempts have been made to view depression from a cognitive point of view, rather than through the psychodynamic model which stresses affective factors. "Cognitive theory assigns a primary role to the cognitive manifestations of depression in contrast to traditional views which hold that all other symptoms are secondary to a basic emotional disturbance."[10] Attention here is focused on certain manifestations of a person's cognitive activities. Cognitively, the depressed person tends to view things from a very narrow, negative perspective. Beck has referred to this constellation of negative perceptions of the self, the world, and the future as the "cognitive triad." In addition to the content of the person's views, Beck has also described typical errors in the form of cognitions:

> These errors include *arbitrary inference,* in which a conclusion is drawn despite inadequate or contrary evidence; *overgeneralization,* or the process of drawing broad generalizations on the basis of a single incident; *magnification* of the importance of a particular event; *selective abstraction,* or focusing on a single detail rather than the whole context of a situation; and *cognitive deficiency,* which refers to disregard for important aspects of the life situations, such as the long-range consequences of drinking or overeating. These typical distortions may affect the patient's judgment concerning only circumscribed areas of experience, especially those relating to his own abilities or prospects.[11]

These errors in conceptualization can be viewed as one resolution of primary process thinking, the primitive, magical thinking characteristic of early childhood.

SOCIOLOGICAL PERSPECTIVES

As we have pointed out, feelings of powerlessness and low self-esteem are prevalent in all forms of depresesion. Certain social situations contribute to development of these feelings. The statuses of minority groups, of women, and of the aging have recently come to be viewed from this perspective. Feminists have identified what they consider to be a "kinship between the subjective feelings of helplessness in depression and the objective helplessness and powerlessness of women in the American society, when compared to the prestige of men in male-oriented professional and business worlds."[12]

Chesler, extending this view, portrays women as "always in a state of mourning from what they never had—namely, a positive conception of

10. Aaron T. Beck and Ruth L. Greenberg, "Cognitive Therapy With Depressed Women," in Franks and Burtle, *Women in Therapy,* p. 118.
11. Ibid., pp. 118-119.
12. Ibid., p. 116.

their own possibilities."[13] Jessie Bernard holds that "depression, among other problems of women, can be attributed to the 'bad deal' they get in marriage."[14]

Bart, who has studied depression in middle-aged women extensively, relates depression at this age to role loss, specifically loss of the maternal role. Women whose lives are almost completely invested in their children are left without a role and without purpose in life when their children leave home. Women who are rigid are particularly susceptible to depression when they lose the maternal role, in that they find it difficult to adapt and find new roles for themselves. Sociocultural influences limit women's adaptability by socializing them into particular roles, namely those of wife and mother.[15] These feminist researchers argue that the low self-esteem and helplessness characteristic of the depressed person are a natural outgrowth of the position of women within the social structure.

Blacks are another minority group whose position in socety is such that they incorporate many negative perceptions of themselves, in terms of both present and future, frequently related to the development of depression. Although the situation is changing, negative stereotypes that have prevailed in the past serve to reinforce this negative self-image in minority groups. It is as though prevailing cultural norms and values provide the same kinds of dynamics we have earlier discussed in relation to parental influences.

A third minority group particularly prone to cultural pressures that may contribute to the development of depression is the aging population. With the aged, the problem is compounded in that all of the factors implicated in depression are accentuated in the aging process. As one ages, one suffers from a series of losses: one loses friends; capacities as a breadwinner or a homemaker are lost or diminished; children grow up and leave the family. In addition, the aged person may suffer loss of mental and physical capacities, frequently is forced to move out of his or her home and into some type of semi-custodial situation, and on all fronts is faced with assaults upon his or her self-esteem.

If a person has had problems coping with losses throughout his or her

---

13. Phyllis Chesler, *Women and Madness* (Garden City, N.Y.: Doubleday, 1972).
14. Jessie Bernard, *The Future of Marriage* (New York: World Publishing, 1972).
15. Pauline Bart, "Depression in Middle-Aged Women," in *Women in Sexist Society,* ed. Vivian Gornick and Barbara Moran (New York: Basic Books, 1971), pp. 99-117.

life and has developed a depressive coping style, it may be anticipated that these problems will be exaggerated with age and that the person will become increasingly depressed. In our youth-oriented culture, little value is placed upon contributions that an aged person can make in society. With current family structure focused on the nuclear family, there is little place for aging grandparents in this schema. Cut off from family, friends, and other meaningful social relationships, the person becomes increasingly isolated and, in many instances, depressed.

DEPRESSIVE REACTIONS

In the past, different types of depression have been considered to be different entities, but currently the tendency is to view them as variants on the same theme. The reader will recall that we have differentiated types of depressions on the neurotic-psychotic dimension according to the four variables of intensity, severity of ego impairment, regression, and precipitating factors. The psychotically depressed person has profound involvement in the first three areas, and a precipitating factor may be difficult to discern. The affect, or mood, is apt to be extremely depressed; the person may cry endlessly or bemoan his or her fate. Delusions are frequent, and generally refer to the person's low self-esteem and/or guilt or to the fear that some catastrophic event is about to take place, such as the end of the world. Common examples are, "I'm the world's greatest sinner, don't come near me," or "I am the most evil, vicious bitch there ever was," or "I can't eat this food, my stomach has rotted away." These types of interactions become problematic when the person refuses to eat or take care of basic bodily needs. The activity level is greatly depressed and movement is a problem. People who are psychotically depressed may sit in the same position for hours, and so develop edematous lower limbs from impaired circulation. Sometimes they lose the will to action and do not take care of themselves in any way. Their intense preoccupation with sadness and despair increasingly cuts them off from more positive forms of interaction. The overwhelming feeling communicated is one of extreme despair and hopelessness; they suffer from an absolute conviction that things are never going to get any better. Ironically, if left alone, these depressions always do improve.

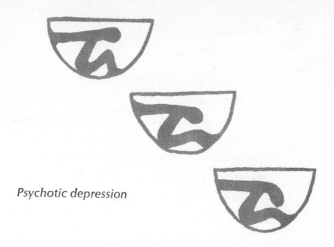

Psychotic depression

One type of affective illness usually placed in the depressed category is the manic-depressive psychosis. Here a relatively short manic phase and a relatively longer depressed phase occur in cyclic patterns. These patterns are varied. It has been known for someone to have one sequence predominantly, but this is extremely rare. The usual case is for people to have several attacks in a lifetime. In the manic phase, the person's mood is elated, thought processes are characterized by flight of ideas and happy thoughts, and he or she is extremely active.[16]

A close correlation is seen between depressed and manic states. While in a manic state, the person engages in a desperate attempt to ward off thoughts that might usher in extreme depression. Degrees of manic behavior may range from hypo-mania, where the person's behavior appears exaggerated; to acute mania, where he or she is in a state of extreme restlessness; to delirium, in which he or she is disoriented and in an extreme state of agitation. The falseness of the manic person's gay mood may be seen in the rapid shifts to extreme irritability and rage when he or she is confronted by any frustration in the environment. People are frequently somewhat intimidated and fearful of the manic person's rapier tongue and unpredictable outbursts of anger.

The manic's feelings are elation and exuberance. Thought processes are rapid, reflected in speech in what is called flight of ideas, or skipping rapidly from topic to topic. The person in a manic phase talks incessantly,

16. Silvano Arieti, "Manic-Depressive Psychosis," in *American Handbook of Psychiatry*, ed. Silvano Arieti (New York: Basic Books, 1959), p. 427.

may become incoherent, and may also sing and shout. If a manic's thought disorder progresses to the point of delusions, they will be delusions of grandeur about wonderful accomplishments or plans for the future. One woman, for example, maintained that she spoke five languages, had ice-skated and played concert piano with world-renowned performers (whom she named), and had business plans that would make her thousands of dollars. There was no evidence that any of this was true.

The manic's behavior is characterized by excess. He or she is constantly in motion, flits from project to project, and can scarcely take time out to eat or sleep. The person may become exhausted; in fact, before tranquilizing medications were available, some manics died of exhaustion. The person in a manic state is extravagant with money and may waste his or her life's savings; he or she tends to be sexually overactive, sometimes becoming promiscuous. The manic is very outgoing and treats everyone like an old friend, but can become belligerent if not given his or her way. In this form of disorder, a manic phase is always followed by a depression.

Some people do not seek help in the manic phase unless they run into trouble with other people in their environment. They can enjoy the good feelings and elation they have during this phase, but as they feel it waning, they usually seek help since they know of the inevitability of the depression that will follow. It is much more usual for the person to experience a depressed phase after a manic phase than vice versa, and this is one of the facts supporting the view of the manic phase as a defense against the person's basically depressive orientation. This cyclic sequence is effectively managed through the administration of lithium, a drug which is discussed in Chapter 9.

INVOLUTIONAL DEPRESSION

Depressions that occur during middle or late middle life have commonly been called involutional, since they mirror the physical changes of of the climacteric or menopause. There are commonly two types described: agitated and paranoid. The usual involutional depression takes the agitated form, in which the prominent symptoms are gross motor activity and anxiety. The contents of the person's mood are the same except that instead of sitting in a retarded manner, the person generally speeds up bodily movements. Somatic complaints are frequent, as they are in the more classic nonagitated depressions. Frequently, persons suffering from an involutional depression will spend days walking back and forth in a hospital corridor, wringing their hands, with an extremely pained expression on their faces, complaining about physical symptoms and bemoaning their sinfulness.

The less common type is the paranoid form. Occasionally persons start out a depression with agitated features and change to a more paranoid orientation. The hallmark of this form of depression is the paranoid ideology, although the predominating feature is the depressed mood. These persons tend to be delusional, usually with a persecution content to their delusions.

SUICIDE

Perhaps more than other manifestations of depression, the possibility of suicide as an outcome is one of the most serious problems associated with this particular coping style.

Suicide is a major public health problem and a particular risk when one is dealing with depressed individuals. It is among the ten leading causes of death in this country, accounting for at least 25,000 deaths per year. In addition, for every completed suicide, there are seven or eight nonfatal attempts.

The incidence of suicide increases with age. Persons over sixty-five, though they comprise only 10 percent of the population, account for 25 percent of the suicides. Though the incidence of suicide increases with age, it is also a significant problem among young people. Suicide before the age of fifteen is extremely rare, but in adolescents it is the fourth leading cause of death, and among college students it is the second most frequent cause of death. Among college students, it is surpassed only by accidents, and some of these are probably intentional.[17]

Suicide rates are also related to sex, marital status, and race. Men are 70 percent of the suicides, though women outnumber men in nonfatal

---

17. Earl Grollman, *Suicide: Prevention, Intervention, Postvention* (Boston: Beacon Press, 1971), pp. 50-52.

attempts by three to one. Men commit suicide most often by shooting and hanging themselves, whereas women choose more passive means, such as sleeping pills, poisons, and gas.[18] Suicide is less frequent among married persons than among those who are single, divorved, or widowed, except for young married persons. In married persons under twenty-four years of age, the incidence is higher than for single persons; the difference is most noticeable in persons under twenty. Under age thirty-five, the incidence of suicide is higher in widowed than in single persons, but over thirty-five the reverse is true. Divorced persons have a higher suicide rate than undivorced persons of the same sex.[19]

The incidence of suicide is low among black persons in the South, about half that of southern whites.[20] The situation is different in the North, however, where in the last ten to fifteen years, the incidence of suicide among young black males in urban areas has risen alarmingly. Among blacks, the incidence of suicide is highest in the teens and twenties. Unemployment, which comes first to the young black male, is a source of emotional as well as financial stress and may precipitate suicide and other types of aggressive behavior that result in self-destruction. A particular problem for black males, considering their status as an oppressed minority group, surrounds the socially accepted avenues for the expression of aggression. The high rates of homicide and suicide are perhaps a reflection of this problem.[21]

CLUES TO SUICIDE

About 80 percent of those who attempt suicide give some clue to their intentions. Most persons who attempt suicide are in a state of crisis and are ambivalent about dying: they wish to escape their plight and view dying as their only workable means of doing so, but they also wish to be rescued and given the help they need. Someone who recognizes the clues that are present can reach out to a troubled person and help him or her find ways other than suicide of dealing with problems.

---

18. Ibid., pp. 47-48.
19. Ibid., pp. 49-50.
20. Ibid., p. 60.
21. Gene Lester and David Lester, *Suicide: The Gamble With Death* (Englewood Cliffs, N.J.: Prentice-Hall, 1971), pp. 99-100.

Grollman classifies the clues to suicide as

—previous attempts
—verbal threats
—behavioral or nonverbal clues
—situational clues.[22]

The most serious clue to suicidal intent is a *previous attempt*. Eighty percent of those who kill themselves have made at least one previous attempt. Dublin estimates that there are about two million persons with a history of one or more nonfatal suicide attempts, and that at least 10 percent of these will eventually kill themselves.[23]

Verbal warnings of suicidal intent may be direct and/or indirect. For instance, the person may say directly that he or she wants to die or is thinking of suicide, or he or she may communicate this indirectly through such statements as, "I can't stand much more of this," "My life seems so hopeless," or, "I don't think I'll be here next week." Suicidal intent is also communicated through *behavioral or nonverbal clues,* such as making out a will, giving away possessions, or a sudden, inconsistent change in behavior, representing a departure from the person's usual behavior. The obsessively neat housewife who announces that this year "there's no need to put away the winter clothes because you can never tell about the weather" may be making a statement about her not being around much longer.

Sometimes the person's *situation* itself may be considered a clue. Situations that contain a variety of stressful elements and in which emotional support from others is not forthcoming are particularly suspect.

Chronic or fatal illness or a long, painful sickness, and all that these imply, may be more than a person can bear. Death may seem preferable to a drastic change in one's self-image, the inability to work or care for one's family, or to prolonged suffering. One study of completed suicides showed that 70 percent had evidence of acute illness at the time of death.[24] Farberow et al. state that the greatest number of suicides occurring in general medical-surgical hospitals are in persons with long-term, serious illnesses, such as cancer and respiratory and circulatory diseases.[25]

---

22. Grollman, *Suicide,* pp. 72-83.
23. Ibid., p. 6.
24. Lester and Lester, *Suicide: Gamble With Death,* p. 26.
25. Norman Farberow et al., "Suicide Among Cardiovascular Patients," in *The Psychology of Suicide,* ed. Edwin Shneidman et al. (New York: Science House, 1970), p. 369.

Economic distress, such as loss of employment, bankruptcy, or inadequate income, is another factor associated with suicide. Financial insecurity implies that the individual's basic needs for food, shelter, and clothing may not be met. It is also a blow to one's self-image as an adequate person and a continual source of uncertainty and anxiety.

Loss of a loved one through death may be more than one can endure, and death may be seen as a relief from unbearable loneliness and pain. Denial of the loss, prolonged grief reactions, and other signs of failure to resolve the loss are indications that the person is not adapting and may be desperate.

It was noted earlier that the incidence of suicide is highest in older persons. It is appropriate now to point out how frequently the situational factors discussed thus far occur in the lives of older people. They are often afflicted with chronic, debilitating diseases, such as hypertension, heart disease, and cancer, in addition to sensory losses of vision and hearing. Many older persons are poor, struggling to live on inadequate or barely adequate incomes. Also, older persons experience many losses through death—spouses, relatives, friends, and sometimes their children. Many older people are alone and isolated, sick, and poor, with nothing to live for or look forward to. It is no wonder that they frequently choose to die.

The fourth situational clue is domestic difficulty, for example, divorce, separation, and the broken home. Divorce is a blow to the self-image and may arouse feelings of failure and guilt. If there are children in the family, the situation is compounded for both parents and children. A suicidal person may be expressing a family disturbance or crisis. An important factor to consider in relation to these situational factors is not only the factor of loss associated with all of them, but also the ties the person may have to others which help him or her to sustain the loss. In situations in which someone has few strong interpersonal ties, and these few relationships are lost, the person may conclude that "there is nothing to live for." Suicide is viewed as the only solution, given the person's isolated position.

Besides the above verbal, behavioral (nonverbal), and situational clues, the person's emotional and mental condition must be considered. Most persons who contemplate or attempt suicide do so after they have begun to improve. This is attributable to different factors. A depressed person may suddenly improve because he or she has made a decision to end his or her life and, once having made the decision, feels better. Also,

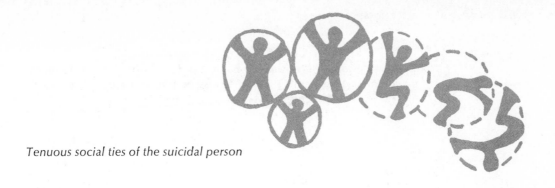

Tenuous social ties of the suicidal person

persons who are deeply depressed, though they may think of suicide, do not have the energy to plan and carry out a suicide attempt while in the depths of a depression. Thus, when their depression improves somewhat and their energy increases, they are more suicidal.

Other factors sometimes associated with suicide are dependence on alcohol, bromides, barbiturates, and hallucinogens.[26] A person is also more likely to commit suicide if there is a history of suicide in his or her family, but the reason for this is unclear.[27]

Small and Opler summarize the factors most frequently associated with suicide:

> Included in the high-risk group we have in our culture are the older white male, very often physically ill and a widower; retired or older people with the "empty nest syndrome," where the children have grown up and moved away, leaving the parents alone in their home in isolation; patients who have had psychiatric illnesses and who have been subsequently discharged; alcoholics; homosexuals; addicts; older persons with terminal illnesses, especially where these are painful; and persons with prior suicidal behavior, particularly where there has been a pattern of suicide within the family. Within these groups there are especially dangerous times, such as anniversaries of births, deaths, and marriages; certain holidays, like Christmas, which is a family holiday and often leads to reminiscing; and cheerful holidays when lonely individuals feel all the more depressed by comparison with the surrounding

26. Grollman, *Suicide,* pp. 79-83.
27. Lester and Lester, *Suicide: Gamble With Death,* p. 39.

all-pervasive jollity. Physical illness, loss of loved ones by death, separation, divorce, loss of one's fortune, loss of job, retirement, and so on can also serve as precipitating events for suicidal attempts.[28]

SUICIDAL PERSONS AND HEALTH PERSONNEL

The nurse will encounter suicidal persons in a variety of settings, sometimes within the hospital and sometimes outside of it. A study by Litman and Farberow suggests the relative frequency of suicide in different hospital settings. In Los Angeles County during the years 1963 and 1964, there was a total of 2,284 suicides, 44 of these occurring in hospitals. Of the forty-four, twenty occurred in nursing-convalescent units, twelve in general medical-surgical units, and twelve in psychiatric units or hospitals.[29] Worth noting from these statistics is the fact that most suicides in hospitals were committed by persons hospitalized for long-term, chronic disabilities. Also worth noting is that there were as many suicides on general medical-surgical units as on psychiatric units.

The number of persons who commit suicide after discharge from a hospital or treatment by a physician is much higher than those who commit suicide while hospitalized. Three-fourths of those who commit suicide have consulted a physician within the four months prior to their death.[30] In the Litman and Farberow study referred to above, more than 150 persons committed suicide within two months of discharge from general medical-surgical units, compared with the twelve suicides that occurred on the units. The incidence of suicide in persons who were on pass or had run away from psychiatric units was also three times higher than the rate in persons still within psychiatric units.[31]

Litman and Farberow studied the characteristics of the persons who committed suicide in a hospital to determine whether there were any commonalities. Knowledge of commonalities can alert hospital personnel to which patients are more likely to be suicidal. In the general medical-sur-

28. S. Mouchly Small and Marvin Opler, "Suicide: Epidemiologic and Sociologic Considerations," in Organizing the Community to Prevent Suicide, ed. Jack Zusman and David Davidson (Springfield, Ill.: Charles C. Thomas, Publisher, 1971), p. 16.
29. Robert Litman and Norman Farberow, "Suicide Prevention in Hospitals," in Shneidman et al., the Psychology of Suicide, p. 463.
30. Grollman, Suicide, p. 72.
31. Litman and Farberow, "Suicide Prevention in Hospitals, pp. 466-468.

gical units, eleven of the twelve patients were male. Their median age was sixty-seven, and their median hospital stay was three days. They were hospitalized for a variety of reasons. All of them were depressed or confused, and their suicides appeared impulsive rather than planned. Ten of the twelve killed themselves by jumping out of a window. The other two took pills or poison.[32] The composite picture then, shows an older male, depressed or confused, who has been hospitalized for only a short time and who impulsively kills himself.

The implications for the nurse and other staff relate to observation and protection. Observation is essential to detect the danger signs of depression or confusion. Protective measures should be instituted when necessary. They will vary depending on the situation and may include constant surveillance by staff or relatives, protective screens or glass, and removal of potential means, such as belts, medication, and sharp objects. A psychiatric consultation or referral may be indicated. Consistent interpersonal relationships with the nursing staff are also helpful.

The number of persons who commit suicide while hospitalized on general medical-surgical units is small compared with the total number of persons admitted to such units. This should be the cause, however, for more, rather than less, alertness to the problem. Something that happens infrequently is not so likely to be in the conscious awareness of hospital personnel as a frequent danger is, and if staff are not aware of the possibility of suicide, they may overlook the danger signs.

The characteristics of persons who committed suicide while in convalescent-nursing hospitals differ from those in general hospitals in several important respects. They were older, the median age being seventy-six; their hospital stay was measured in years rather than days; and they suffered from chronic diseases—tuberculosis, diabetes, cardiac disease, arteriosclerosis, multiple sclerosis, and cancer. Many of them were severely depressed, communicated their suicidal intent, left suicide notes, had made previous attempts, and were chronically suicidal. Most committed suicide by taking an overdose of medication or by cutting themselves.

Litman and Farberow say that many of their informants raised the question of why persons who are old, incurably ill, lonely, and unwanted should be prevented from taking their lives. They point out, however, that

---

32. Ibid., p. 463.

such persons who do commit suicide are a small minority of those in similar circumstances, and that the suicidal persons seemed to have an inability to adjust to their environment. These persons constantly complained, tried to change things, and aroused antagonism in the staff. Perhaps, with such persons, an effort should be made to adjust the treatment plan.[33] Protective measures, psychiatric consultation, and attempts to provide meaningful relationships are also indicated.

The individuals who committed suicide on psychiatric units were younger, with a median age of forty-four, and had been hospitalized for varying periods from a day to several years. Hanging was the method most frequently used, and many had made prior attempts. The number of persons who commit suicide in the hospital is relatively small, but, as mentioned above, three times as many killed themselves while on pass or after running away. The greatest suicide risk exists in those persons who have just been admitted or discharged. In a study of the Los Angeles area, 7 percent of the suicides had recently been discharged from a psychiatric hospital. Another 15 percent had received, but not followed, a recommendation for psychiatric hospitalization a few weeks before their deaths.[34]

The above statistics and statistics quoted elsewhere in this chapter emphasize the fact that many persons who commit suicide are or have recently been in the care of medical and mental health personnel. The fact that suicidal persons are seen in a variety of settings emphasizes that nurses and other health personnel can be key figures in the prevention of unnecessary deaths.

■ *Relationships.*   Regardless of the setting, establishing a relationship with the suicidal person is crucial in intervening. In a study of hospitalized patients, Farberow and McEvoy state that staff interest and concern are crucial in preventing suicide.[35] In the treatment of out-patients who are suicidal, Litman says, a prerequisite for successful treatment is establishing and maintaining a relationship. This is basic to the patient's asking for help and the therapist's perceiving and responding to the patient's need.[36] Grollman, too, emphasizes the importance of a relationship in which the

---

33. Ibid., pp. 466-467.
34. Ibid., pp. 467-468.
35. Norman Farberow and Theodore McEvoy, "Suicide Among Patients With Anxiety or Depressive Reactions," in Shneidman et al., *the Psychology of Suicide,* pp. 345-368.
36. Robert Litman, "Treatment of the Potentially Suicidal Patient," in Shneidman et al., *Psychology of Suicide,* pp. 405-413.

troubled person can feel understood, accepted, and supported. "To one who feels unworthy and unloved, caring and concern are great sources of encouragement."[37]

Of all the measures nurses might institute, establishing a relationship is the most basic and most important. A relationship can convey to the suicidal person that the nurse believes he or she is a worthwhile person and cares about him or her. Nurses must attempt to understand the patient's feelings and convey that they understand; in this way, they can begin to reduce the patient's intense feelings of isolation and aloneness. A person intent upon suicide will find some way of attempting it, regardless of preventive measures. A relationship, on the other hand, is the means through which he or she can begin to discover a reason to live, something a seriously suicidal person lacks.

The relationships that a nurse encourages the suicidal person to establish are not only with nurses and other staff, but also with his or her family and friends. This is true whether the person is in a hospital or another setting. Suicidal persons are frequently alone and isolated. Sometimes their depression has caused them to neglect social ties, or their depression and suicidal crisis may be the result of loss of significant persons. Whatever the cause, the re-establishment of former relationships or the establishment of new ones is necessary for eventual rehabilitation. The nurse and other staff might help a person during this time of acute need, but they are no substitute for normal social relationships. The element of relationships outside the treatment setting, then, is a factor to be planned for from the first contact with a suicidal person.

■ *Observation.* Another general area of intervention, whether or not a suicidal person is hospitalized, might be called observation, including both verbal and nonverbal behavior. It is important and serious because most suicidal persons give some warning or clue before they attempt suicide, but if one misses a clue, there may not be another chance. Verbal and nonverbal clues were discussed earlier in this chapter. Detection of them requires attentive listening to what is said as well as what is implied, along with astute observation of the person's situation and behavior.

For persons who are hospitalized, observation includes frequent checks. Even on a secure ward, suicidal patients can find ways to harm

---

37. Grollman, *Suicide,* p. 89.

themselves. It is important *not* to follow a regular schedule (such as every half hour), however, because patients will quickly notice any pattern. Checks must be at frequent but irregular intervals. Dangerous times on a unit are those times when all the staff are occupied, such as report at change of shifts or other staff meeting times. Many suicidal attempts are made when patients know the staff are busy. A suicidal patient should be placed where he or she can be easily observed, for example, in a room close to the nurse's station.

▪ *Protection.*   The third general measure, protection, applies to patients who are hospitalized, particularly on a psychiatric unit, though the measures would also be appropriate for suicidal persons on a nonpsychiatric ward. Patients can be protected by making the means of suicide as unavailable as possible; for example, keeping the patient on a locked ward, supplying locked razors, controlling the use of sharp objects, removing belts and ties, and making certain the patient swallows medications so he or she cannot accumulate them for an overdose.

Such measures are useful in that suicide is more likely to occur if the individual has the means at hand when the impulse strikes. The nurse should not find unwarranted security in them, however, for it is impossible to remove all potential weapons, and patients who are intent upon suicide can find some means of attempting it. This fact serves to emphasize once again the original point made in caring for the suicidal person, namely, that the best prevention is to provide the patient a relationship through which he or she can begin to find a reason to live.

▪ *Crisis Intervention.*   Most suicidal persons are in a state of crisis and are suicidal for a relatively short period of time.[38] Crisis intervention, as described in Chapter 10, is an appropriate form of treatment for the individual in a suicide crisis. Suicide prevention centers, established throughout the country, aim to help persons through the crisis period. The attempt is to involve significant others with the suicidal person, that is, to try to help him or her re-establish personal and social ties. Another goal is to assess the seriousness of the risk and make referrals if necessary. Sometimes listening and acceptance are sufficient to reduce the immediate crisis. Grollman cautions, however, that further treatment may be necessary, and the matter should not be dropped when the crisis subsides. Half

---

38. Litman and Farberow, "Suicide Prevention in Hospitals," p. 462.

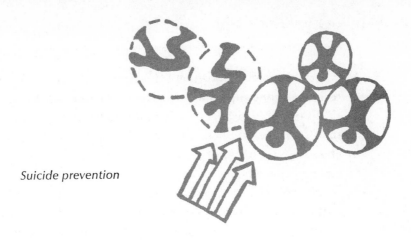

Suicide prevention

the persons who commit suicide do so within ninety days after the precipitating crisis. Sometimes a basic problem remains after the crisis has passed.[39]

To illustrate the central themes found in depression and suicide, let us go back to Mary, one of the young women described earlier in this chapter, who was disappointed when her boyfriend broke off their relationship. We left her at a point when she was feeling despairing and hopeless and had difficulty envisioning that the future would hold any happiness for her. As her somatic difficulties persisted, she continued to have difficulty sleeping as well as intermittent abdominal pain and tightness in the chest; she went to the health service. She feared she might fail her final exams because of her inability to sleep, which she felt was causing her difficulty in studying. At the health service, the doctor who saw her was sympathetic and kind. The doctor did ask her how things were going, in an attempt to account for her symptoms, but concluded that it was just the usual kind of stress everyone might experience at exam time plus the added stress of losing a boyfriend. Under these circumstances, it was only reasonable that she would have these symptoms. The doctor gave her a two weeks' supply of Seconal to get her through exam week. Mary did, in fact, get through exam week, and although her grades were not as good as they had been, she did pass her courses.

39. Grollman, *Suicide,* pp. 100-101.

Mary made a decision at this time to change her major from chemistry to home economics. She felt that it was a field she could be useful in and that she would probably learn a number of things that would be helpful in the future. In chemistry, she had always been in predominantly male classes, and in this setting she was always in competition with them; home economics would be a change from this situation, as well as a chance to make new acquaintances. Her former boyfriend was also a chemistry major, and it was too painful always to have to see him in class; this was a way out of that situation. Besides, her mother had always suggested that home economics was a good field for women and had wanted her to major in it. Although Mary had previously resisted this idea, she increasingly concluded that her mother had been right and that she could have been spared some problems had she followed her mother's advice.

Mary did well in her home economics courses although she missed the excitement and challenge of chemistry. Sometimes she imagined herself in a laboratory instead of the kitchen setting where she usually worked. Her social life in the past year was much better than she could ever have imagined following her break-up, and she dated two or three men intermittently. Although she did not develop a particularly close relationship with any of them, she had some good times and enjoyed herself.

At graduation, Mary again found herself in turmoil over future plans and with her parents. She received an unusually good job offer from a major magazine in a large metropolitan area. The particularly appealing aspect of this job was that it offered an experimental cooking situation where she could combine her interests in chemistry and home economics. Also it would take her to a cultural center and she was excited, though fearful, at the prospect of broadening her horizons. When she went home to relay this good news to her parents, she was surprised by their response: "That's halfway across the country. How are you ever going to manage by yourself? Besides, where will you be when we need you?" "Why don't young people have more concern for their parents after all the sacrifices they make for their children?"

This scene reactivated some of Mary's own fears about moving so far from home, and the more she thought about it, the more afraid she became of taking this step. She remembered how, in the past, she had gone to Girl Scout camp and had to come home because she was so homesick. She also thought of the times when she could rely on her parents to help her out of a situation; once, when she was in school, she had gotten in trouble with a teacher and they had come to "bail her out." She worried that if she were far away they could not do that. As she thought about what her parents were saying, she had to agree that it was true, they had been awfully good to her and maybe she had not appreciated them enough. She still was somewhat resentful that they were unwilling to let her try out something on her own and felt that if she did not appreciate them, they certainly did not seem to appreciate her either. Although she had these thoughts, she certainly would never express them to her parents and found that the feelings gradually subsided as she reached what she thought was a good compromise decision. Mary accepted a job in the small county seat, a town thirty miles away, as a dietitian in a small hospital. She found a small apartment which her mother was delighted to decorate for her. Being so close to home, Mary now planned to spend the weekends with her parents, and knew that they were not far away and that she could call on them if she needed them.

Mary now has become involved in a new relationship with Ted, a drug detail man whom she met in the hospital. After two months of a rather intense relationship he moved into her apartment, and she continued her earlier patterns of behavior, being concerned about pleasing him in every instance and troubled about how she might explain the relationship to her parents. In fact, her parents are the one point of contention between them. She finds that her involvement with Ted makes her work go easier because she has something else to think about rather than concentrating so much on her work. He helps her look at situations that she tends to take too seriously in a new light and points out that nothing is that important. As time goes on, she finds she cannot imagine what life would be without him; sometimes she becomes upset when she senses that he does not seem to be similarly invested in her.

In his work Ted travels a lot and often does not call her when he has said he will; she calls him, a practice that annoys him. She has wondered about the advisability of getting pregnant as a means of strengthening the relationship. This area of conflict between them continues, with Ted coming to feel more and more that Mary is not the girl he thought she was. He really likes her domestic, submissive qualities, but is troubled and cannot account for what he considers to be her leaning on him for everything. He reaches the decision that change is impossible for them and coincidentally finds himself wishing for other relationships. Eventually Ted becomes involved with another girl. Since he really has not been too open with Mary about his increasingly negative feelings regarding their relationship, he wonders how she will take the news that he wants to break off. The only time this subject had been broached, she seemed to overreact, saying that that sort of thing was not going to happen to her again, that life was not worth living if it was all a series of heartbreaks, with men taking advantage of her.

The relationship with the new girl, however, impels Ted to do something about breaking up with Mary, and so one day he announces his departure, saying that things really have not worked out between them. Ted advises Mary not to take things too seriously, telling her that one of her troubles is that she gets too intense with people. Mary experiences a recurrence of the depressive reaction she had earlier, but this time it is intensified. She uses this experience as confirmation of her earlier fears that she will never find happiness.

Having the same type of somatic problems as on the previous occasion, she seeks out a pharmacist to give her some medication to help her sleep. In the course of the conversation he mentions that he is going on vacation the following day, to which Mary replies, "I'll never have a vacation." He thinks that she is referring to being a relatively new employee, not yet entitled to vacation time, and does not really think anything of it. In the diet kitchen others have noticed that she is not quite herself, particularly since she has been late to work every single day, something which is very unlike her previous work pattern. One day she comments to Nellie, the salad girl, "You've always been so good to me; I want you to have my cat. I can't keep him any more." Mary has overheard a conversation in which Nellie was talking about moving and how she wanted to get a cat.

The pharmacist who supplied the pills gave her a month's supply because he was going to be on vacation. After being talked to by the chief dietitian about her tardiness, Mary goes home and takes the entire bottle of sleeping pills. When Nellie comes to get the cat, she finds the door ajar and looks in to find Mary dead, hand on the telephone receiver. Thus ends the career of Mary, although any one reading this history can imagine points at which crisis intervention might have precluded this tragic outcome. At least two times Mary made approaches to getting some sort of help, but each time the depressive nature of the problem was not identified and dealt with. Although nothing can be done to help Mary at this point, is it likely that her suicide will create a crisis for a few people: for her parents, Ted, and perhaps her fellow workers. They are likely to feel particularly guilty and concerned about their lack of understanding of Mary's situation. The usual aftermath for immediate family members is recriminations about whose fault this was and how the act of the deceased is seen as a reproach to the family.

SUMMARY

The prototype for depression is found in basic grief reactions, a process that attends all losses. Grieving follows a pattern of physical and psychological distress over the loss of anything that was valued by the person; it results in a restoration of a sense of completeness when the person finds some way of replacing the lost object and restructuring his or her life. Many people feel that the basis of depression is a short-circuiting of the grief process. When the person does not work through the grief, there is a later, more exaggerated reaction in which the symptomatology of grief is heightened and sometimes distorted. In this frame of reference, depressions are viewed as reactive. Other people argue that while reactive depressions follow this pattern, there are other depressions in which the symptomatology is severe and seems to stem from some physical or genetic, organic source (endogenous) as opposed to a situational loss (exogenous). Although there are these two different views about the source of depression, people generally agree that the symptomatology or the severity may differ.

Discriminations between diagnostic categories within this general area are ambiguous and generally seem to rest on four distinctions: (1) severity of ego impairment, (2) intensity of mood changes, (3) degree of regression, and (4) presence of precipitating factors.

The most commonly identified endogenous states are involutional depressions and manic-depressive psychoses. Although behavior during the manic phase is quite the opposite of that in the depressed state, it is posited that it represents a massive denial of the underlying depression.

Perhaps the most serious consequence of depression is the possibility of suicide, which is among the ten leading causes of death in this country.

Suicide more frequently occurs when a person is either going into or coming out of a severe depressed state, since a person in these stages can muster up enough energy to complete the act. The key element is that the person sees himself or herself as without hope. In trying to establish the seriousness of a suicidal possibility, it is necessary to assess the reasonableness of the person's plan for completing the act, the lethality of the means, and his or her connections to a social network.

The chief issue in the treatment of both depressions and possible suicidal behavior is to help the person in some way redefine his or her situation so that it is more hopeful and conducive to a reasonable self-esteem.

FURTHER READINGS

Anderson, Nancy. "Suicide in Schizophrenia." *Perspectives in Psychiatric Care* 11, no. 3 (1973): 106-112.

Ayd, Frank. *Recognizing the Depressed Patient.* New York: Grune & Stratton, Inc., 1961.

Bodie, Marilyn K. "Bridge to the Mainland." *Perspectives in Psychiatric Care* 3, no. 4 (1965): 8-27.

———. "When a Patient Threatens Suicide." *Perspectives in Psychiatric Care* 6, no. 2 (1968): 76-79.

Crary, William, and Crary, Gerald. "Depression." *American Journal of Nursing* 73 (March 1973): 472-475.

Crumb, Frederick W. "Limited Social Recovery—Further Discussion of a Depressed Behavior Pattern." *Perspectives in Psychiatric Care* 4, no. 3 (1966): 26-30.

———. "A Resonance of Agony." *Perspectives in Psychiatric Care* 1, no. 6 (1963): 16-18.

Fallon, Barbara. "And Certain Thoughts Go Through My Head . . . ." *American Journal of Nursing* 72 (July 1972): 1257-1259.

Fitzgerald, Roy, and Long, Imelda. "Seclusion in the Treatment of Severely Disturbed Manic and Depressed Patients." *Perspectives in Psychiatric Care* 11, no. 2 (1973): 59-64.

Grollman, Earl. *Suicide: Prevention, Intervention, Postvention.* Boston: Beacon Press, 1971.

Jackson, Pat. "Chronic Grief." *American Journal of Nursing* 74 (July 1974): 1289-1291.

Jourard, Sidney. "Suicide: An Invitation to Die." *American Journal of Nursing* 70 (Feb. 1970): 2694.

Kicey, Carolyn. "Catecholamines and Depression: A Physiological Theory of Depression." *American Journal of Nursing* 74 (Nov. 1974): 2018-2020.

Lester, Gene and Lester, David. *Suicide: The Gamble With Death.* Englewood Cliffs, N.J.: Prentice-Hall, 1971.

Mendels, Joseph. *Concepts of Depression.* New York: John Wiley & Sons, 1970.

Risley, Joan. "Nursing Intervention in Depression." *Perspectives in Psychiatric Care* 5, no. 2 (1967): 65-76.

Schwartz, Morris, and Shockley, Emmy. "The Patient is Suicidal." *The Nurse and the Mental Patient,* pp. 167-181. New York: John Wiley & Sons, 1956.

Shneidman, Edwin. "Preventing Suicide." *American Journal of Nursing* 65 (May 1965): 111-116.

Shneidman, Edwin; Farberow, Norman; and Litman, Robert. *The Psychology of Suicide.* New York: Science House, 1970.

Ujhely, Gertrud B. "Grief and Depression: Implications for Preventive and Therapeutic Nursing Care." *Nursing Forum* 5, no. 2 (1966): 23-35.

Vollen, Karen, and Watson, Charles. "Suicide in Relation to Time of Day and Day of Week." *American Journal of Nursing* 75 (Feb. 1975): 263.

Westercamp, Twilla. "Suicide." *American Journal of Nursing* 75 (Feb. 1975): 260-262.

CHAPTER SEVEN

RETREAT AS A FORM OF COPING

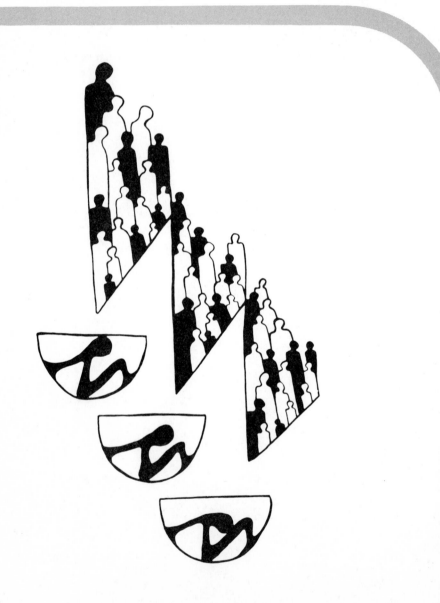

The repertoire of coping styles is almost endless. Retreat as a form of coping is another broad pattern which has a variety of forms. Although they have many points of difference, the patterns of behavior so categorized have in common the refutation in some way of the boundaries set by society. In this style of coping, the anxiety-managing behavior both allows and requires one (however one chooses to regard it) to ignore, or to refrain from incorporating as part of oneself, certain societal norms that most people have come to accept. For this person, these norms do not serve as the usual motivating force in shaping behavior.

To account for the development of a retreat pattern, let us once again consider our earlier model (page 000), which focused on the connection between anxiety and evolving behavior. We referred to a person in a situation that was anxiety-producing because it presented a problem that he or she was unable to resolve with ease. The satisfactory resolutions that most people eventually achieve under these circumstances entail their mastering the problem in such a way that they gain the approval of the significant others in their lives and are reinforced in their wish to adhere to the standards of these important people.

For instance, the child who incurs her mother's rather alarmed disapproval when she tries to stick a fork into a wall socket will experience a lot of anxiety. Typically, children learn to resolve situations like this so that they acquire the norm of leaving wall plugs alone. They may not notice wall sockets. They thus selectively ignore a stimulus that will get them into trouble; they may point to them and say, "No-no" or "That's for lamps," and thus indicate their incorporation of parental norms; they may go through any number of maneuvers, but the end point will look the same: the child does the socially accepted thing and regains the mother's approval. But the child who develops a pattern of retreat will solve this problem in such a way that she does not incorporate the notion of "don't touch the plug." She could do this in a number of ways, but essentially she is not incorporating the usual societal norms about avoiding wall plugs as mediated through her mother.

Usually the first pattern, the assumption of norms, happens because relationships with important people in the child's network provide sufficient structure; these relationships satisfy the child to the point that they become of key importance in mediating the culture. The important point to remember is that these relationships provide enough consistency, predictability, and emotional warmth that the child can attach himself or herself and be strongly influenced by them in all dealings with his or her environment.

The second pattern—not adhering to cultural norms—usually accompanies some difficulty with important people in the child's life. For whatever reason, relationships with these people have not provided sufficient staying power to command the child's entire loyalty and trust, and so they do not have as much positive influence in the child's acquisition of values. An obvious example is one in which parental figures have been absent or constantly changing during early periods of a child's life. In this situation, the child has not experienced enough predictable gratification to make it worthwhile to attempt to gain their approval by fitting into their version of the prevalent societal norms. In other cases, a child has not experienced enough emotional or affective responses from significant parental figures to make it seem worthwhile to seek their approval. In still other situations, the child receives contradictory responses to his or her behavior; affective responses come in such an inconsistent fashion that he or she cannot reliably predict what response to expect, and thus the child tends to withdraw from people rather than engage in behavior designed to gain their approval. In all these examples, the child is likely not to develop a consistent pattern of incorporating societal norms, for he or she cannot associate them with predictable rewards that would be a basis for adopting them. In fact, the child may come to feel that the norms are fraudulent and not to be trusted because of their contamination by his or her experiences with important people. In this sense, norms become a way to handle some of the difficulties with these people; if the child cannot directly defy people, he or she can defy the norm and thereby get back at them.

Viewing these types of maneuvers from the framework of coping styles, we may say that the child develops a pattern of changing the premises of the problem. Going through the usual problem-solving pattern does

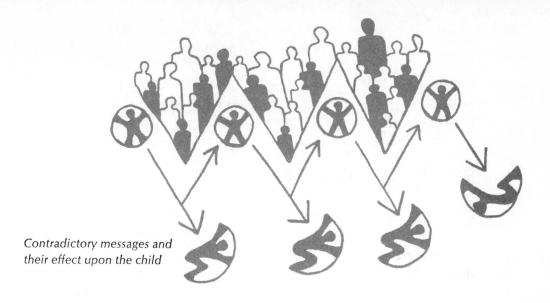

Contradictory messages and their effect upon the child

not yield the usual results because the child and his or her significant people fail to form the necessary matrix. The child then redefines the premises of the problem and either solves a different problem from the one he or she started with, or steps outside the problem and thus avoids anxiety. The child either has not experienced sufficient attachment to people to acquire their norms, or he or she actively rejects their norms as a way of protecting himself or herself from inconsistent and otherwise anxiety-provoking contact with them. Since the child does not care about the norms, he or she does not experience anxiety through violating them. In fact, the reverse is usually true, and the person experiences anxiety whenever her or she becomes tied into fitting into the norms, because this is associated with closeness to people and immediately becomes tied to the difficulties he or she has had in these types of relationships.

The pattern of difficulty with significant others associated with retreat from norms is commonly elaborated in one of two ways: it can take the form that leads to a schizophrenic style of life or it can follow patterns that many people consider less disruptive—deviant life styles. Deviant life styles themselves are varied, and the term applies to a range of people, from the quiet unassuming person who shares intimacy and sexuality with a companion of the same sex to a "Jack the Ripper" type. The common theme is that of people opting to step outside the usual societal norms. In this chapter we will attend primarily to schizophrenia, but will first discuss briefly other deviant life styles which fall into the framework of a basic pattern of retreat from usual societal norms.

DEVIANT LIFE STYLES

While the retreat typically seen in schizophrenia is massive in nature and results in severe distortions in the usual patterns of social interaction and thinking, the retreat characterizing certain deviant life styles is quite different in its origin and behavioral manifestations. Indeed, it sometimes seems more like a sidestepping of norms than a retreat from them.

How can we account for rule-breaking and the failure to accept usual societal standards as guides for behavior? People disposed to rule-breaking behavior have in many cases not experienced sufficient attachments to others to acquire their cultural norms; while in other instances they actively reject norms as a way of protecting themselves from inconsistent and otherwise anxiety-provoking contact with significant others. Children who experience inconsistent patterns of reaction from their parents, including considerable unpredictable anger and rage as well as unpredictable disinterest, are likely to develop maneuvers designed to protect themselves against too close involvement in such a relationship. Similarly, children who have experienced frequent separations from significant others develop protective maneuvers to defend against the feelings of abandonment. These protective maneuvers usually involve a failure to invest in other people.

In children, this may take a couple of forms, one being that the child appears as if he or she care for no one, another being that he or she appears to care for everyone too easily. The child who goes to anyone without any sign of discrimination between friend or stranger is an example of the latter. Children who have been bounced from foster home to foster home frequently appear as if they care for no one but themselves. People become identified as objects for them to use in gaining their own ends, whatever they may be. These patterns sometimes persist into adulthood and are carried on with minimal revisions. The Casanova male who seduces innumerable women, the charming psychopath who uses other people to achieve his or her ends, and the promiscuous woman are types of this form of relatedness. The connotation of "deviance" for these forms of behavior usually arises from the nature of the norm-breaking that occurs.

Persons socialized into these patterns of "deviant" behavior do not have the usual sense of norm-breaking because they have not become sufficiently attached and hooked into social relationships that it makes any difference to them if someone disapproves. Their point of reference is themselves and whatever provides them with satisfaction, even though temporary, rather than the responses of "significant others" and a longer range concern for maintaining these relationships. A further characteristic is that they see other people simply as objects to provide gratification for their immediate needs rather than becoming involved in any long-term obligations. Depending upon the particular norms the person tends to break, society may or may not get involved in the usual correctional processes. If the person violates norms that have to do with killing other people, most certainly there will be some type of societal response. In contrast, if a person chooses to set up a number of quasi-romantic involvements that he or she subsequently abandons, the abandoned person is frequently pitied, but relatively little is done to correct the "fickle" person. Occasionally one's status may even improve as a result of what could be termed "sociopathic" behavior. The financial tycoon who profiteers through breaking a few rules is generally admired for doing so.

Generally the forms of sociopathic behavior that we are aware of in our society are handled through the judicial system. Persons get into trouble because of lawbreaking behavior and, as a consequence, have to pay the usual societal penalties. Correction usually consists of locking them up, which does little to alleviate the basic problem. Occasionally, however, a person labeled as having a character disorder is admitted to a psychiatric hospital rather than jail, usually through a legal maneuver.

A few characteristics of persons who employ this form of deviant life style as a way of coping are worth noting in planning for any type of treatment. The time orientation of people so labeled is predominantly toward the present; the past is of little concern and the future is not considered. The absence of guilt for violation of norms is noticeable. Cause-and-effect relationships have little significance. As can be imagined, treatment is fraught with problems, the primary one being that persons so involved have little motivation for treatment. It is usually someone else involved with them who wishes them to receive treatment. Most situations in which treatment would ordinarily be given can be used only too well by such people for perpetuating the patterns that got them into trouble in the first place. For treatment to succeed, such a person would have to be placed into a situation where he or she would be forced to develop some attachments to people. There have been some reports of successful treatment in which people with this type of problem have been placed in a group living situation isolated from the usual amenities of society and in situations where they must depend upon one another for survival. Under this type of living situation, they are forced to develop new patterns of relatedness.

SCHIZOPHRENIC LIFE STYLES

Schizophrenia has long been considered a paramount problem in the field of mental health, since so many of the people residing in psychiatric facilities or treated as out-patients have, at one point or another, been diagnosed as schizophrenic. Beyond the diagnosis, however, controversey about the meaning of schizophrenia is rampant. People disagree about whether it is a disease entity, after the medical model, or a pattern of adjustment to difficult life situations, taking a more socio-psychological frame of reference. They also disagree about whether it is one discrete entity or a multiplicity of types of deviant behavior for which we have no appropriate name, lumped together under the rubric schizophrenia.

Since there is no agreement about what schizophrenia is, there is also no agreement about its causes. Some view schizophrenia as a physiological or genetic problem and seek causality in isolating particular biologic processes. Those with a psychological perspective look to early disruptions of relationships leading to a faulty ego structure as the underlying cause. Sociologists look not to the individual but to the society for an understanding of the forms of behavior which become identified as deviant. They trace causality to a societal structure to which the individual is responding, rather than to factors within the individual.

HISTORICAL OVERVIEW

The early theories about schizophrenia were primarily descriptive in nature; that is, the symptoms manifested by patients were simply de-

scribed and categorized into nosological entities. Kraepelin is usually cred-
ited with the first attempt to make a comprehensive list of the symptoms
and to develop a categorization of varying types of schizophrenia. He felt
that "dementia praecox" was one disease with many subtypes which was
attributable to some unknown metabolic disorder.[1] Whatever the differences might be among subtypes, they all started relatively early in the person's life and led to a more or less inevitable deterioration.

Eugene Bleuler, another early theorist, followed Kraepelin's model of
categorization and saw schizophrenia primarily as an organic problem, but
used psychological terms to describe the disease entity. In 1911 he coined
the term "schizophrenia" and described its basic manifestations as disturbances of thought and feeling. In coining the word schizophrenia, which
means "split personality," Bleuler called attention to the splitting of various psychic functions, which resulted in a lack of coherence in the patient's
personality but did not necessarily lead to dementia.

The next developmental step was that of advancing psychological explanations for the cause of schizophrenia. These explanations did not replace earlier views but provided alternatives that were found useful by
some theorists. These psychological explanations consider schizophrenia
as a reaction to a life situation, involving faulty or distorted mental functioning, which can be understood by studying the person's individual history. Adolf Meyer and Harry Stack Sullivan are examples of such theorists.
Although there are many differences between their theories, both focused
primarily on life patterns a person evolves over time and believed that the
key to treating schizophrenia was to alter these life patterns.

Although Freud commented on certain features of schizophrenic behavior, he did not get involved, to a great degree, in the treatment of
schizophrenia. The psychoanalytic theories that he formulated, however,
have been applied extensively to the problem of schizophrenia. Federn was
the first psychoanalyst to consider schizophrenia specifically as a disorder
characterized by weakness of the ego. It was common for the early psycho-
analysts to hold the view that because of ego deficits, schizophrenic patients
could not maintain a sufficiently stable relationship with a therapist to
allow for personality restructuring. These views have changed markedly

---

1. Frederick C. Redlich and Daniel X. Freedman, *The Theory and Practice of Psychiatry*
(New York: Basic Books, 1966), pp. 459-460.

since that time. Schizophrenia is now considered treatable on an intensive basis over a long period of time.[2]

Current views of schizophrenia build on these historical origins. The descriptive framework is still commonly used. An explanation is then sought for the origin and meaning of the symptoms so categorized, which the purely descriptive view did not incorporate.

The biological point of view focuses on altered physiological functioning as the primary cause of schizophrenia, though there is no consensus about organic factors underlying altered physiology. Treatment from the biological perspective involves correcting the person's organic functioning. The sociological view emphasizes the individual as a reactor to social forces that mold his or her behavior. Treatment within this context necessitates the restructuring of societal factors impinging on the individual. The most common characteristic of the psychological view is its emphasis on the psychic structure of the individual in accounting for behavioral events. Treatment from this perspective entails some alteration in psychic functioning.

DESCRIPTIVE VIEW OF SCHIZOPHRENIA

If one adopts a descriptive view of schizophrenia, one is likely to focus on certain aspects. In 1911, Bleuler labeled certain manifestations of schizophrenia as either *fundamental,* meaning basic symptoms that are present to some extent in every person with schizophrenia; or *accessory,* symptoms that may or may not occur commonly. A similar categorization of symptoms of schizophrenia is still recognized by most current theorists, although slightly different names and definitions may be attached to them, such as "primary" and "secondary." The primary or fundamental symptoms are considered to be the major flaws or areas of difficulty that schizophrenics have; they are felt to give rise to lesser or secondary symptoms. These primary symptoms are four in number, and generations of behavioral practitioners have learned the "4-A's"—association, autism, ambivalence, and affect.

---

2. Harold F. Searles, *Collected Papers on Schizophrenia and Other Related Subjects* (New York: International Universities Press, 1965).

ASSOCIATION AND AUTISM

Perhaps the central problem in schizophrenia is disturbance in association. This disturbance, involving the cognitive realm, means that the person's thoughts are not logically connected. All cultures teach their members how to think in a way that is shared by other members of the culture. There are rules about how ideas can be associated with one another, constituting the cultural definition of logic. It is quite usual for people identified as schizophrenic to fail to follow this logic in their thought processes and to make connections based on some private or symbolic meaning that is not readily apparent to an observer.

This disturbance in association, as well as some others, is considered by some to occur because of "regression." In the face of insurmountable stress or conflict, the person abandons his or her current mode of mature functioning, reverting to an infantile mode in which the rules are the unsocialized primitive, magical kinds of symbol manipulation that normally precede what we usually regard as thinking. This early symbol activity is called primary process thinking, and it gradually becomes transformed into a more mature rational process called secondary process thinking. Primary process thinking is never entirely eliminated. The most common example of its occurrence is probably the phenomenon of dreaming.

Others, such as Sullivan,[3] argue that the person subject to schizophrenia has never achieved a mature level of development from which to "regress." They feel that the person adopted a mode of behavior to gain the approval of significant others without truly mastering the developmental tasks involved. In the face of insurmountable anxiety, the façade crumbles, leaving a person who appears to have shifted from a higher level to a lower level of functioning. All agree about the primitive or immature, unsocialized nature of the schizophrenic person's thought processes, and it is generally felt that some of the content of these thoughts is related to experiences from the person's past which he or she has found anxiety-provoking and, therefore, has kept out of his or her conscious mind.

Autism is the other primary symptom (in addition to the disturbance in association) that involves the cognitive sphere of activity. Autism is

3. Harry Stack Sullivan, *Schizophrenia as a Human Process* (New York: W. W. Norton, 1962).

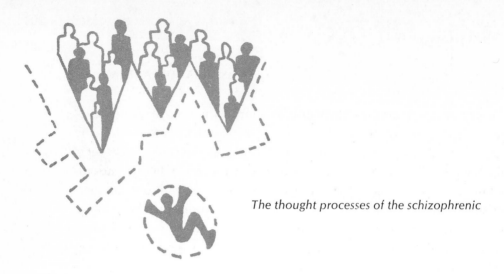

The thought processes of the schizophrenic

commonly used to refer to both the person's state of being, or feeling, and his or her cognitions. The term refers to the schizophrenic person's propensity to use his or her inner, private self as the only referent while moving through life in an unconnected way. Autistic thought, for instance, is entirely subjective and does not rest on the culturally shared meanings of symbols that one usually derives from connectedness with other people. As we have mentioned, much of the content of these thoughts originates within the person, with the unconscious mind usually thought of as a prolific source of stimulation.

Autism, referring to the person's state of being or feeling, as opposed to his or her cognitions, connotes an extreme preoccupation with the inner self and an accompanying withdrawal from external connections or interests, including people. The common instances in which people labeled schizophrenic seem to have no interest in eating, dressing themselves properly, or otherwise caring for themselves are usually attributed to autistic preoccupation with internal stimuli, fantasies, delusions, or hallucinations.

Delusions and hallucinations are examples of secondary or accessory symptoms related to the fundamental problems of association and autism. A hallucination is considered to be a false sensory perception without apparent basis in reality. Auditory hallucinations are the most common; that is, the person hears voices or other sounds. These voices frequently are threatening or hostile to the individual, but they may also be pleasant and comforting. Typically, hallucinations start out as unpleasant, as repressed thoughts and feelings are expressed through this medium, but over time they sometimes become incorporated into the thought processes as a pleasant and expected companion. Hallucinations occasionally affect the senses of vision, taste, smell, and touch. The presence of hallucinations can often be inferred, even though the person does not talk about them, from the fact that he or she seems to be attending to something other than the immediate surroundings, for example, apparently listening to someone talk.

Delusions are beliefs that are not culturally shared. The most common types of delusions are those of persecution, grandeur, and reference. Individuals with delusions of persecution believe falsely that they have been singled out for persecution. They may believe, for example, that someone is spying on them, plotting against them, or trying to harm them. Delusions of grandeur are the belief, again false, that one is an important person or has some special powers. For instance, one may identify oneself as an important political, military, or religious figure, or maintain that one has power to change or destroy the world. Delusions of reference mean the individual believes falsely that certain happenings relate to himself or herself; for example, that a television show relates to his or her personal life, or that a group of people are discussing him or her.

Delusions and hallucinations develop through the process of projection. Projection was defined earlier as a mechanism in which unacceptable thoughts and feelings are attributed to someone else rather than accepted as part of one's own personality. For example, hostile feelings toward others may be denied and repressed because of prior experiences which have led the person to conclude that any expression of anger is wrong or dangerous. The pent-up anger demands some relief, so it is attributed or projected onto others in the form of perceiving them as trying to harm him or her. One important thing to note about delusions, in particular, is the cyclic type of action-reaction that is set up, which serves to reinforce what becomes described as delusional behavior. In studies of persons considered to be delusional, it has been found that there usually is some reality base to their delusions. An example is the woman office worker who thinks others are talking about her. This may in fact start out as a true perception; but the person who senses gossip may tend to withdraw from the usual social networks of the office. This in turn leads to further talk about her peculiar behavior in the office. She becomes increasingly alienated from others and angry, leading to more projective thinking and further difficulty in relating to others.

Commonly, as a person increasingly fails in relationships to other people, he or she concentrates on internal processes rather than external relationships. As he or she does this, communication with others becomes disrupted, sometimes even to the extent of the person's developing a private language that has meaning only to himself or herself, combining several words into one (condensation), or inventing new words (neologisms). One of the frequent difficulties in working with those who are considered to be schizophrenic is that their speech does not follow the usual rules of logic and appears to be bizarre and disconnected. These patterns of speech are sometimes referred to as "word salad." A frequent response of those who become involved with patients who communicate in this manner is to take the position that it is impossible to understand them; and thus their connections with others are further severed. However, in many instances, as these people come to feel safe in a relationship, it is possible to explore with them the meanings of their communications and achieve understanding.

Other accessory or secondary symptoms related to the cognitive problems (which may or may not be present) are clang associations, in which words are strung together because of how they sound and not what they mean; and blocking, in which verbalizations come to an abrupt end, with the speaker seemingly unable to proceed.

AFFECT AND AMBIVALENCE

The disturbances of affect and ambivalence have more to do with feeling states than with anything else. A disturbance of affect means that the person experiences distortions in feeling responses. In schizophrenia, this distortion usually involves some blunting of emotion. The common term used to describe this phenomenon is "flattened affect." The person may be experiencing very strong feelings about something at the same time he or she looks totally unaffected. Another commonly used term is "inappropriate affect," which describes the lack of match between the person's affect and his or her thought processes, for example, a person who is thinking about the death of his mother but is smiling.

The important thing to note is that one cannot tell what a person is thinking or feeling from his or her obvious, observable behavior. Frequently we use our own standards of what is reasonable behavior to judge the behavior of others. When someone's behavior does not fit within these norms, we become uncomfortable. A frequent way of handling this discomfort is to ignore the "inappropriate" behavior, with the end result of cutting off communication and leaving the person in an increasingly alienated position.

Note the curious dilemma in the interaction between affect and autism; in a sense the cardinal symptoms of the patient flow from his or her inability to absorb and make his or her own the usual social and cultural forms of expression and meaning. Instead, he or she substitutes primary process unsocialized thinking. The people who try to communicate with him or her in the process of "helping" have absorbed the usual cultural norms. The "patient," who has adopted this form of communication, clings to it as a protective maneuver and a way to disguise his or her feelings and thoughts from others. From the patient's point of view, this is the only way to maintain distance and control. The "helpers," on the other hand, are in a position in which they must be able to shift from what they have incorporated as their socially approved reality to reach into the "patient's" world and learn a whole new set of ground rules. Frequently, instead of the "helper" reaching into the patient's world, they engage in power struggles with one another. The therapist is attempting to draw the "patient" into his or her world, while the "patient" tries to maintain himself or herself through a unique form of communication.

Coming to the last of the "four A's," ambivalence may be defined as the simultaneous presence of opposite feelings toward some person or goal. While these feelings are common to us all, they tend to become exaggerated in the "schizophrenic," and he or she does not incorporate or respond to them in an integrated fashion. Most of us are aware of having feelings of affection and anger toward the same person, such as a parent, but it does not become an overwhelmingly disruptive experience. People who are "schizophrenic" do not have as many bounds on the degree of feeling; not only are their feelings not integrated, but they are also extremely intense. On the one hand, a person may idealize his mother as a saint, and on the other, despise her as a devil. These strong and contradictory feelings toward the same person frequently tend to immobilize the person so that he or she becomes frozen in expressing any feeling at all. He or she has strong and compelling needs to be close to others, but equally strong fears of the dangers inherent in closeness. He or she may fear being engulfed or destroyed by the others.

Another problem of people labeled schizophrenic is some variable level of difficulty in discriminating the exact boundaries between their own selves and anyone or anything else, a problem commonly referred to as "poor" or "inadequate" ego boundaries. This difficulty, related to the primary symptoms just discussed, represents a major developmental failure, since the process of differentiating between oneself and others should be well underway before the infancy period of development is over. This lack of differentiation frequently interferes with accurate communication, particularly with people who become closely involved with the "schizophrenic" person. Both parties to an interaction may be using pronouns that actually mean different things to them without knowing about that difference. "We" to the nurse may mean "Mrs. Brown to whom I am talking and me," but to the person with ill-defined ego boundaries, it may signify "This nurse, God, my mother, me, the six other people I see out of the corner of my eye, and the dead butterfly on the window sill." The example may sound exaggerated, but confusion of this order does exist. This confusion is heightened by the lack of stability and predictability of the boundaries. They are not simply faulty but unstable, in contrast to delusions, and may vary from situation to situation. A common manifestation of this difficulty can sometimes be seen in the interaction of the family of a schizophrenic person, in which one person may answer a question directed to another or report a feeling belonging to another without consulting the other, as though there were no difference between himself, or herself and that person.

Many people with a schizophrenic coping style experience the feeling of depersonalization, though this phenomenon is not limited to schizophrenia. It can accompany severe anxiety states and is sometimes frightening to the anxious person, who may incorrectly view it as confirmation that he or she is "going crazy." Depersonalization is experienced subjectively as a state of being isolated or removed from the reality surrounding oneself. The reality is experienced as strange and alien and not truly connected to oneself. Common descriptions are "like watching a movie," or "I was watching myself go through the motions," or "My kitchen didn't seem real to me." Many theorists consider that depersonalization serves a defensive function, in that it is a distancing maneuver undertaken as a means of avoiding intolerable anxiety. People who are "schizophrenic" sometimes experience this phenomenon about parts or all of their own bodies. In this instance, the connection between defective ego boundaries and depersonalization is quite clear.

TYPES OF SCHIZOPHRENIA

In addition to identifying major characteristics of schizophrenic behavior, numerous attempts have also been made to classify varying forms of the "disease" entity. One differentiation is according to whether the onset appears to be in reaction to a specific event or is more insidious, manifested through an overall "disease" process. A second way of classifying schizophrenia is by whether it is an acute episode or a chronic process. Schizophrenia is further divided into diagnostic categories of simple, paranoid, hebephrenic, catatonic, schizoaffective, and undifferentiated. The usefulness of these designations applied to a given patient is that

Acute and chronic schizophrenia

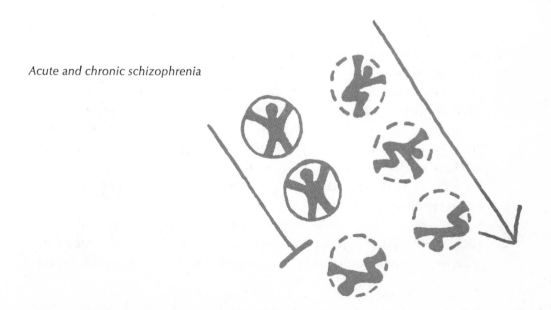

they indicate some information about the major manifestations of his or her "illness" at that particular time, about the onset, and the expected response to treatment.

It is important to note how categorization functions in respect to schizophrenia. It is commonly noted that the tendency to categorize arises out of ambiguous situations. For instance, in state hospitals where there are a large number of persons defined as schizophrenic, diagnosticians are inclined to devote considerable effort to categorize types of schizophrenia. Although this occupies considerable time, there is little agreement between diagnosticians; in fact, some studies report as low as 20 percent agreement.[4] It may be conjectured that expending considerable time and energy in the diagnostic process is an attempt to bring some organization and predictability for the therapist into viewing schizophrenic behavior; insofar as relating to the schizophrenic "patient," these categories have little use. However, since much of the language of those who work within psychiatric hospitals uses these descriptive labels, it is important for the nurse to understand what they attempt to communicate.

The *reactive/process* distinction refers to the onset of the disturbed behavior and the probable response to treatment, or prognosis. *Reactive* schizophrenia supposedly develops suddenly as the result of acute stress in individuals whose coping styles were such that they appeared to be functioning in a relatively healthy manner. That is, they were able to fit into the usual societal definitions of acceptable behavior. Because of their prior patterns, it is suspected that after a brief period of disorganization they will return to their usual coping patterns and once again "fit in." *Process* schizophrenia has a more insidious onset. The person was probably always considered to be a little peculiar. Since this has been his or her usual pattern, it is not likely that this person will ever be "normal" as defined within our culture. The *acute/chronic* differentiation means almost the same thing, with acute being equivalent to reactive and chronic to process.

Simple schizophrenia is characterized by apathy, flat effect, withdrawal from social relationships, and associative looseness. There are none of the more flamboyant symptoms of other forms of schizophrenia, and the per-

---

4. R. Arnoff, "Some Factors Influencing the Unreliability of Clinical Judgments," *Journal of Clinical Psychology* 10 (1954).

son appears to be a "born loser," one who has never quite made it all the way along. Delusions and hallucinations are not apparent.

Paranoid schizophrenia. The main distinguishing feature of paranoid schizophrenia is the presence of delusions of persecution or grandeur. As might be expected, the person is hostile and suspicious in relations with others and shows some of the primary symptoms of schizophrenia. People who have a well-defined set of delusions but are otherwise in good contact with reality (meaning that when their delusions are not involved, they appear as normal as anyone else) are sometimes categorized under "paranoia" instead of paranoid schizophrenia.

Hebephrenic schizophrenia. The hebephrenic type is characterized by "early onset, massive disturbance of behavior that is clearly regressed, fragmented, and silly."[5] This type is generally considered the "end of the line" in the sense that the regression is pronounced and the level of functioning is limited. The prognosis is poor.

Catatonic schizophrenia is divided into two subtypes—catatonic stupor and catatonic excitement. Stupor is characterized by extreme withdrawal and hypokinetic symptoms, sometimes to the point of complete immobility. In contrast, catatonic excitement is characterized by extreme overactivity and lability. In such a state the person may become destructive and assaultive.

Schizoaffective schizophrenia. Schizoaffective disorders have a pronounced mood component of elation or depression in addition to the basic thought disorders of schizophrenia.

Undifferentiated schizophrenia means that the person's behavior does not fit into any of the above classifications, though he or she has a thought disorder and poor interpersonal relationships.

Descriptive theorists hold that the same person usually shows symptoms characteristic of more than one of these types in the course of his or her illness, usually progressing through a catatonic state to some form of paranoid manifestation. The hebephrenic form is usually manifested rather late in the sequence. There are marked differences in the way people proceed through these stages; some move through certain ones in a very transitory manner, while others tend to become fixated at a particular point, such as a paranoid state, without moving to other states.

---

5. Redlich and Freedman, *Theory and Practice of Psychiatry,* p. 479.

THEORIES ABOUT THE ORIGIN OF SCHIZOPHRENIA

BIOLOGICAL THEORIES

A considerable amount of biological research has been directed toward the identification of genetic factors that might relate to the development of schizophrenia. Researchers have noted that there is a greater likelihood for a person to become schizophrenic if one parent has been schizophrenic. Other studies have identified a greater incidence of schizophrenia in monozygotic twins. Although these studies seem to indicate that there are genetic factors related to schizophrenia, researchers as yet have been unable to identify specific factors and have no idea of how this influence works across generations. These problems are further compounded by the lack of certainty about the nature of schizophrenia and by the implication of other factors in the development of the schizophrenic process. Kallmann's studies done through the 1930s, 1940s, and 1950s clearly demonstrate the strongest evidence in support of the genetic position.[6] Two of the problems geneticists struggle with are (1) if there is a factor, how is it transmitted; and (2) granted a genetic factor, how can one discriminate between it and the contamination of psychological and societal overlays?

There have been many approaches toward the study of physiological or biochemical factors that may be implicated in schizophrenia.[7] Metabolism studies have been done on amino acids, tryptophane, and epinephrine, to mention but a few. Anomalies in carbohydrate metabolism are more prevalent in schizophrenic populations than in normal groups, and it is hypothesized that this factor may leave the person with less energy to respond to stress. A considerable amount of research has been directed toward the neurological system and brain processes. Attempts have been made to identify either the presence of some factor that should not be there, or the absence of a factor that should be present. Neurological studies attempt to account for failures to process experiences in an accurate way. The enzyme serotonin is frequently identified as important to study. Serotonin is an enzyme in the brain that acts as a catalyst; it was first no-

---

6. David Rosenthal, "Genetic Research in the Schizophrenic Syndrome," in *The Schizophrenic Reactions*, ed. Robert Concro (New York: Bruner/Mazel Publishers, 1970), pp. 45-47.

7. Redlich and Freedman, *Theory and Practice of Psychiatry*, p. 491.

ticed when researchers discovered that hallucinogens, such as LSD, blocked its effects. Heath and his coworkers have carried out a number of studies to determine the effect of taraxein, a protein substance isolated from the blood of schizophrenics which is not found in nonschizophrenic individuals. In one study, when taraxein was injected into normal volunteers, they developed temporary schizophrenic symptoms. Rosenbaum, however, points out the methodological weakness of studies such as these and stresses the need for replication.[8]

The big problem with such physiological studies is that, though varying substances have been noted in certain schizophrenic conditions, it can be argued that the symptoms of schizophrenia could alter the physiology, rather than altered physiology being the cause of schizophrenia.

Recent biological research has taken a new direction. As an offshoot of the interest in biofeedback, it has been noted that the galvanic skin responses of schizophrenic patients differ from those of a normal population in that they have a diminished response to external stimuli. It is as if the person with little skin reactivity does not deal adequately with the input of outside stimuli and is therefore more likely to respond in a schizophrenic fashion. Biofeedback then becomes a part of the treatment, to help the person identify more clearly the things that make him or her anxious, and thereby build up protective mechanisms.[9]

Although physiological research to date has been generally inconclusive, a large number of the treatment approaches focus on altering some biological aspect of the schizophrenic. Medications and shock therapies are directed toward altering neurological functioning, thereby cutting down on some of the more troublesome symptoms of schizophrenia. Psychosurgery is based on a claim that certain mental illness, behavior disorders, and emotional disturbances can be cured by destroying particular portions of the brain. Considerable controversy surrounds the use of psychosurgery, with those who are for such an approach pointing to the possibility of dramatically altering behavior. Those who oppose its use raise the issues of side effects and of the moral and ethical ramifications of using such an approach to alter behavior.

---

8. C. Peter Rosenbaum, *The Meaning of Madness* (New York: Science House, 1970), pp. 189-200.
9. Marvin Karlins and Lewis M. Andrews, *Biofeedback: Turning on the Power of Your Mind* (Philadelphia: J. B. Lippincott, 1972).

■ *The Need-Fear Dilemma.*   One psychological view that attempts to explain both the developmental and the functional aspects of schizophrenia is presented by Burnham et al., who view schizophrenics as being particularly plagued by what they term a "need-fear" dilemma.[10] Because of faulty ego development, these people have inordinate needs for others with whom they can be close and who will perform some of the ego functions they lack. At the same time, they have just as strong fears about the dire consequences of getting into these relationships. These authors argue that as a child begins life within a family situation, he or she uses the ties with parents in the first stage of development to complete some fundamental ego-development tasks. First, the child has to differentiate himself or herself from his or her surroundings, a task that requires a clear sense of his or her own identity. This involves the capacity to distinguish inner from outer events and the symbolic structuring of reality.[11] The second aspect of this differentiation is that of inner organization, so that he or she can be discriminating and specific about feelings, instead of having massive generalized states. The first phase of differentiation occurs as the child distinguishes aspects of the external world and separates himself or herself from his or her environment. Internal structure becomes differentiated in that the child grows from having the global responses to stimuli, commonly seen in newborns, to having very specific responses. This differentiation contributes to a clear sense of personal identity and a separateness from the people and things within his or her environment.

A related task is integration. "Integration is the process by which differentiated parts or functions are brought together into a coherently articulated and harmoniously functioning whole. Differentiation and integration are related in that with differentiation into specialized parts there can be no integration of parts into a whole."[12] Difficulty or inability in differentiating or integrating results in a poor capacity for autonomy, an inability to form reliable representations of reality, and "a central system of control

---

10. Donald L. Burnham, Arthur I. Gladston, and Robert W. Gibson, *Schizophrenia and the Need-Fear Dilemma* (New York: International Universities Press, 1969).
11. Ibid., p. 19.
12. Ibid., p. 19.

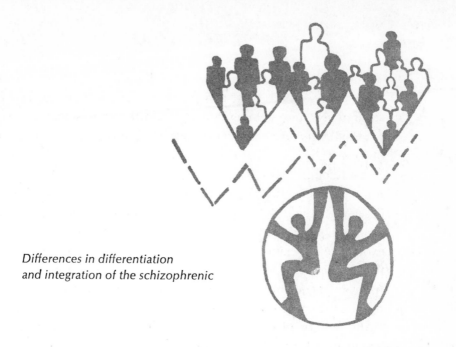

*Differences in differentiation
and integration of the schizophrenic*

and personality organization (ego) which is so weak and easily disorganized as to limit the ability to aim and focus behavior purposefully."[13]

It is as though the infant needs to acquire a blueprint for categorizing his or her experiences and for directing behavior toward useful goals. To acquire this blueprint he or she needs a very stable, secure relationship with parenting figures who, through the external structuring of the child's experience and consistency, facilitate his or her capacities for developing internal structure. If a person does not develop an autonomous, integrated personality, he or she is highly vulnerable to disorganization. People who are prone to schizophrenia have such poorly developed abilities. They become easily upset and, once upset, they lack the necessary balancing mechanisms to get back on an even keel.

As we have noted, persons experience crises when they encounter problems for which their usual problem-solving mechanisms no longer work. The person with poorly developed capacities for autonomy and integration will have a problem-solving style that reflects this lack of internal

13. Ibid., p. 16.

organization. As Burnham and his colleagues point out, this person "has both an inordinate need and an inordinate fear of objects. His lack of separateness and self-regulatory structure renders him dependent upon external structure and extraordinarily susceptible to the influence of objects."[14]

In coping with their problems, such persons frequently get into a number of difficulties in an attempt to solve the need-fear dilemma. Those beset with these difficulties in relationships try, in some cases, to avoid objects as a way of avoiding the fear attached to these relationships. Their avoidance may take the form of silent withdrawal or verbal assaults upon people. However, they will very soon run into the difficulty that comes from having no one who can assist them in their internal structuring, a function they are unable to manage by themselves. An alternative to avoidance is the pattern of clinging to objects that may substitute for persons to whom an individual fears getting close. The use of substitutes is a compromise maneuver aimed at solving the need-fear dilemma. The substitute objects a person might cling to are such things as pets, books, or treasured personal effects. They may also be abstractions such as political causes or social or religious ideologies. The person may also cling to stereotyped words and phrases. In some instances the person's own body may be treated as a substitute object.[15] The person treats these substitute objects as he or she relates to people, at times clinging to them, at times denying dependence on them by discarding or destroying them.

A third maneuver sometimes employed is the redefinition of significant objects. Usually people develop a rather constant view of others, unrelated to their dominant feelings at the moment or to the person's presence or absence. In the person who has not developed this constancy,

> . . . his perception of the object changes according to the feeling of the moment. If love and need predominate, the object appears good, desirable and approachable; if fear and hate, the object appears noxious and only to be avoided or destroyed. He may even perceive the object's entire identity as having changed from one time to another, and tends to attribute these changes to unreliability of the object rather than to instability within himself.[16]

---

14. Ibid., pp. 31-32.
15. Ibid., pp. 35-36.
16. Ibid., p. 37.

This changeability makes for lack of stability and constancy in so-cial relationships which again serves to compound the person's problem. Sometimes redefinition of objects takes the form of idealizing certain people and vilifying others. The degree to which any of these solutions work is a tenuous matter at best, since the person is likely to re-experience disequilibrium. The disequilibrium will be attributed to the substitute objects, which will then be viewed as unpredictable, and the persons will have to again reshuffle his or her relationship.

FAMILY THEORIES

Much of what we have been describing takes place within a family con-text and therefore has been either wittingly or unwittingly supported. The effects of some patterns of early child-rearing are so detrimental as to raise the question of why parents allow such distortions to occur. Per-sons who work in facilities that treat schizophrenics commonly have had such difficult experiences in their contacts with families, particularly mothers, that they often wind up with very derogating views of them. The predominant view is that the interaction between their schizophrenic charges and family members, particularly mothers, is so damaging that continuance of the relationship is equivalent to continued schizophrenia. Some treatment programs go so far as to sever all family ties, hoping that the person will form new relationships and thus relearn in a more posi-tive manner the early lessons that were so mismanaged in his or her family or origin. In any event, the family is often seen as an adversary in the treatment process.

The other approach, based on the same premise, is that the schizo-phrenic person cannot be treated apart from his or her family. A number of family studies provide some data on certain features of families in which there is an identified schizophrenic member. Most of the writers on this subject have described families that, because of the parents' personalities, are grossly deficient in one way or another in providing the kind of devel-opmental matrix that children require to achieve the personality growth we have just described. These writers have noted that, basically, the parents are unable to view their children as independent persons in their own right, but instead relate to them so that they will undo or make up some of the parents' own deficiencies or unmet needs.

■ *Skewed and Schismatic Family Configurations.* Lidz et al., in a study of seventeen families of schizophrenic patients, described the families as belonging to one of two major types of distorted family patterns— skewed or schismatic.

> In the skewed family the focus of attention is apt to fall upon the mother who is called "schizophrenogenic," a mother who is impervious to the needs of other family members as separate individuals and is extremely intrusive into their child's life. Yet, the very poor model the father provides his son and his inability to counter the mother's aberrant ways in rearing the children are also critical. Although the mother has serious difficulties in being close and maternal to her son when an infant, she soon becomes overprotective, unable to feel that the child can even exist without her constant concern and supervision.[17]

The family pattern is thus one in which the mother is over invested in her son as a fulfillment of things she feels have been denied her, while the father is withdrawn from involvement in the relationship; it is as though the father has abandoned the son to this intense relationship with the mother. In this type of relationship, the mother opposes any move toward autonomy by the son. She cannot mediate between the infant and his environment as the infant attempts to form some reliable notions of what he himself is like and of what that environment is like. Her own wishes and fantasies, in which the infant son plays a major role, keep interfering with an accurate perception of reality. Families of these types may be viewed as somewhat different within the community context, but usually only when the offspring set forth into the larger environment is social attention brought to bear on the family because of the child's strange behavior. It is mainly from these types of families that male schizophrenics emerge.

In contrast, schismatic family paterns are more closely related to the development of schizophrenia in females.

> The schismatic family is characterized by continuing overt conflict between the spouses with each undercutting the worth of the other to their children, and usually competing for the loyalty of the children. The mother not only has little self-esteem as a woman and is insecure as a mother, but her position and value as a wife and mother are constantly undermined by her husband's contempt and derogation of her.

---

17. Theodore Lidz, *The Origin and Treatment of Schizophrenic Disorders* (New York: Basic Books, 1973), p. 31.

Although the mother usually struggles against her husband, she cannot hold her ground against a man who may be overtly paranoid. Markedly insecure in their masculinity, these men need to have their narcissism bolstered by constant admiration. Many marry passive women whom they believe will docilely cater to their wishes, but find themselves tied to women who need support from a husband to be able to function adequately. Poorly organized, the mother usually conveys a feeling of the meaninglessness or the hopelessness of life and cannot provide her daughter with any maternal warmth.[18]

The daughter in this type of relationship becomes caught up in the problems of her parents. The mother's insecurity is particularly pronounced as the daughter moves into adolescence and thereby becomes increasingly threatening to the mother's own self-definitions. The father's need for approbation and admiration extends to the daughter, and it is difficult for her to work through certain aspects of development dealing with sexuality.

We can see that in these patterns almost every level of development from infancy on would be accompanied by problems. The child does not have a stable environment on which he or she can depend to develop trusting relationships. He or she learns not to trust his or her own perceptions and abilities and relies on others' definitions, but even these definitions will be problematic. The push toward autonomy in this type of family structure is seriously hampered. The parents have strong needs for the children to accept their definitions, and seriously interfere with the children's becoming autonomous beings in their own right. The children retain a distorted view of the power of the parents. Such a view presents particular difficulty as the child moves into the Oedipal stage. Not only are the parents perceived as overly powerful, but the child is unable to achieve a realistic identification with the parent of the same sex, which is the usual basis for the final resolution of the conflicts of this stage. With this shaky foundation, the child has difficulty making subsequent transitions that would lead him or her to becoming a person in his or her own right.

▪ *Pseudomutuality.* Other family theorists have focused on similar types of themes within the families of schizophrenic persons. Lyman Wynne and his colleagues have described the suppression of communicative exchanges that leads to problems of differentiation of family members.

---

18. Ibid., p. 43.

The differentiation of a personal identity or distinct individuality on the part of a family member was considered impossible in such families because of the consistent use of interpersonal techniques by members that prohibited or strongly sanctioned the articulation of such individuality or personal independence within any interactional episode.[19]

These families demonstrated communication patterns characterized by what Wynne et al. describe as pseudomutuality; that is, all areas of disagreement or potential conflict were masked so that families appeared, on the surface, to epitomize all the stereotypes of the "happy" family. This appearance was maintained at the expense of individual members achieving individuation.

■ *Double-bind communication.* Another approach used in studying families is that developed by Bateson, in which he focused on particular characterizations of communication in families with a schizophrenic member. Bateson and his colleagues propose a double-bind theory of communication as characteristic of these family networks.

> The necessary ingredients for a pathogenic double-bind situation were seen to be (1) two or more people, (2) repeated experience, (3) primary negative injunction enforced with threats of sanction, (4) secondary injunction conflicting with the first at a more abstract level and accompanied, like the first, with signals threatening survival, (5) a tertiary injunction prohibiting escape from the intercommunicative field, and finally (6) the stage is attained in which the victim perceives his universe of social relations in double-bind patterns, and the entire interactional ingredients are no longer necessary.[20]

The main feature of double-bind situations is that the person perceives conflicting messages being sent to which he or she must respond or suffer severe consequences. He or she cannot escape from the situation, and the person sending the messages is of great significance. Faced with these incongruencies, the person becomes very skilled in sending double-bind messages to others and thus engages others in the same communicative pattern.

Being adept at this form of communication, the schizophrenic patient

19. Lyman Wynne et al., "Pseudomutuality in the Family Relations of Schizophrenics," *Psychiatry, Journal for the Study of Interpersonal Processes* 21 (1958): 2-5-220. Quoted in Jeff Coulter, *Approaches to Insanity* (New York: John Wiley & Sons, 1974), p. 44.
20. G. Bateson et al., "Toward a Theory of Schizophrenia," *Behavioral Science* 1 (1956): 251-264. Quoted in Coulter, *Approaches to Insanity,* p. 48.

Pseudomutuality

is quite capable of placing staff into double-bind positions, something they frequently do not see at first. In fact, the difficulty in dealing with persons who respond through a schizophrenic mechanism is the reciprocal nature of the interactions that quickly become established. Caught in the need-fear dilemma, the patient, in attempts to preserve himself or herself engages in the same maneuvers that he or she used in the past. Frequently the person engaging in these maneuvers establishes the same type of relationship with the hospital that he or she is familiar with in the family network. In fact, one of the arguments raised in response to family studies is that of causality: which comes first, the family network that produces the schizophrenia, or the behavior of the person whose ways of coping create social networks like those seen in families of schizophrenics? In any event, the patterns of action-reaction that are established in networks surrounding the person identified as schizophrenic serve to reinforce this particular pattern of coping.

SOCIOLOGICAL THEORIES

In contrast to psychological theories which look to the origins of schizophrenic behavior in the individual's structuring experiences, sociological theories look outside the individual to factors within society that are considered to be causally implicated. Three general categories of theories look to societal factors as of prime importance: (1) epidemiological studies, (2) symbolic interaction and labeling theories, and (3) existential philosophical explanations.

▪ *Epidemiological Approaches.* Epidemiological studies, unlike other sociological theories, accept the incidence of schizophrenia as a given. Studies conducted from this perspective attempt to identify ecological relationships that might have etiological significance. By counting the number of schizophrenics within certain geographic areas, it is possible to identify areas where the incidence is high. Epidemiologists then attempt to identify social and cultural factors in specific areas that might contribute to this increased incidence of mental disorder. The criticism of studies [21] done from this perspective centers on the issue that the number of persons identified as schizophrenic in a community may not be a true indicator. This figure may reflect the readiness of family and community to extrude those who are identified as troublesome, whereas other groups might tend to be more protective and encapsulate deviance among community and family members.

▪ *Symbolic Interaction and Labeling Theories.* Some research related to schizophrenia has been based upon the theoretical foundations laid by George Herbert Mead; Herbert Blumer called this approach "symbolic interactionism." One theory emerging from this perspective closely relates to some of the family studies. It holds that a person's conception of "self" arise from a series of complex interactions with significant others. One achieves a definition of self through an intricate process of acting, seeing others respond to one's performance, trying out new behaviors, watching others' responses, and eventually imagining, or carrying on a dialogue with oneself about expected responses to certain forms of behavior. Now it is easy to see how an individual employing this perspective, who does not receive consistent and predictable responses, may have difficulties in developing a clearly delineated concept of "self." Bannister[22] has suggested that thought disorders of schizophrenic patients are the end result of a certain mode of socialization in which they are exposed to serial invalidations of themselves as persons. Employing this frame of reference, the focus is on identifying societal factors that are implicated in the development of schizophrenic behavior.

---

21. A. B. Hollingshead and F. C. Redlich, *Social Class and Mental Illness* (New York: Hafner, 1960); R. Faris and H. W. Dunham, *Mental Disorders in Urban Areas* (New York: Hafner, 1960); J. A. Clausen and M. L. Kohn, "The Ecological Approach in Social Psychiatry," *American Journal of Sociology* 40 (1954): 140-149.
22. D. Bannister, "The Genesis of Schizophrenic Thought-Disorder: Retest of the Serial Invalidation Hypothesis," *British Journal of Psychiatry* 111 (1965): 377-381.

A second perspective growing out of symbolic interactionism relates to the societal reaction to deviance. These are generally referred to as labeling theories. Edwin Lemert, the pioneer of this view, suggested that many symptoms may be an outgrowth of a societal reaction. From this point of view, a person for some reason becomes identified as deviant, and from this time, his or her set of interactions is based on this definition. "A person begins to employ his deviant behavior or a role based on it as a means of defense, attack, or adjustment to the overt and covert problems created by the consequent societal reaction."[23] Lemert's original work was based on observations of paranoid persons in whom he observed the processes of exclusion and reinforcement described earlier in this chapter.

Becker, building upon Lemert's earlier work, points out that a person's identity frequently becomes constructed around a particular deviant label; a person labeled deviant will tend to play out the expected deviant role.[24] From this point of view, becoming a mental patient is a socially constructed role and not a result of a disease or illness process. Scheff, carrying this argument further, considers mental illness to consist of residual forms of deviance for which we have no other name.[25] Persons labeled as deviant have broken certain societal rules. Once identified as deviant, they tend to play out these roles. A frequent criticism of these points of view centers on the lack of explanation for why persons initially engage in rule-breaking behavior. Nonetheless, in these arguments, as in the psychological ones, the effects of reinforcement and of action-reaction between the individual and those who compose his or her social networks are common features.

■ *Existentialist Views.* Although not sociological theorists per se, R. D. Laing and his associates view society as the prime causal factor in the etiology of schizophrenia. Working from an existential, philosophical frame of reference, they argue that a schizophrenic life style is the only rational way to live, given the irrationalities of our society. Their original work, based on extensive observations of families of schizophrenics, advances the argument that the behavior of the person identified as psychotic is perfectly understandable within the context of his or her family net-

---

23. Edwin M. Lemert, *Social Pathology* (New York: McGraw Hill, 1951).
24. Howard S. Becker, *Outsiders* (New York: Free Press of Glencoe, 1963).
25. Thomas Scheff, *Being Mentally Ill: A Sociological Theory* (Chicago: Aldine Publishing Co., 1966).

work. The schizophrenic experience is viewed as an inner voyage to self-discovery, a breaking loose from the constriction placed on the individual within society as mediated by the family.[26] Employing this perspective, the therapist, instead of attempting to intervene in the psychotic process, is expected to facilitate this internal exploration. In contrast to the persons who are involved in a schizophrenic experience, all others are considered to be engaged in lives that are basically caricatures: people playing stereotypic roles rather than relating to others on significant interpersonal levels.

One of the criticisms leveled against sociological theories, particularly by those oriented toward more psychological explanations, is of the interpretation of hallucinations and delusions. For those who have worked with those labeled "schizophrenic" and have become involved in trying to communicate about their delusions and hallucinations, the presence of these factors seems a very real and pervasive aspect of the person's personality. Those who advance sociological explanations, however, argue that delusions and hallucinations are perfectly understandable phenomena. Some argue that we all experience some form of hallucinatory experiences, although we do not commonly recognize them. In essence, the sociologists contend that whether or not one has hallucinations or delusions is solely a function of the norms of one's reference group. Wherever people are identified as having hallucinations, careful study reveals that such behavior is normative in the group to which the person feels most closely tied. These theorists go so far as to point out that many things that are considered nondelusional and social or cultural artifacts, such as belief in God, could just as easily be considered delusions. They are not so conceived because there is majority agreement about them.

Evidence for this position is garnered chiefly from commonplace observations, some from a historical perspective, others from a cross-cultural view, and still others based on current practices in certain segments of our society. Szasz advances the argument that much of what is now encompassed under the rubric of mental illness was in another time and place construed to be a form of demon possession. Witches and witchcraft were the equivalents of therapists and psychotherapy. Disordered behavior was frequently viewed from a religious perspective.[27]

---

26. R. D. Laing and A. Esterson, *Sanity, Madness, and the Family, vol. 1, Families of Schizophrenics* (New York: Basic Books, 1964).
27. Thomas Szasz, *The Manufacture of Madness* (New York: Harper & Row, 1970).

Anthropologists have made extensive observations about practices in other cultures that, were they carried forth in ours, would be construed to be evidence of mental disturbance. For example, the Haitian voodoo leader who communicates with the dead would most likely be viewed as slightly "mad" within the context of American society. Similarly, methods for dealing with evil spirits in other cultures may, in many ways, be equated with some of our forms of psychotherapy. In some African cultures, the person who is demon-possessed is taken to a remote area by the witch doctor, and over an intensive two- or three-day period of time, the evil spirits are cast out. On closer examination, the methods employed by the witch doctor, although based on cultural practices, in many aspects parallel some of our treatment practices. The important difference to note is that persons who have been purged of the demons that possess them return to the tribe after a period of time, whereas in our pattern persons are sent to mental hospitals, frequently never to return to the same position within their social networks. The label "mental patient" in our society carries with it the connotation of irreversibility; the person's subsequent interactions with others, either in the family or in a work setting, are muted for fear that he or she will have another "nervous breakdown," which usually implies some associated fear that the person will go out of control and be dangerous. Similar connotations do not hold in other cultures, and one may only question whether persons have "relapses" because they are expected to. In our society, people tend to relate to the person who has been labeled "mentally ill" primarily on the basis of his or her identity as a former patient.

A final observation relates to some common practices within our own culture that, within another context, are not considered to be evidence of mental illness. For example, speaking in tongues, seeing visions, and praying to God are accepted practices in certain religious groups in this country. This same behavior, outside the restricted context of certain churches or with people who are unfamiliar with its religious basis, is apt to result in the person's being identified as mentally ill.

Taking all these points of view into consideration, it is reasonable to conclude that "schizophrenia," whatever it may be—a physical disease entity, a result of inadequate psychological structuring, or a creation of society—poses a great dilemma within our society. In reviewing the literature, we are struck by its volume and by the lack of research support for any of the theoretical positions. It is difficult to relate some of these abstract views to the real dilemma of being schizophrenic, both for the person and for those to whom he or she relates.

CASE STUDY

Consider Girard, a nineteen-year-old eldest son, with a sixteen-year-old sister and a brother of thirteen. His parents are of European origin, both sets of grandparents having come from Europe. The father is of Italian descent, the mother, French. Girard's father, Guy, is manager of a hardware store. Guy's father ran a fruit market, and his family had wanted Guy to go to college so that he would not have to work in a store like his father. He was a freshman in college when he met Anna, Girard's mother. Although Guy followed his parents' wishes in going to college, he found it boring and was unable to manage the work. He stayed in college, though, not wanting to become like his Uncle Gino, who was considered the family black sheep. Uncle Gino had never succeeded in any task he undertook, was considered "queer," and was institutionalized for mental illness by the time he was twenty-five.

Anna was the youngest member of her family, an only daughter with two older brothers who she felt were given all the advantages and thought much more worthwhile by both parents. Anna's father considered himself to be an inventor, always tinkering around, but never quite hitting on any acceptable invention. He claimed to come by the talent naturally, since his grandfather was a tinkerer. He resented his wife's reminders that an eccentric recluse like his grandfather was hardly a good model. To support the family he took odd jobs, but never worked for an extensive period of time with one company. The family did not talk about the times when Anna's father took janitorial positions, which he was frequently forced to do to support them. Anna's mother continually nagged the father to make something of his life, dreaming of the day when he would hit upon his great invention and they would be able to advance in the social hierarchy. Anna's mother always perceived herself to be somewhat better than her father. This myth was kept alive in the family by her talk of a great-great uncle who had been a count and therefore of "royal" blood.

The all-pervasive theme underlying most of their family interactions was "quality doesn't always win out." Anna's mother had given up on her father, sensing that he would probably never really make it, and turned her attention to the children. Anna's brothers were pushed to go to college and become something, while the expectation for Anna was that she would marry well. The tragedy of Anna's young life was her feeling that the only way to get her mother's attention was to be a man; faced with this situation, her only alternative was to find a man who would meet her mother's standards. For Anna to develop a self-identity that would be of worth in and of itself was never a possibility; the only path open for her was to live in the shadow of a man who could bring her this sense of identity.

When Anna was sixteen, she decided to join the Universalist church as a means of meeting a better class of young people, since she did not get along particularly well with any of the young people in the neighborhood. She became involved in a young people's group and there met Guy, who struck her as possessing all the desirable characteristics she had dreamed of in a man. He was handsome, his father was a store owner, rather than a ne'er-do-well like her father, and he was going to college, which surely meant that he was going to make something of his life. He seemed to have a superior air, which stood out even on first meeting. Guy was swept into Anna's orbit by his appreciation for the fact that she found him so marvelous, in contrast to the messages of not measuring up that he had previously received in his family. He felt that Anna was very approving and did not even seem to mind his lack of social facility. It never occurred to him that his awkwardness in mingling and interacting with people was interpreted by Anna as an air of superiority.

Similarly, he thought Anna was a "salt of the earth" type who would not be concerned with some of the artificial things he thought his family was preoccupied with. As he and Anna started to spend more time together, he frequently found himself, while in Accounting II (a class that he was repeating with difficulty after having flunked it once), daydreaming about being in his own home with an adoring Anna preparing a meal in the kitchen. Anna's fantasies, in contrast, were of walking down the street on the arm of a Guy who is obviously a great success. As they go down the street, others nod and bow in deference to this handsome couple. Their courtship was highly formalized and brief; Guy, dissatisfied with school, became increasingly preoccupied with thinking of marriage, and Anna, wishing to escape her nonentity existence, saw marriage as her way out of an unhappy relationship within her family. They married on Anna's seventeenth birthday, and Anna left her senior year of high school to become Guy's wife.

The first three years of their marriage were characterized by a few stormy scenes as it became apparent that neither one was fulfilling the other's expectations. Guy had dropped out of college and gone to work as a clerk in the neighborhood hardware store, an occupation far removed from what Anna had envisioned. Anna, in turn, had never mastered the skills associated with housekeeping. Her days were spent watching the soap operas and fantasizing how it would be to be a doctor's wife. Their personal resolution to these dissatisfactions was to become increasingly distant from one another, with little attempt to work out common goals.

Guy worked long, hard hours in the hardware store, and as a reward for his diligence, he received a raise. This momentarily rekindled Anna's dreams of success, and at that point Girard was conceived. The pregnancy was basically uneventful, although she was fearful and worried about both her own state of health and the well-being of the baby she carried. As the pregnancy progressed, she found herself thinking more and more of how much better her life would be after the baby arrived, and began to look on the baby as her means of making life what it should be, rather than continuing to focus on Guy. Guy, on his part, was both relieved and distressed. He was relieved that the nagging had stopped, although somewhat jealous at having been replaced in his wife's eyes by the baby-to-be.

This theme continued after Girard's birth. Anna's days were filled with tasks and concerns related to the baby's well-being. She became, in effect, a super-mom, never letting anyone else care for Girard, always sterilizing things, preventing drafts, changing his clothes, bundling him up lest he catch cold, and in general, insulating him against any outside influences. When Girard was six weeks old, Anna left him with her parents while she went shopping. Her mother criticized her for keeping the baby too warm and said that he did not seem to be quite right. After this experience, Anna did not leave the baby with her parents, for it stirred up her nagging doubts about her abilities to be a good mother.

Guy left all the childcare to Anna because of her zeal to be a good mother. He sometimes thought that she protected Girard a little too much, but he did not interfere. He thought, "It's all right when he is a baby," but he did not want the boy to grow up to be a sissy. As Girard grew up, Guy had the feeling that Anna did not want the boy to do too many of the things that he, Guy, liked to do, such as carpentry work. She said that such activities would never get him any place in the world, but Guy felt that she did not want Girard to become as involved with him as he was with her. It was as though Anna did not really want him to get too close to his son.

Girard's sister, Annette, was born when he was three years old. This was a time when his parents had another period of renewed hope about their future. Guy's aunt had died, leaving them a small inheritance and her house. Again they reached an impasse, in which Anna wanted to sell the house, take the money, and buy a house in a better neighborhood in the suburbs. Instead Guy insisted that they move into the house and use the money to "fix it up"; after all, the aunt had been his favorite, and the least he could do would be to keep her house. As Guy became increasingly involved in working on the house, Girard was interested in following him around and helping. Anna did not have as much worry and concern about her mothering role with Annette; it seemed to others that Girard remained the "apple of her eye," and she continued to devote much of her energies and attentions to providing him with the environment and influences she thought he should have. She was somewhat unhappy at his interest in copying his father, fearing that he might get too involved in manual labor, while she wanted him to appreciate the "finer," higher class things in life. She often thought of him as a brilliant trial lawyer who would win the esteem of the community, and she did not want him sidetracked by becoming too interested in manual skills such as carpentry.

After her routine with Annette settled down, Anna decided on a program to counteract Girard's involvement with Guy's house repairs. She bought books and sat down with him to read; she tried to provide interests for him in the house so that he would not pester her to go out into the neighborhood to play with other boys, since she did not consider them a good influence. This became a real source of contention between Anna and Guy, who thought his son should be out playing with other boys rather than sitting around the house. Anna would always throw it back to Guy that if he had not insisted on living in this house instead of moving to another neighborhood, Girard would have had many good friends to play with. Did he want his son to be influenced by the ruffians around them?

Guy always retreated from these verbal interchanges, usually to his work at the hardware store or to his home repairs. In fact, as the years went by, Guy seemed to be at the store more and more. One day when Anna was there, she met the new bookkeeper, a very attractive woman. Anna became suspicious about Guy's working evenings, particularly after one of the neighbors mentioned having seen Guy and the bookkeeper at dinner one evening when the store was open. Guy enjoyed his wife's fears and did nothing to dissuade her for several weeks. He felt that maybe if she were worried about him, she would be more admiring rather than taking him for granted. Finally, after he felt she had worried about this enough and might carry stories outside the family, Guy told her that there were women who thought he was attractive, but he surely would not do anything to sully the family name. In another attempt to consolidate the marriage, the third child, Alfred, was conceived.

When Girard entered school, he had really never learned to play with other children his own age; he was timid and shy and overly tied to his mother. The teacher was somewhat concerned because he did not seem to be able to play with the other children as she thought a six-year-old boy should; rather he preferred to stay inside or by himself. On the other hand, he was not any trouble, so maybe she need not worry about it. Girard did average work in school, but was not exceptionally bright; he spent a lot of time drawing geometric designs, highly structured and self-contained. He was always rather fearful and hesitant about anything new, had to be pushed to get into it, and was never able to take much of the rough-and-tumble activities expected in the gymnasium. The teachers at the school felt that Anna's husband was henpecked and that she was difficult to deal with.

Anna tried to arrange a number of meetings with the teachers to tell them how the school should be organized so that Girard might do a little better. She was critical of the discipline in general, feeling that they were hard on Girard but generally too tolerant of unruly behavior that they certainly should have squelched. On the one hand, she seemed to wish Gerard to succeed and do well in school, but on the other seemed fearful of his branching out and of risking the chance that school might have any influence on his life. She gave many mixed messages along this line, such as, "Girard, I want the best for you; I want you to do all these things that the boys do and have fun while you are in school"; while at the same time letting him know that she thought these activities were dangerous and he should not get involved. She impressed on him that he should never lie to his teacher, but then would criticize him severely when he reported something about his home that was true. She said things to encourage him to notice things, such as, "Be observant! How are you going to be a lawyer if you don't notice things?" But if he happened to comment upon something that was upsetting to her, she would chastise him, saying (for instance) that he had a dirty mind.

All in all, Girard would have to be considered a loner. His classmates considered him a little odd; he did not share many of their interests and ways of doing things and was regarded as fair game for teasing. He was a fairly gentle boy, and he did gradually earn a certain kind of esteem among his classmates because of his manual dexterity. He spent much of his time building model airplanes, which he shared with his classmates and thus made up somewhat for the fact that he did not like the rough-and-tumble of boys' sports. He did not have any close friends; this was largely because the boys never knew where they stood with him. At one point he would seem distant, and then the next thing they knew, he would bring a model airplane for them to play with; they never knew what to expect. This pattern continued through grammar school and into high school. As other boys his age began to date girls, Girard did not have much to do with them. He was exceedingly shy, and the girls did not seem to pay any particular attention to him; he seemed to fade into the background.

A major problem during his first year of high school centered on his flunking composition. He did poorly in most subjects, but was particularly weak in anything having to do with literature and English. He did somewhat better work in math and science courses, but the big problem was that he spent all his time tinkering and did not get involved in studying as he might. He flunked the composition course after his mother had made him drop the shop course, which he dearly loved, and had insisted that he stop building model airplanes at home so he could spend more time on his homework. His mother made a big fuss about this, and at that point his teacher suggested that counseling would be in order, because she thought there was a family problem. Of course, Anna would not hear of this, and Guy did not particularly want it either. He did not want the stigma attached to having a problem in the family, and by that time he was relatively detached from it all. Guy personally thought that Girard was very talented with his hands, but he left all matters having to do with the children's schooling to Anna.

When Girard started to fail other subjects, the counselor, after enlisting Guy's support, was able to convince Anna to let him be transferred to the local vocational school, where he could continue to follow his basic interest, mechanics. Anna rationalized this on the basis that he had to get out of the other high school, where he was doing so poorly, because he really had to get better grades if he was going to be a lawyer. She spent a great deal of time criticizing the high school and the teachers, attributing Girard's failure to the poor school. She persisted in her fantasies that he was going to make it as a lawyer. Any attempts on his part to dissuade her from this belief were greeted with an outburst of rage: "Of course you'll make it." Eventually Girard avoided this type of scene by just not talking about it. He found a great deal of enjoyment in his mechanical work and knew he could never make it as a lawyer, as his mother wished, but he could not convince her of this and so stopped trying. Consequently, he felt something of a fraud and had difficulty enjoying his new-found feelings of competence. However, in some ways he acted out his mother's fantasies by writing away to law schools for information about their programs and avidly shared in viewing with Anna all the lawyer shows on television. This kept Anna's fantasies about Girard alive and postponed the catastrophic day when reality must be confronted.

In the vocational school Girard did very well; he was intensely involved in his work, to the exclusion of all else. While the others tended to joke as they worked, his involvement was all-encompassing. In fact, one of the students commented that when they walked by Girard, it sounded as though he was talking to the engine—not cursing as some of them did when things didn't work out right, but actually talking to it as though it were real. The other students recognized his abilities to solve difficult problems, and if they had trouble with an engine that they could not solve, frequently they came to Girard for help. In one of the parent conferences, a counselor expressed some concern about Girard's single-minded concentration on automobile engines to the exclusion of relationships with other people. Anna became upset at this and stated that Girard had always worked hard in school, and after all, weren't his studies the most important thing? He was not like some of these other guys, out running around with girls and messed up with dope—her Girard was a good boy.

As spring of his senior year came, the students had a class concerned with placing them in jobs and discussing aspects of job-finding. Girard was sent out to one of the best garages in town for a job interview and, on the way home, stopped at the library to check out a book titled *How to Get Into Law School*. The week following this interview, Girard slept poorly; in fact, Guy found him at 4:00 one morning reading the book about law school. Guy expressed some concern about Girard to Anna, but she had not noticed anything that was problematic. She did get him some vitamin pills and fixed some special stew that he liked particularly well, because "Maybe he isn't getting the right food in that school he is going to."

On Monday morning Girard discovered that the engine he had worked on for two months had been dismantled, and all of the parts were lying in a jumbled heap. He ran into the principal's office shouting, "My engine, my engine, why did you let them do this to my engine? Was my mother here?" The principal told him to sit down and calm down: "Now, Girard, you knew that these engines weren't going to be here forever; you're taking this much too seriously. We have to get ready for the next class. You boys will be out working within the month and we have to get ready for the summer session." Girard seemed hardly to hear him, abruptly got up, slammed out of the office, and went back to the workroom where he stood guard over his dismantled engine. Others tried to talk to him, but he totally ignored them. Finally they called his parents to come and get him. As Anna walked in, he muttered, "And who are you, the Virgin Mary?" She threw her arms around him and said, "My boy, my boy, what have they done to my boy?" He was heard to respond, "No, you're an evil trollop. You wanted them to wreck my machine." After much encouragement, Girard finally went home with Guy and Anna, but went to bed and would not talk to anyone. Anna plied him with all of his favorite foods and tried in every kind of way to get Girard to talk to her. He acted as if she were not there. Guy came in and told him, "You'd better shape up. Get out of that bed."

The following Monday, when Girard still would not get up to go to school, Guy and Anna had a long argument and finally admitted that something was wrong. Guy threatened to go into Girard's room and drag him out to go to school, while Anna shouted, "Leave him alone! A week of home cooking and my taking care of him and he will be all right." Guy responded, "Anna, you've babied the boy all his life and look how he's turned out. He doesn't need home cooking, he needs sternness." This argument led to recriminations between the parents about how each one had failed the other. They did agree that if Girard had not returned to his usual state by the next morning, they would call their family doctor. The family doctor, when he was consulted by phone on Monday morning, thought privately that the boy might have had a catatonic break and referred them to the local mental health clinic.

TREATMENT ISSUES

When faced with a situation such as the one described in the case study of Girard, those who work in places such as local mental health clinics are faced with a number of difficult decisions. The first is probably what to do with the person—in this case, Girard. The most common decision would usually be hospitalization, although it is not necessarily the preferred mode of treatment. This decision would hinge on how serious they thought the crisis of his illness might be, both to Girard and his family. Issues such as whether he will commit suicide or dissolve into rage and kill his mother are paramount factors to consider. Another factor involves an assessment of the current struggle in the family; that is, to consider the possibility of modifying the family interactions in such a way that Girard might shift out of his current pattern of withdrawal to some form of behavior that would yield better results in solving the conflicts he faces. What are the assets of the family that might serve as counterbalances in the system? For instance, what might the position of Annette and Alfred be? Could they be of some use in assisting the parents in making a new form of détente? Or, if Girard were taken out, would they become the next victims of this family network?

The advantage of having Girard at home would be twofold. First, it would allow the total social network, which contributed to the development of Girard's problem, to be dealt with as a whole. Since the family is now in crisis, there would be more chance of promoting beneficial change in the whole network. Second, if Girard is kept within the family rather than taken to the hospital, the labeling process is diminished, in that he is not admitted to a psychiatric hospital where he would be likely to learn the sick patient role. Further, if he is maintained within the family, they do not have the opportunity to extrude him from the social network. Many times when a patient enters the hospital, the family system closes in such a

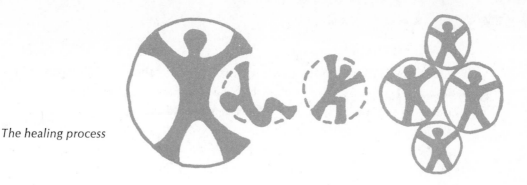

way that it becomes almost impossible for the "patient" to re-enter the family system.

On the other hand, the advantage of having him in the hospital may be that it will protect him from noxious influences that are rapidly locking him into a deviant pattern within the family. His inability to deal with the conflicts and the continual bombardment of pressures that he can no longer avoid must be considered. His breakdown, from this perspective, can be seen as a "cry for help"; removing him would permit some strengthening of his defenses so that he could cope more effectively. It is sometimes felt that the only salvation for people in Girard's position is for them to acquire some other base of attachment and growth besides this damaging family of origin. This view may be particularly pertinent in instances where the symbiotic bond between the child and one parent is such that no independent growth is permitted. Hospitalization is sometimes felt necessary as a way of relieving the family of a problem that they can no longer manage. In any event, whether the person is hospitalized or not, considerable attention needs to be paid to the family; this family is at an optimum point for change in that they are in crisis, and the unfortunate solutions of the past are now open for some different resolutions. It is not unusual, provided they receive the proper type of support at a time like this, for the marital pair to reach a better realignment of their relationship than they have achieved in the past.

Those who work with people who have adopted the coping mechanisms described as common to schizophrenia face some particular problems. First, they are dealing with a person whose primary mode of coping has been through isolation and who is only tenuously connected to others.

He or she is prepared for disaster in relation to other people and is therefore fearful of any type of close interpersonal contact. The loneliness and isolation that the person experiences is all-pervasive. Those who attempt to engage such a person in therapy are confronted by some basic problems.

The primary treatment issue that first confronts the therapist is that of establishing a relationship with someone whose primary mode of operating has been to avoid such relationships. This is compounded by the underlying need-fear dilemma we have previously described, in which the person sorely needs such a relationship but fears that he or she will be destroyed by entrusting himself or herself to it. The therapist, aware of the intensity of the person's feelings, sometimes responds in a similar fashion. Sensing the patient's tremendous need for meaningful interpersonal relationships, the therapist fears that these needs may prove overwhelming, and sometimes he or she inadvertently responds by distancing maneuvers. Because of the patient's problems of ambivalence, related to the way he or she uses objects to avoid noticing his or her structural problems in managing the world, the patient often treats the therapist as another object. The therapist becomes the recipient of anger, rage, and adoration in unpredictable serial sequences. Frequently the person's emotional responses to the therapist seem to have no connection to anything that is going on within the relationship at that particular time. To prove oneself trustworthy in this situation is not something that is accomplished overnight. The therapeutic course is frequently long, with many ups and downs; the person who has developed this particular style of relating has considerable difficulty in even trying alternative patterns because of the double-bind predicaments of his or her past, when there was no acceptable solution other than the one already chosen—complete withdrawal. Therapeutic maneuvers should be directed toward providing a relationship in which the person can begin to experiment with new patterns of relating.

As described earlier, the person with this style of coping has had considerable difficulty receiving any input from others to help him or her structure relationships with them and with the environment so that, in turn, his or her internal structure could be developed. A critical part of the treatment process, then, is structuring the person's experience so that this development can be now accomplished. The developmental work needs to proceed in all areas that should have been accomplished earlier in life. The development of the capacity to trust others, the usual social role reciprocities that will yield more positive results than those of the past, the ability to take in and interpret with some degree of accuracy what is going on with other people, and a development of a sense of personal identity are all part of the treatment goals.

To accomplish these goals a combination of treatment modalities is probably desirable. The need for change has to occur at a number of levels: first, there is the need for restructuring the person's way of relating. Second, there is a need for shifts in family patterns of relatedness to free up the situation so that the person is not forever caught in irresolvable conflicts. Third, the person's relatedness to a wider world outside of the family must be accomplished. Treatment, therefore, should be related to all these different levels of desired change. Considerable individual work is usually thought to be an essential part of the treatment process, to accomplish the internal restructuring for the initial stages of developing trust and learning responsibility, and to experience safety in taking the initiative.

As we have already pointed out, work with the family is advised because of the present crisis and the possibilities of promoting change within the system that will allow the person to make these personality shifts. Usually the particular type of treatment in which the person is involved shifts according to his or her functioning at any given time. Because of the nature of the family network, it is not possible to predict at what points their therapeutic work can proceed most productively. It is always advisable to do some family work at the point of crisis. No matter how damaging the family may appear, other family members are equally distressed and are sincerely concerned that the person be helped. For instance, as we have pointed out in the case of Guy and Anna, they have experienced a series of disappointments in one another that they never had any help in resolving. They did not maliciously set out to do in Girard; in fact, Anna is particularly pained by Girard's condition because she saw him as her only way out of her own personal disappointments. She will probably be terribly concerned if Girard is hospitalized. She has every reason to suppose that she knows more about her son's sensitivity than other people and will genuinely feel that hospital personnel would not understand him. Instead of seeing the family as an adversary, it is important to employ them as allies in the treatment process.

In addition to individual and family work, group work is an important part of the treatment program. In Girard's situation, one can readily see his limited facilities in relating to groups. Certainly part of the reso-cialization process consists of gaining necessary experience in relating to groups under various conditions. Girard has never learned the give-and-take of social relationships that people usually acquire from their peers in the growing-up years. Whether in a hospital milieu or in a work-type pro-gram outside, an important facet of the treatment process is to provide opportunities for more productive patterns of relating to others, which also contributes to the vital restructuring process. Girard's capacities to work with his hands should be encouraged as a medium through which he can make the bridge to other forms of relatedness.

SUMMARY

In summary, retreat as a form of coping is a pattern that essentially involves a retreat from or a disregard for the usual normative rules that govern behavior. A variety of deviant life styles consist of patterns of be-havior that actively violate the usual societal rules. Frequently persons who behave in this manner become involved with the judicial system because of the nature of their rule-breaking. It is argued that persons employing this type of coping pattern do so to keep significant interpersonal relation-ships encapsulated, thus preventing themselves from becoming too closely attached and consequently vulnerable.

A second form of retreat is that commonly labeled schizophrenia. Schizophrenia is one of the more frequently identified forms of "mental illness." Explanations as to its cause are plentiful and contradictory, rang-ing from those based on biological or genetic factors through various intrapsychic or interpersonal causes to broad-ranging sociological variables. Typical patterns have been noted, particularly in relationship to thinking and emotional processes. Various arrangements of these symptom patterns result in a typology of schizophrenia as of six types: simple, paranoid, hebe-phrenic, catatonic, schizoaffective, and undifferentiated.

One of the central problems identified is the tenuous interpersonal relationships of the person labeled schizophrenic. This inability to estab-lish stable relationships is associated with the isolation and loneliness schizophrenic people commonly describe; it becomes a key issue in any kind of therapeutic endeavor.

FURTHER READINGS

Arteberry, Joan. "The Disturbed Communication of a Schizophrenic Patient."
    Perspectives in Psychiatric Care 3, no. 5 (1965): 24-37.

Braverman, Shirley. "Homosexuality." *American Journal of Nursing* 73 (April 1973):
    652-655.

Chrzanowski, Gerald. "Cultural and Pathological Manifestations of Paranoia."
    Perspectives in Psychiatric Care 1, no. 4 (1963): 34-42.

Cleckley, Hervey. *The Mask of Sanity.* 4th ed. St. Louis: C. V. Mosby Company, 1964.

Courtade, M. Simone. "The Challenge of Becoming." *Perspectives in Psychiatric Care*
    7, no. 1 (1969): 34-38.

Donner, Gail. "Treatment of a Delusional Patient." *American Journal of Nursing* 69
    (1969): 2642-2644.

Field, William, and Ruelke, Wylma. "Hallucinations and How to Deal With Them."
    American Journal of Nursing 73 (April 1973): 638-640.

Gerber, Claudia, and Snyder, Deanne. "Language and Thought." *Perspectives in
    Psychiatric Care* 8, no. 5 (1970): 230-233.

Green, Hannah. *I Never Promised You a Rose Garden.* New York: New American
    Library, 1964.

Mellow, June. "The Experiential Order of Nursing Therapy in Acute Schizophrenia."
    Perspectives in Psychiatric Care 6, no. 6 (1968): 249-255.

———. "Nursing Therapy." *American Journal of Nursing* 68 (1968): 2365-2369.

Moser, Dorothy Hale. "Communicating With a Schizophrenic Patient." *Perspectives
    in Psychiatric Care* 8, no. 1 (1970): 36-41.

Roberts, Sharon. "Territoriality: Space and the Schizophrenic Patient." *Perspectives in
    Psychiatric Care* 7, no. 1 (1969): 28-33.

Rosenbaum, C. Peter. *The Meaning of Madness.* New York: Science House, 1970.

Rubin, Theodore Isaac. *Lisa and David.* New York: Ballantine Books, 1965.

Schizophrenia Bulletin. A periodical published by the National Institute of Mental
    Health since 1969.

Schwartz, Morris, and Shockley, Emmy. "The Patient is Hallucinating, Delusional, or
    Self-Preoccupied." *The Nurse and the Mental Patient,* pp. 113-138. New York:
    John Wiley & Sons, 1956.

———. "The Patient is Withdrawn." *The Nurse and the Mental Patient,* pp. 90-112.
    New York: John Wiley & Sons, 1956.

Sherrill, Lattice. "Nursing the Patient Who Expresses Concern for Self-Identity."
    Perspectives in Psychiatric Care 2, no. 2 (1964): 24-30.

Stankiewicz, Barbara. "Guides to Nursing Intervention in the Projective Patterns of
    Suspicious Patients." *Perspectives in Psychiatric Care* 2, no. 1 (1964): 39-45.

Stevens, Helen. "A Distracting Experience." *Perspectives in Psychiatric Care* 5, no. 1
    (1967): 47-51.

Wildman, Laura. "Reducing the Schizophrenic Patient's Resistance to Involvement."
    Perspectives in Psychiatric Care 3, no. 3 (1965): 26-32.

Will, Gwen Tudor. "A Sociopsychiatric Nursing Approach to Intervention in a
    Problem of Mutual Withdrawal on a Mental Hospital Ward." (Reprint)
    Perspectives in Psychiatric Care 8, no. 1 (1970): 11-35.

SECTION 2

INTERVENTIONS

INTRODUCTION

In earlier chapters we discussed how each person develops his or her own repertoire of coping behavior in confronting life's problems. For some, the coping styles developed bring little personal satisfaction and, indeed, prove to be costly in that the person must spend so much energy in either avoiding problems or engaging in unsuccessful problem-solving maneuvers; any one of the basic patterns described has the potential of becoming a crippling restriction on the development of a more open coping style.

In some people, psychosomatic illness develops and is incorporated as an integral part of their coping pattern. The illness becomes an important factor in the way they structure relationships with others. With this as a foundation, the person has little opportunity to develop warm, trusting interpersonal relationships based on himself or herself as a true person. Many times, significant persons seem to cater more to the particular problems generated by the psychosomatic disorders than they do to other aspects of the individual. An example of this is the wife who carefully prepares her husband's ulcer diet, but seems otherwise impervious to his sense of well-being. Her husband, in turn, can derive satisfaction from the care given, but could never allow himself to enjoy being "cared for" without the excuse of his ulcer. The two of them are thus locked into relating to one another through the ulcer, and the husband may not know whether his wife truly cares for him as an individual of worth or merely sees that his physical needs are met out of a sense of duty. Further, he cannot accept a view of himself as having needs to be "cared for," but must constantly maintain an image of self-sufficiency and independence. A considerable amount of one's life becomes structured around the presence of a psychosomatic illness, and as long as this is so, one has little experience in, first, developing a view of oneself as a person of worth in one's own right, and second, entering into a series of interpersonal relationships that are a reflection of the "true" person, with all his or her supposed foibles and human weaknesses.

Neurotic coping styles can also serve as a restrictive and isolating force to the people who engage in them. In such instances, this pattern of living reflects a series of maneuvers such people employ to avoid anxiety and thereby maintain safety. Their lives, to a greater or lesser degree, become involved in attempts to preserve themselves. Their life styles, whether involved in obsessive-compulsive, phobic, or hysterical behavior, reflect the rigidity of their behavioral repertoires. Their interpersonal relationships become structured around their particular form of neurotic behavior, and thus they are deprived of positive relationships that are based on mutuality developed out of a sense of truly knowing themselves and the other. Life becomes a series of maneuvers to keep the true self hidden, lest it be destroyed.

Others use chemical substances as a crutch as they face life's problems. Instead of actively attacking problems and reaching resolutions, they rely on drugs, such as alcohol, to escape having to tackle their problems. When the effect of the drug wears off, the problem still remains, and the anxiety over inability to cope often increases; the drug again becomes the solution to avoid and numb their awareness. A vicious cycle of drug-taking develops. While some drugs serve to sedate a person and make him or her temporarily less aware of problems, other drugs serve to alter the person's self-perception. The male college student who sees himself as a failure because he can never measure up to his father's expectations, who is not adept at sports and perceives himself as less successful than others, may take drugs so that he can experience the effect of feeling as though he could "conquer the world" and be the kind of man he would like to be. Although the drugs temporarily make him feel better, constant use will make him even less capable, and so the vicious cycle goes. Social relationships become structured around drug usage, rather than on a deeper interpersonal level. The person becomes the captive of a coping style developed over time and reinforced by the network of social forces surrounding the use of drugs.

Still other people depend upon others to solve their problems, but in the process perceive themselves to be martyrs or victims. They experience life as a series of losses and they go through life in a depressed state. This particular coping style may develop early in life when a child learns that the only way of garnering the approval of parents is to acquiesce at every turn.

Compliance becomes an early pattern of life. As the person experiences losses, either real or symbolic, he or she is stripped of any way of "fighting back" in response to them. The angry feelings that arise when this person experiences a loss must be suppressed, for to express them would result in further abandonment and loss. Unable to express his or her feelings, the person is never able to truly work through the grieving process and goes through life in a chronically depressed state. Facing further losses, he or she has no resiliency in meeting these circumstances and becomes increasingly depressed. Others, sensing the person's withdrawal from active involvement in living, increasingly take over in making decisions and running his or her life. A Suicide attempt, either actively, as by taking an overdose of drugs, or indirectly, as in being accident-prone, represents both the state of the person's despair and the inability to express anger openly to those who now hold him or her "captive."

As in all coping styles, the individual and those within his or her social network play reciprocal and reinforcing roles. The depressed person becomes increasingly incapable of handling his or her affairs, to which others respond by taking over increasing amounts of responsibility for him or her. This in turn makes the person feel increasingly worthless, and so the cycle continues. Once more the person is captive and is unable to "break loose," for fear the tenuous hold on others will be broken, and he or she will be totally "lost."

Still others' lives demonstrate patterns of retreat. Some have never formed a solid base of trust that enables them to enter into stable, satisfying relationships with people. Lacking this initial bonding, their lives are lived in constant norm-breaking behavior in the sense that they do not adhere to the prevalent norms for interpreting their world and relating to people. Indeed, the person labeled schizophrenic, instead of relating to people on an affective level, may at times relate to "voices," inanimate objects, animals, and to himself or herself as an object. Other people frequently attempt to bring him or her back to reality, a task they consider accomplished when the person fits into the societal norms that he or she has been ignoring. Since past experience with reality has been troublesome, the schizophrenic person frequently resists these efforts, even at the expense of being considered a nonperson. It is noteworthy that certain people or circumstances in the environment may be instrumental in helping this person maintain his or her rule-breaking definition of reality.

Others violate societal norms in different ways. The homosexual person violates the norms for sexuality in our society, while those people labeled as "character disorders" or "sociopaths" are not bound by the norms of right and wrong, and thus elicit the censure of others. Even though people with these types of coping styles are norm-breakers in the usual sense of the word and theoretcially may be considered free of some of the constraints that normally serve to control people, frequently they too are bound by their need to violate the rules. Their lives are lived in defiance of those significant others, and in their own way, they are as enchained as others we have described. In their attempts to retreat from societal bonds, they become enmeshed in their need to live their lives in defiance and in this way are captives of this particular style of coping.

In our earlier discussion we pointed out that, although people develop a general style of coping, these patterns are not fixed; and in the course of the usual daily problems, a person at times shows personal growth in his or her ability to problem-solve and at other times experiences difficulty that is reflected in a maladaptive coping style. Through repeated difficulties in meeting life's crisis situations, people may become increasingly circumscribed in the coping styles they employ to counteract anxiety. They become "locked in," so to speak, and their repertoires of role behavior are increasingly rigid and confining. These persons are unable to truly be themselves, but find themselves captive of the roles they must play in order to maintain a sense of self. They become locked into the roles, and as they play them, they increasingly lose any sense of who they are separate from these roles.

The person with a neurotic, dependent, depressive, or retreatist coping style employs his or her particular style of coping to deal with anxiety. He or she engages in a set of behaviors that protect him or her, rather than entering freely into interpersonal relationships based on mutual feelings of trust and respect for others. All of his or her energies are expended in defensive maneuvers, leaving little energy for the enthusiastic experiencing of life.

GOALS OF THERAPY

The therapeutic task, given people with these rigid and costly coping styles, becomes one of finding ways to help them to be free from their chains of anxiety. These interventions may occur at any point in the continuum; at best, people will be assisted early in their problem-solving endeavors so that they do not become locked into maladaptive coping styles. But even if intervention is late, experimentation with alternate styles of problem-solving, and consequent changes in the behavioral repertoire, are always possible. Interventions may be either with the individual or with his or her social networks. Remember that a person never acts in isolation; those surrounding him or her play reciprocal roles that serve to reinforce a particular coping pattern. Interventions at the individual level are aimed at generating change within the person, which is then reflected in an alteration of behavior as he or she interacts with the environment. It is also possible to intervene with the environment, changing the input the person receives. When the social network is altered, the person reciprocates by changing accordingly. Frequently the interventions for any one person involve a mix of both (individual and environment), and it is impossible to separate out the effects of one from the other.

METHODS OF INTERVENTION

Some methods are designed to help individuals gain insight into the basis for their particular style of problem-solving, as well as the meaning and function of that pattern in their lives. They are encouraged to explore their early set of significant relationships in the quest for an explanation of their current problems. Another method is to help people understand the nature of their current precipitating problem and to develop more adequate problem-solving approaches. By developing improved problem-solving, it is argued, these persons will also resolve some of their underlying problems. Still a third treatment strategy is to modify a person's behavior without working toward an understanding of the basis for his or her problems. This type of behavior modification is achieved through manipulating reinforcers; the end result is that the person, through a modification of behavior, will have an altered set of social relationships and thus may experience positive gains.

This second section of the book consists of seven chapters, all touching on the treatment, in one way or another, of people characterized by the restricting coping styles just discussed. Chapter 8 outlines some of the treatment approaches in common use. Included is a discussion of therapies that rely heavily on an exchange of meaning, primarily but not exclusively verbal, between the person to be treated and the therapist. Although the medium of all therapy of this kind may be "talk," there are a number of variants. In our discussion, such therapy is categorized as *insight psychotherapy* and *brief psychotherapy*. *Behavior modification* techniques represent another area of treatment. These techniques are based on some formulation of stimulus-response behaviorist theory. *Chemotherapy* is another widely used treatment; it sometimes is the primary mode of treatment and sometimes is used as an adjunct. Still another form of therapy, less widely encountered but definitely in common use, is the category of *somatic therapies*. Perhaps the most common of these is electro-convulsive therapy, or E.C.T. Insulin coma is still being practiced in some areas and is mentioned briefly.

In Chapter 9, the nurse's relationships to patients are discussed. Therapeutic use of self, the nursing process, and phases of the nurse-patient relationship are considered.

In Chapter 10, anticipatory counseling and crisis intervention are presented. This is a particularly fruitful area for the nurse, who has a broad base of contact with people in crisis, when they are particularly susceptible to change.

Chapter 11 describes the family as a social system and attempts to elucidate how certain variables in that system relate to some of the problems in living that members of the family have. Nursing intervention with families is then discussed.

Chapter 12 focuses on groups, rather than on an individual or family. Here, group interaction is the means by which behavioral change is achieved. It occurs on a small scale, as in making use of the dynamics of small groups, and on a larger scale, as in making use of the therapeutic potential of a ward milieu.

Chapter 13 describes the therapeutic community as an example of applying a wide range of treatment approaches.

Finally, Chapter 14 points up some of the moral or ethical issues that are very much a part of the current mental health scene.

CHAPTER EIGHT

TYPES OF TREATMENT INTERVENTION

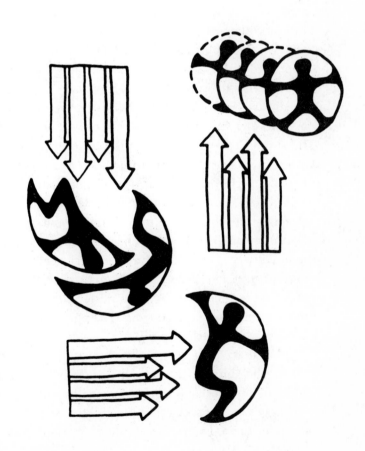

The point has been made that people frequently become locked into coping patterns that prove costly in terms of the amount of energy invested in behaviors developed to defend themselves. Since most of their energies are tied up in varying forms of defensive maneuvers, they tend to become captive; their behavior, as a consequence, becomes rigid, with little spontaneity, and they rarely experience moments when they are free to be truly themselves. In fact, many people tied to ineffective coping patterns have, in a sense, become the roles they repeatedly play, rather than "true" persons who experience themselves as worthy of respect and cherished by significant others because of what they are as individuals.

For example, the woman who copes by withdrawing and becoming depressed rarely is free to entertain the idea that her husband might love her for who she is as a person. Her worth, from her point of view, becomes predicated on how well she fulfills her roles as wife and mother, and she assumes her husband shares this view. She spends her life carrying out these roles as best she can in the way she thinks others require. Of course, other people in turn structure their own roles and their expectations of her in a reciprocal fashion. Her life is spent in a frenzy of chauffeuring children to school and other activities, getting her husband off to work, cleaning the house, cooking, washing, and mending. In her mind, her worth depends on how well she performs these tasks. Tied up in this constant activity, the woman rarely experiences any feelings of worth in her own right, of herself as a person apart from these roles she plays. She may even find it difficult to envision herself separate from her family. Her feelings of worth are derived from the approbation of others, placing her in a particularly precarious position.

What frequently happens is that her performance in the roles of "wife" and "mother" receives little positive affirmation, since it is taken for granted. The husband assumes she will maintain the house in the manner he has grown to expect, and the children expect their mother to do everything for them. Even worse, if she is for some reason unable to perform as

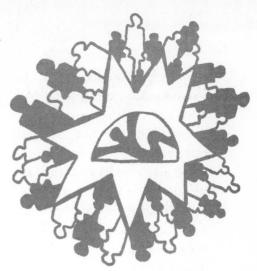

*The person tied to
ineffectual coping styles*

everyone has grown to expect, she receives considerable negative feedback. The husband may complain that the house is not cleaned, his shirts are not ironed right, and dinner is not ready. The children may similarly complain. Given this state of affairs, the woman, retreating into a common pattern of depression, ruminates, "No one loves me . . . . They are a bunch of ungrateful people . . . . I'm just a doormat for everyone to walk over . . . . And I really am not worth much as a person if I'm treated in this manner." The low self-image of this particular mother is further compounded because she dare not express any of these angry feelings, lest her fears that no one cares for her be confirmed by their angry retaliation.

Frequently a woman such as the one described in this example runs into difficulty when something occurs that disrupts the usual patterns of relationships in her immediate social system. Physical illness, for example, might interfere with her performing her usual role behaviors, which in turn upsets the equilibrium in that system and exacerbates her natural inclinations to depression. The nurse caring for such a patient in a hospital setting may be struck by the pessimistic, "blue" outlook this woman has and feel that it is out of proportion to the seriousness of the physical condition that brought her into the hospital in the first place. Most frequently, nurses working general hospital settings, in public health situations, and in other places outside the traditional psychiatric setting encounter persons who are experiencing pain not only from physical causes, but also from the coping patterns they have developed over time. All too frequently, nurses define their role in the limited framework of providing care for immediate problems, particularly related to physical care. The nurse may wonder about the degree of the woman's depression, but rarely feels that it is any of her or his business to explore patients' psychological problems. In our view, nurses are in a key position to identify persons who are experiencing difficulties in their patterns of living; moreover, because these routinized patterns that have become a way of life are temporarily disrupted by the presence of physical illness, these persons are at a point where they are probably more amenable to change than at any other time. Therapeutic interventions are not limited to the psychiatrist's office or to the psychiatric ward and are not the private domain of psychiatric nurses or other kinds of therapists. The nurse with a knowledge of human behavior may do much to help people question the conceptions that they take for granted about themselves and that play a large part in their role relations with others. Nurses can carry the process a step further, helping people to question these role relationships and to consider alternatives. In this way, the person trapped by a particular form of coping can move toward more personally rewarding ways of viewing the world, solving his or her problems and relating to other people.

In some instances, the nurse may not be the primary therapist, but someone who is supportive to the overall treatment regime. In either case, it is important to understand some of the basic rationales underlying varying treatment approaches.

"TALKING" THERAPIES

Varying forms of "talking" therapies have been used to help people with "problems in living." Talking therapies vary from the analytically oriented, which have personality reconstruction as their goal, to short-term supportive types designed to help people through temporary difficulty. Verbal exchange is the primary medium in this treatment process. The goal of therapy is to free people from stereotyped behavior so that they may experience the freedom of being themselves. This is accomplished through enlarging their range of behavior, increasing their satisfaction potential, and bringing behavior more under their control. The end goal is increased personal autonomy.

It is important to keep this in mind, for often persons come into therapy because they are causing trouble to others around them. When this is the case, it is easy for therapy to be used as a tool to try to get them to "fit in" better in their social relationships. Getting someone to act more appropriately in the context of social groups may do nothing for his or her development of autonomy, and indeed may accentuate his or her problematic coping style.

For example, consider the twenty-year-old college sophomore who is in college because his father wants him to take over the family business. He begins to get failing grades, particularly in subjects relating to the business. However, he has become interested in sociology courses, in particular, the area of social problems. In the process, he grows increasingly concerned with problems of the poor and minority groups in our social structure. He is becoming identified with a group of students who share the same interests, and they constitute an important reference group for him. At the semester break from school he goes home, bringing with him a report card that indicates failing grades in two of his business subjects, but A's in the two sociology courses he has been taking. On seeing the report card, his father begins to shout, as has been his pattern in the past: He can't understand how his son has changed, since he has "always been such a reasonable boy," and now he is not only failing his most important subjects, but "insists on wasting his talents on a group of losers." The boy is greatly distressed. He really wants to oppose his father this time, but is very anxious about doing so. He toys with the idea of dropping out of school altogether.

Now assume that the conflict between father and son blows up into an incident that brings the son to the attention of some authority outside the family, such as the police or the emergency room staff. Assume that counseling is suggested, and the father agrees, hoping that someone else will be able to help his son regain his happy, sensible former self.

What will the therapist in this situation do? If the goal of therapy is to make one a more autonomous individual, capable of making decisions for oneself, the therapist will probably direct the therapy in this direction. Through talking with the therapist, the young man will carefully examine his notions about the kind of person he wishes to be, in himself, not as a reflection of his father's wishes. He will examine the factors involved in his getting "turned off" by the business courses and "turned on" by other areas of study that represent the exact opposite of what his father had in mind for him. Is he becoming interested in these "forbidden" areas of thought as a way of rebelling against his father, as an expression of his "true" self, or as some combination of both? Why is opposing his father so fraught with anxiety for him? Having sorted through the answers to these questions and become more aware of the significance of his behavior patterns, the young man can go on to make decisions about his future and the further courses he may wish to take. He will have difficult decisions to make, but he will make them free of his prior propensity to make only decisions that others wish him to make.

In contrast to this end goal of psychotherapy, it frequently happens that someone like this comes into a therapy situation that becomes focused on his or her fitting into the standard norms and aspirations of society, a viewpoint also held by the significant others with whom the person is having difficulty. This frequently happens subtly and certainly may not be the intent of the therapist. The therapist may not deliberately set out to apply this kind of pressure; it may happen unwittingly. By focusing on the problems this student is having with a particular course, for instance, rather than on a broader view of what the course represents in terms of his total life pattern, the therapist may be helping him master the course as a means of achieving academic success. As part of the counseling process, the student may be provided tutorial assistance on the assumption that his failure in the course demonstrates a learning problem. What may be lacking is a recognition that the student may have a problem in the way he relates to his father, and that his very presence in the course of study is a manifestation of that problem, which he is experiencing as such for the first time. Therefore, the therapist or counselor may unwittingly participate in pushing the student through the course of study that will prepare him for the role prescribed by his father, rather than considering what is best for him as an individual.

Although ethical issues such as these will be further explored in Chapter 15, another word may be in order at this point about the ways in which the therapy process may be used not to provide greater autonomy for the individual, but to coerce him or her into "fitting" the societal mold. Suppose the therapist in this situation is appraised of the long-range career implications of the decisions this student might make. Suppose she (the therapist) views the boy's opportunity to follow his father into a business in which he would have a ready-made position of power and wealth as the obvious good choice, since he has much to gain in this position and much to lose if he opts for the lower status, low-reward arena of social problems. Or we could make the opposite assumption: Assume the therapist views a career dealing with social problems as more ennobling and sees the business world as cutthroat and mercenary.

In either event, the therapist may again inadvertently push the student toward the "good" choice, from her point of view. Too often a therapist moves into a parental role, assuming that she or he knows what is "best" for a person, thereby pushing her or his own value system onto the clients, rather than helping them reach their own conclusions based on a thoughtful exploration of the ramifications of their particular choices.

Although it may be obvious that some people do not employ the most effective means of coping, they do not always wish to change their coping styles, and therapists need to guard against superimposing their ideas of what would be "better" for their clients, who are relatively content the way they are. The individual is the one who ultimately determines if he or she wishes his or her life to change; and if he or she does not express the desire for change, the therapist who superimposes his or her will is only adding to the patient's difficulties. On the other hand, it is important for those, such as nurses, who work closely with people at times of personal upheaval to be alert to the ways in which people ask for help and then be prepared to offer them the type of assistance that might help them find a freer, more rewarding pattern of living. With these cautions in mind, let us turn, then, to the types of interventions that might be employed in assisting people with their problems.

INSIGHT THERAPY

Insight therapy refers to the broad category of therapy in which the goal is for the client to gain an understanding of his or her coping style in terms of the origin of the pattern and how it functions in his or her daily life. Varieties of insight therapy range from the prototypical, most formal, Freudian psychoanalyst to shorter, much more limited encounters between therapist and client, in which the goal approximates the one stated above,

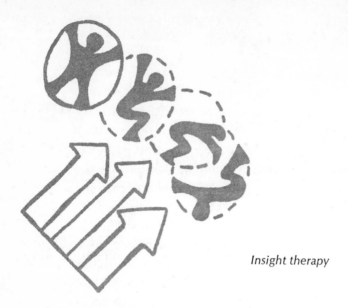

Insight therapy

rather than symptom relief, support through a stress period, or problem-solving in the "here and now."

The person experiencing symptoms and deciding on a course of insight therapy would be expected to gain an understanding both of the meaning of those symptoms in terms of the past and of their function in maintaining his or her current coping style. In other words, the person would learn about the conflicts in his or her past that led to the current symptoms and would understand the role those symptoms now play in his or her difficulties.

The person would be likely to attain this information through exploring the past and present in depth, seeking connections between the two. Paramount to this exploration is a consideration of the feelings that arise in the therapy situation about anything, including the therapist, since one of the basic tenets of this therapy is that whatever conflicts and distortions the person has picked up through life experiences will be re-experienced in the process of therapy. For example, the patient would be expected to endow the therapist with qualities of important people in his or her past, and to experience the therapist as carrying out his or her role in the same way as those important people in the past carried out theirs. The conflicts a person acquired from the relationship with his or her father, for instance, may be expected to show up as he or she responds to the therapist as though the therapist were behaving like that father. Becoming aware of such reactions is an important help for people in uncovering the conflicts of their past and in discovering how that past evolved into their current coping styles.

Three assumptions are readily apparent in this view. The first is psychic determinism: all behavior has meaning. Underscored here is the notion that behavior never happens randomly; it is caused and has some coherent meaning and in turn, contributes or leads to subsequent behavior. Thus, anyone's symptoms can be understood by unraveling his or her past to determine what caused them. The second assumption is that insight into behavior frees one from the necessity to blindly reproduce that behavior. The third assumption, sometimes referred to as the"pleasure principle," states that behavior is designed to produce pleasure and avoid pain. The second and third assumptions interact to support the notion that once one becomes aware of how and why he or she is locked into certain patterns, which cause considerable anguish, one will no longer be captive and will automatically choose more productive or pleasure-producing modes of reacting.

- *Psychoanalysis.* The founding father of the genre, so to speak, psychoanalysis deserves special mention. In addition, because of its historical position, its principles have colored the practice and premises of insight therapy. It is the oldest formalized type of psychotherapy. Prior to Freud's development of psychoanalysis, people sought help for their personal problems primarily from the clergy. Psychological problems were interpreted largely in moralistic terms until Freud and his disciples translated them into another framework. Persons who were labeled "insane" were sent to priests to have the evil spirits exorcised or, failing this, were sent to prisons for incarceration. Those with problems of lesser magnitude were provided little assistance in solving their psychological problems.

Freud, a neurologist by profession, began to recognize a large number of patients who had no physical basis for their symptoms. When they participated in hypnosis and later free association, these patients reported incidents from their pasts that they were ordinarily unaware of. Sometimes these incidents seemed factual and other times seemed to be fantasy. In any event, they turned out to be closely related to the symptoms of the patient. This discovery of a level of mental functioning of which people were ordinarily unaware was further elaborated into the concept of the unconscious, and Freud decided that it was this psychic level which gave rise to many of these symptoms that had no physical basis.

Freud originated the concept of psychic determinism; following this line of reasoning, one's early relationships become the bedrock upon which his or her subsequent life was built. Current problems are but manifestations of and re-identifications of difficulties experienced in the early years of life, usually before age five. Equally important to this theory is the position of the unconscious. All the early happenings that have faded from consciousness are not lost, but remain in the unconscious where they are constant factors in determining behavior. Thus each person is viewed as a product of his or her past, since his or her patterns have been set by early events, even though they can no longer be recalled.

From these theoretical premises, psychoanalysis and some insight therapy focus on the person's gaining insight into the basic early conflicts that resulted in the particular patterns of behavior in his or her life. To accomplish this end entails an exploration of one's past, part of which will be unconscious. One's symptoms are regarded as manifestations of underlying unconscious conflicts, and therefore are seen as clues rather than as central problems in their own right. The point of the therapy lies in ascertaining the nature of the basic conflicts that underlie the person's patterns of living, and then working through or gradually resolving these conflict areas so that they lose their potency in his or her coping style.

As one communicates with the therapist, one tends to begin to relate to the therapist as one does to significant others in one's social constellation. One particularly tends to relate to the therapist as he or she did to parental figures in early childhood. As this occurs, it is said that the person develops a transference to the therapist; that is, he or she transfers to the therapist the feelings, both negative and positive, from earlier relationships, particularly those with parents. As the therapy proceeds, the person works through the ambivalent feelings about his or her parents, not the therapist, and eventually grows to respond to the therapist in terms of the therapist's own qualities.

- **Working Through.** The process of working through is regarded as central to all forms of insight therapy. Having learned the common denominators of their difficulties and the ways in which they act and react, persons in therapy are encouraged to try out new forms of behavior and work through a new way of relating to people. As Bellak and Small describe the process:

> Working through, therefore, is a process whereby the patient applies the newly acquired insight to a variety of situations for which the same patterns hold true. His awareness of his manifest behavior and its causes are thus increased. This is essentially a learning process through which the patient's behavior is changed.[1]

In other words, as they apply their insights about the way they interact with others, patients begin to change their behavior. As their behavior changes, they experience changes in their relationships to others and, in our terms, their abilities to problem-solve are increased. Instead of being locked into recurrent patterns of behavior that have developed out of repeated coping maneuvers, they discover new forms of behavior that free them. And as they experience this freeing process, they no longer are hemmed in by the feelings of guilt that for so long have kept the cycle of relationships going in a set pattern.

In summary, the goal of insight psychotherapy is to free the person from repetitive patterns of relating that have developed since early childhood. Through an analysis of current difficulties, usually involving a retrospective examination of how these difficulties evolved over time, the person achieves an understanding of how he or she arrives at the particular individual style of relating. As the person gains insight into the meaning of his or her current patterns of behavior and of the basic conflicts underlying that behavior, he or she can begin to modify the behavior and experience more personally satisfying ways of relating to others.

BRIEF PSYCHOTHERAPY

An alternative approach is emergency or brief psychotherapy. Here the focus is the patient's here-and-now predicament. A basic assumption is that the current problem reflects more generalizable patterns of coping and that helping the person increase his or her capacity to resolve current problems will help improve his or her overall patterns of coping. Brief psychotherapy, then, begins with an assessment of the person's current coping patterns.

---

1. Leopold Bellak and Leonard Small, *Emergency Psychotherapy and Brief Psychotherapy* (New York: Grune & Stratton, 1965), p. 18.

Assessment includes an evaluation of how realistically the person perceives his or her reality situation and how well he or she is functioning. This assessment includes such areas as emotional lability, relationships to others, rationality or logic of thought processes, and defensive maneuvers employed under stress.[2]

Let us imagine the depressed woman described earlier as a patient in a medical-surgical unit. She has come to the hospital for a general medical checkup after her husband insisted that she go to her doctor. Her husband complains that she no longer seems able to manage as she has before—she spends long periods of time brooding, and he has occasionally found her crying for no reason. The general practitioner has suggested that she enter the hospital for a thorough checkup to see if there is anything physically wrong. The nurse on the unit is concerned because, while the patient's physical findings have been within normal limits, she seems so depressed. She sits alone in her room staring out the window, is convinced she has cancer and the doctors are not telling her about it, will not eat, spends much of the night pacing the halls, and periodically is found weeping in her room.

■ *Evaluation.*   For illustrative purposes, imagine an assessment interview with this patient. First let us assess perception reality.

> *Nurse:* Could you tell me a little about the situation at home? Has there been anything there that is different, or can you describe anything that might be troubling you?
>
> *Mrs. Adams:* I don't know. It's just like life is over now, with the children gone to college and my husband going away on business trips. I've lived my whole life for them, and now what does it matter?
>
> *Nurse:* Can you tell me how things go for you at home these days?
>
> *Mrs. Adams:* Well, I just sort of sit around; I don't have the usual things to do. My children are gone and I don't have them to care for, to cook for and clean up after, and my husband, he says we don't need to eat fancy meals. He's afraid of cholesterol and he's been trying to diet. I just don't have anything to live for any more. I don't hear from my children, and I guess I'm just not of any use to anyone. (She starts to cry.)

Mrs. Adams has experienced a major shift in her life. Since the children are grown, they are no longer dependent upon her. Her husband is away more than usual, so he, too, appears to have a lessened need for her

---

2. Ibid., pp. 22-29.

to perform what she considers to be the role of wife and mother. She has been unable to adapt to these changes by making shifts in her life style and so finds herself locked into feeling that she is worthless and that life has passed her by, with no one truly appreciating her. Underlying these feelings is the thought that since her family no longer need her, they have no further use for her, and rejection is on the way.

> *Nurse:* You seem to feel that no one really appreciates you any more. Has anyone, your husband or your daughters, said anything that would lead you to think that?
>
> *Mrs. Adams:* Well, you could never ask them; I can just tell. They just don't consider me at all. I'm a drag—they only come to visit me because they feel that they ought to. I hate being a burden to them.
>
> *Nurse:* In what way do you think you are a burden to them?
>
> *Mrs. Adams:* Well, being in the hospital and all that. They have to take time away from their studies to come and visit me. My husband has had to stay home from a business trip to New York, and what for? I'm just a burden.
>
> *Nurse:* Have you ever asked them how they feel?
>
> *Mrs. Adams:* I couldn't do that. I know how they feel. If I asked, they'd only lie.

Despite evidence to the contrary, Mrs. Adams persists in her view that she is a burden to her family. Even though her daughters and husband come every day to visit and bring her gifts, she cannot perceive accurately the reality that they truly care for her as a person, but persists in her belief that they are doing it only out of a sense of obligation.

Throughout the interview the nurse notes that Mrs. Adams cries repeatedly and has little control over her emotions.

> *Nurse:* I notice that you are crying a lot. Can you tell me why you cry?
>
> *Mrs. Adams:* I don't know. That really bothers me. I can be sitting at home, or in a crowd of people, and all of a sudden I find myself crying. I just can't control myself.

In assessing the degree of difficulty people are experiencing in managing to cope, it is important to note their ability to control various drives. For our purposes, drives may be regarded as basic tension states that impel people to action. (Some writers use the term "impulse" to mean roughly the same thing.) In the case of a depressed person, it is of particular importance to evaluate his or her potential for committing suicide as a result of limited drive control. Another important factor in making this assessment is the strength of the person's relationships to other people. In Durkheim's study of suicide, and other studies that followed in this tradition, it was found that the suicide rate is higher among persons with minimal attachments to others.[3]

> *Nurse:* Can you tell me a little bit about yourself and your husband? Would you describe yourself as close to one another, or what?
>
> *Mrs. Adams:* I've always thought of us as being close to one another until just recently. He's been away so much, and I feel lost since I don't have my girls to take care of any more. We've been through a lot. I lost one of my babies—the only son we ever had—and my husband helped me a lot then. . . . We've always done things together, but now I feel that it would be better if I just weren't such a burden to everyone.
>
> *Nurse:* Do you feel that you can talk to your husband about some of the things you are feeling?
>
> *Mrs. Adams:* He doesn't want to hear how rotten I'm feeling, and then he's away so much. I don't want to burden him. . . . But he always asks, and then he insisted that I go to the doctor to get a check-up.

In this case, Mrs. Adams has experienced a dramatic shift in her usual role relationships. She is not sure of the strength of others' attachments to her, and since she sees herself as relatively worthless, she feels that no one can truly be attached to her.

The degree of a person's disturbance is often measured by the extent of disruptions in his or her thought processes. Assessment should therefore include such an evaluation.

> *Nurse:* What do you do to occupy your time? Do you read, or watch television, or sew, or what do you do?
>
> *Mrs. Adams:* I used to like to read. I'd read mysteries but now I just can't seem to concentrate. I can't follow the plot. And with television, I watch the soap operas and that just gets me thinking about my problems, and I can't follow them. I get so wrapped up in wondering what I'm going to do. Then I tried to knit a sweater for my daughter and I just got it all mixed up. I dropped the cable stitch, and had to tear up the whole front. It's like I just can't do anything anymore. All I do is worry about what's wrong with me, and if I'm going to die . . . . (She begins to cry.)

The obsessive thoughts of impending doom flood in upon Mrs. Adams so

---

3. Emile Durkheim, *Suicide* (New York: The Free Press, 1951).

that she cannot concentrate; all her energies are tied up in the insoluble nature of her problem. Note, however, that her fears have not reached the point of being delusional.

A final element in making an assessment is to determine the types of defensive maneuvers the person consistently employs. In some instances the person's usual defenses no longer work, and he or she is overwhelmed by stimuli against which he or she has no defense. As part of the assessment process, it is important to check out the person's usual patterns. Mrs. Adams, for instance, has traditionally used compulsive behavior to bind her anxiety. The obsessive activity has helped her repress any of the troubling thoughts breaking through from her unconscious. But now she can no longer maintain the repression, and as these thoughts break through she becomes increasingly disorganized and depressed.

This initial assessment of Mrs. Adams would most likely lead the therapist to conclude that she has been able to manage tolerably well thus far, although her general prior behavior indicates a rather rigid and neurotic life style. She has maintained her marital relationship and has successfully launched two daughters.

■ *Treatment Goals.* In deciding what treatment is most appropriate for someone like Mrs. Adams, it is important to consider a number of factors. First is the degree of personality disorganization the person demonstrates: Mrs. Adams is obviously experiencing considerable difficulty at this particular time. Second, the length of time the person has been experiencing the difficulty: Mrs. Adams has had an acute problem for a relatively short period of time. Although one can reasonably suspect that she has been chronically depressed over a long period of time, the acute episode is related to her daughters' leaving home and her husband's being away on business. A third factor, implied in the second, is the ability to identify a precipitating event a "last straw." Fourth, the person's relatedness to other significant figures who could be supportive in helping work through the problem: Mrs. Adams obviously has interested daughters and a husband who is deeply concerned about helping his wife. Considering all of these factors, Mrs. Adams would probably be a good candidate for brief psychotherapy.

Brief psychotherapy is directed toward the "removal or amelioration of specific symptoms; it does not attempt the reconstitution of personality except that any dynamic intervention may secondarily, and to a certain

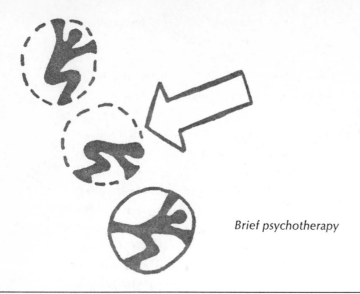

Brief psychotherapy

extent, autonomously lead to some restructuring."[4] In the case of Mrs. Adams, the goal would be to relieve her present acute depression. Even though it is obvious that she has a long-standing neurotic problem, the goal of brief psychotherapy is not to change this basic coping style. However, as we have spelled out before, if Mrs. Adams learns new ways of coping with the current situation, it is likely that she can transfer this learning to other aspects of her life, thus creating more pervasive changes in her life style.

■ *Phases of Therapy.* The initial phase of brief psychotherapy consists of taking the history, both the history of the present problem and a more comprehensive view of the person as he or she sees himself or herself. The goal of the initial interview is to ascertain how the person identifies his or her problem, and then to place this current problem in the larger perspective of the patient's whole life. It is of particular importance to note the gaps that may appear in the person's own "story." Mrs. Adams is likely to tell a great deal about her patterns of living—how hard she has worked and how little anyone appreciates her—completely excluding any information of a positive nature about her husband and daughters. Information of this nature provides a clue to some of the underlying issues; in the case of Mrs. Adams, to some of the unresolved feelings of anger surrounding her perceptions of herself as being "used."

---

4. Bellak and Small, *Brief Psychotherapy,* p. 9.

The second phase consists of formulating the nature of the problem. Drawing on the definition of the problem the therapist begins to formulate a plan for undoing the problematic behavior. As in longer term psychotherapy, one way of facilitating undoing of the symptoms is for the person to gain insight into the meaning of his or her behavior. Sometimes this is facilitated by the use of interpretations.

■ *Interpretations.* In the case of Mrs. Adams, the therapist will probably become aware of the underlying anger that she has been unable to express. Even though the therapist is aware of this, it is important that the interpretation be timed appropriately and worded so that the patient can "hear" the message and begin to process it. Too often therapists impute certain feelings to patients without checking out or validating that the person is able to make these connections at the time. For example, a nurse, knowing the dynamics of depression, might see Mrs. Adams crying and, without too much advance preparation, deliver the message, "You must feel pretty angry about the way your husband and daughters are treating you." If the groundwork has not been prepared, and if this interpretation does not naturally arise out of the information the person is giving, the response might well be, "How dare you, a stranger, attack my family? You don't really know anything about me." The person at this stage is likely to become defensive and not be able to process the information, even though the nurse's interpretation may be accurate.

On the other hand, the nurse could make almost the same statement in a different context. Mrs. Adams has told her the story of her life, most recently the history of her depression. She has told how hard she has worked, how she has always hoped that her children would not suffer the deprivations she felt as a child, and her feelings that her daughters do not appreciate all she has sacrificed for them. In response to this story, the nurse might say, "You know, I can understand what you're saying. I sometimes feel angry when I feel that people don't understand that I'm trying to help them." Identifying with the feeling that the patient is expressing, and acknowledging that the nurse, too, gets angry at finding herself in a similar situation, makes it permissible for the patient to entertain the idea that it is all right to feel angry. Instead of having to deny as a method of defense, a response such as this often serves to open communication on an affective level.

Having identified some of the underlying feelings, the therapist then goes on to help the person work through the current situation and find alternate ways of resolving the problem rather than the ineffective means she or he has been employing. Sometimes it is helpful for the person to re-enact certain interpersonal transactions to begin to identify problematic situations.

For example, imagine that Mr. Adams has been out of town on a business trip. While he has been gone, Mrs. Adams has spent long hours brooding over her problems. When he comes home he greets her, only to be greeted in return with her complaints about how bad she is feeling. He comments that maybe he should cancel his next trip out of town if she feels so bad, and her reply is, "Don't worry about me. I'm just getting old, and that's the way it is." Instead of talking about how she feels deserted and how she worries that he does not care for her any more, she retreats to physical complaints, making him feel guilty for leaving her. Instead of taking a more aggressive stand, saying that she wishes he would take her with him and stating her true fears that he no longer cares for her, she retreats into passive behavior, against which he has no defense. Unable to help her with her complaining, Mr. Adams may eventually seek out additional trips to avoid feeling helpless. In a situation such as this, role-playing is sometimes effective in providing the person with insight into the effect of his or her behavior upon significant others.

As the person gains insight into the nature of his or her behavior and its effect upon other people, alternate behaviors may be explored. As the person becomes able to identify his or her feelings and explores different ways of dealing with situations, he or she then tries out these new patterns in the actual situation. For example, Mrs. Adams is encouraged to talk openly to her husband about her feelings of desertion when he goes away, and to explore with him the possibility of accompanying him on some business trips. As she experiences his acceptance of this idea, along with his relief at her coming "out of her shell," she may then begin to redefine her own personal worth.

Even though the central issue dealt with in this example of brief psychotherapy is Mrs. Adams's relationship to her husband, it is possible to suggest to her that similar problems exist in her relationship to her daughters. And as Mrs. Adams gains confidence in herself, she then may risk testing out some new behaviors with them. Thus what she has learned in one situation may be generalized to others, and her general style of coping enhanced. Brief psychotherapy, then, is similar in many ways to longer, more intensive, forms of therapy. However, the focus is on the immediate situation that has created problems for the person. If the current situation is untangled, and the person helped to develop more effective coping patterns, major changes can result.

BEHAVIOR MODIFICATION

Various forms of behavior modification, operant conditioning, desensitization, or whatever the variant may be called have recently assumed an important place among treatment modalities. All of these treatment approaches are based on principles of conditioning originally illustrated by Pavlov and more recently refined and expanded by Skinner and his followers. They are based on a view of problems as learned behavior; following this premise, treatment involves unlearning certain problematic behaviors or replacing them with others. This is achieved through providing reinforcers. It has been demonstrated that, other conditions being equal, people tend to repeat behavior that is positively reinforced. Although negative reinforcers have been used as an approach to eradicating problematic behaviors, it has been demonstrated that negative reinforcement for unacceptable behavior is not nearly so effective in modifying behavior as positive reinforcement for approved behavior.

In the usual treatment program using behavior modification techniques, positively valued behavior is reinforced by some sort of tangible reward. For example, autistic children who have been markedly uncommunicative are given a tangible reward, such as a piece of food, for saying a word, such as "mama." In working with reinforcement techniques, it is extremely important that the reward follow immediately upon the production of the desired behavior; if there is too long a time interval, the person cannot make the appropriate association between the behavior produced and the reward for producing it.

In the case of the autistic child, it has also been demonstrated that parents or significant persons in the child's interpersonal network inadvertently tend to reinforce unacceptable behavior. The child who throws a temper tantrum is frequently held and cuddled in an attempt to control the tantrum. In a behavior modification program, parents (or surrogates) are taught to ignore unacceptable behavior—a difficult procedure, to say the least. Coupled with reinforcement of approved behavior, this approach eventually tends to reverse the behavioral balance. On the other hand, unacceptable behavior that is positively rewarded tends to increase in frequency. A problem in this scheme arises when the unacceptable behavior is in itself rewarding and therefore reinforcing. Many behavioral modification plans rely heavily on some authority (parent, staff) having control over the reinforcers. It is a serious complication that such control is difficult, at best, to achieve.

Desensitization is a variant of behavior modification that applies the principles of conditioning to the treatment of neurotic symptoms; it was first used by Wolpe after World War II. The approach is based on the premise that anxiety is learned and that it likewise may be unlearned or extinguished. Through a treatment method he called reciprocal inhibition —which means learning new responses to replace present ones, such as learning to relax rather than feel anxious in response to certain stimuli— Wolpe demonstrated positive results in the treatment of persons prone to anxiety attacks. This treatment approach is particularly helpful if anxiety is specifically attached to something and occurs in response to well-defined situations. For example, a phobia is a type of neurosis that is readily treated using this method, since the stimuli in a situation are clearly defined and the phobia is related to specific instances.

Wolpe referred to the procedure for carrying out reciprocal inhibition as systematic desensitization. It entails constructing, with the help of the anxious person, an anxiety hierarchy, or a list of those situations that evoke anxiety, and then ranking these situations in the order of greatest to least anxiety. The patient is taught relaxation, with or without hypnosis. Then, in a state of relaxation, he or she is guided to think of the lowest item on the hierarchy. The patient does this until he or she can think of it without feeling anxious. He or she then moves up the list until all anxiety responses are extinguished. Wolpe noted that this learning carried over into a person's daily life. He found, after treating several hundred persons, that almost 90 percent were cured or much improved, and that there was no substitution of other symptoms for the ones extinguished.[5] His findings contradict the most common criticisms leveled

5. Joseph Wolpe, *Psychotherapy by Reciprocal Inhibition* (Stanford, Calif.: Stanford University Press, 1958).

against conditioning therapy; that is, that the effects do not hold over time, and that other symptoms tend to be substituted as replacements for those that have been extinguished.

As we have noted before, there is considerable controversy over what needs to be treated. Does one need to change the total personality structure of the person, or to recondition him or her behaviorally and expect some generalization to other areas of life? There are no answers to these dilemmas, inasmuch as tangible research findings that might provide definitive answers are practically nonexistent.

A further complicating factor relates to moral and ethical issues of treatment. In conditioning therapies, as in some others, there is an underlying assumption about the existence of "a proper normality" that should be achieved by everyone. Frequently the therapist is the person who makes the judgment about what "normality" is. When people ask to be desensitized, no moral problem arises, since they themselves have made the decision. But in instances of captive populations, such manipulation of behavior without consent has raised the spectre of "Big Brother," a charge disputed by behaviorists. These issues will be discussed in detail in Chapter 15, but the mention of behavior modification brings them into focus as a consideration of central importance. On the one hand, it has been demonstrated that behavior modification techniques work to change behavior in clear and dramatic ways, something that more traditional forms of psychotherapy have not been able to demonstrate. On the other hand, behavior modification is viewed with trepidation by some who see the relative power position of treator and treatee as even more lopsided than usual, and fear the amount of control they perceive in the hands of the therapists.

CHEMOTHERAPY

Chemotherapy is used either as an adjunct to therapy or as the sole form of therapy. In our medically oriented culture, we tend to accept the view that taking medicine for one's illness, be it psychic or physical, is an accepted form of treatment, and few people question the appropriateness of taking various drugs to treat their psychic problems. As with most other issues in the field of mental health, there is no professional consensus on that issue. Generally speaking, professionals who adopt a largely organic or biologic view of illness are more positively oriented to the place of drugs in treatment. Others argue that although drugs may be used effectively to allay some of the symptoms that result from problematic coping patterns, they do little to resolve the underlying problem. Most professionals, regardless of their position on the cause of illness, agree that a person so treated will be given access to other treatment approaches that will help him or her resolve some of the related or underlying issues that are associated with his or her current problems. Psycho-chemotherapeutic drugs are divided into three main categories—minor tranquilizers, antidepressants, and major tranquilizers.

MINOR TRANQUILIZERS

The minor tranquilizers, used primarily for the relief of anxiety, are divided into three subgroups—the propanediols, the benzodiazepines, and the diphenylmethane derivatives. The common drugs in each group, together with their range of daily doses, are listed in Table 8-1.

The most common side effect of the minor tranquilizers, especially early in treatment, is drowsiness; hence, persons receiving these drugs should be cautioned against driving, operating machinery, and pursuing dangerous activities or occupations. Also, minor tranquilizers should not

Table 8-1   Minor Tranquilizers

	DRUGS	TRADE NAME	RANGE OF DAILY DOSAGE (MG.)
Propanediols:	Meprobamate	Miltown, Equanil	800-1600
	Tybamate	Solacen, Tybatran	750-3000
Benzodiazepines:	Chlordiazepoxide	Librium	15-100
	Diazepam	Valium	5-30
	Oxazepam	Serax	30-120
Diphenylmethane derivatives:	Hydroxyzine	Atarax, Vistaril	75-400

Based on: (1) Nathan Kline and John Davis, "Psychotropic Drugs," *American Journal of Nursing* 73 (Jan. 1974): 54-62; and (2) *Physicians' Desk Reference* (Oradell, N.J.: Medical Economics Company, 1974).

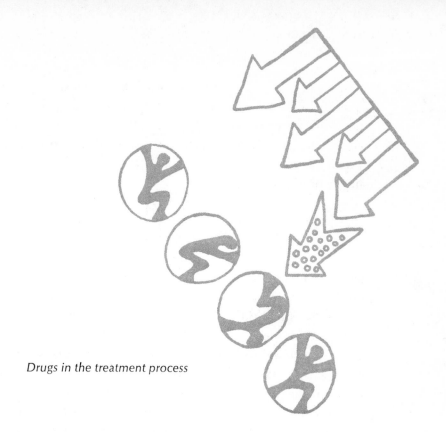

Drugs in the treatment process

be taken with alcohol or other central nervous system depressants, as these substances enhance each other's effects. Other side effects occasionally reported are ataxia, confusion, and paradoxical excitement. The potential for psychological and physical dependence exists for these drugs, and withdrawal symptoms have been reported in persons taking excessive doses of meprobamate (Miltown, Equanil) and chlordiazepoxide (Librium) over a period of time.[6] Minor tranquilizers are indicated for periods of acute anxiety and tension but, because of their potential for dependence, not for prolonged use. As we have already noted in Chapter 5, tranquilizers may be used to relieve anxiety; however, the person who relies on tranquilizers in this way tends to retreat from problems and therefore finds no satisfactory resolution. When the tranquilizer wears off, the person is once again

6. Nathan Kline and John Davis, "Psychotropic Drugs," *American Journal of Nursing* 73 (Jan. 1974): 61.

aware of his or her problems. Faced with this situation, the person frequently takes more tranquilizers, and thus the vicious cycle of drug dependence begins. On the other hand, if the minor tranquilizers are used as an adjunct to therapy, they may effectively reduce the anxiety to a level at which the person may be engaged in the therapeutic process, actively seeking resolutions to problems.

DRUGS USED FOR AFFECTIVE ILLNESSES

There are two major classifications of drugs used to treat persons with affective illness: antidepressants and lithium carbonate. Antidepressants are of two types, monoamine oxidase inhibitors (MAOI's) and tricyclics. The different antidepressant drugs, together with their range of daily dosages, are listed in Table 8-2.

Monoamine oxidase inhibitors. Because MAOI's have some potentially serious effects, they are used only when close supervision is available and other measures have failed to relieve a severe depression. They are long-acting, cumulative, and contraindicated with a number of foods and other drugs. Persons taking MAOI's should not eat naturally aged cheese

Table 8-2   Antidepressant Drugs

DRUGS	TRADE NAME	RANGE OF DAILY DOSAGE (MG.)
Monoamine Oxidase Inhibitors		
Tranylcypromine	Parnate	10-60
Isocarboxazid	Marplan	20-60
Phenelzine	Nardil	45-60
Tricyclics		
Imipramine	Tofranil, Presamine	75-300
Amitriptyline	Elavil	75-250
Desipramine	Norpramin, Pertofrane	75-200
Nortriptyline	Aventyl	40-100
Protriptyline	Vivactil	15-60
Doxepin	Sinequan, Adapin	75-300

Based on: (1) Kline and Davis, "Psychotropic Drugs," pp. 54-62; and (2) *Physicians' Desk Reference.*

or other foods high in tyramine, such as wine, yeast products, yogurt, fava beans, chicken livers, and pickled herring. They should also be cautioned against alcoholic beverages and self-medication. The drugs with which MAOI's should not be given are tricyclic antidepressants, sympathomimetics, narcotics, antihypertensives, diuretics, antihistamines, sedatives, and anesthetics. Taking these drugs or the foods listed above with MAOI's may produce a hypertensive crisis with possible intracranial bleeding, coma, and death. Careful monitoring of blood pressure is necessary for persons taking these drugs.

The side effects of MAOI's are dryness of the mouth and nose, urinary retention, constipation, sweating, tremors, loss of visual accommodation, headache, orthostatic hypotension, dizziness, syncope, drowsiness, and weakness. Side effects generally are an individual matter and can occur early or late in treatment; they seem to be more frequent in women and elderly persons.

Besides hypertensive crisis, MAOI's can cause some other untoward reactions. One of these is hepatitis and liver damage. The others are psychological reactions, namely, confusion, euphoria, or aggravation of underlying schizophenia.

Tricyclics. The second category of antidepressants, the tricyclics, is much safer than the MAOI group. Some of them are better for retarded depression and some for depression with anxiety. Some have an initial stimulating effect, and the actual antidepressant effect does not begin for one to two weeks and sometimes longer. Therefore, suicidal persons taking these drugs may become more suicidal initially, because their energy level is increased before their depression begins to lift. Tricyclics have many of the same side effects as the MAOI's, though they are less severe.

Lithium carbonate. Lithium carbonate (Lithane, Lithonate, Eskalith), a mood normalizer, is used primarily to treat manic patients. Studies indicate that two-thirds of manic patients improve with lithium and that, if taken over a period time, it also exerts a prophylactic effect. One study showed that without lithium, patients experienced a recurrence of their illness on an average of every eight months and spent thirteen weeks per year in a psychotic state, while with lithium they had recurrences every five to seven years and averaged only two weeks per year psychotic.

Mild side effects of lithium are tremor and slight nausea; these are not serious. Signs of early intoxication are diarrhea, increased tremor, and

The effect of tranquilizers

ataxia; signs of serious intoxication are confusion and central nervous system depression with possible coma and death. A normal salt intake is sufficient to control the mild side effects, as lithium excretion is tied in with sodium reabsorption in the kidneys. The person should be instructed to maintain a normal diet and adequate fluid intake. For toxic effects, diuresis or even dialysis may be necessary.

Lithium is given in divided doses, usually three times daily. The usual maintenance dose is 900 mg. daily, although persons in an acute manic state may require twice that amount. Because the toxic and therapeutic levels are close, serum lithium levels must be checked periodically. Furthermore, outpatients taking lithium should be instructed to discontinue the drug and contact their physician if signs of toxicity develop.[7]

MAJOR TRANQUILIZERS

The categories of major tranquilizers currently in use are phenothiazines, butyrophenones, and thioxanthenes. Of these, phenothiazines are the most frequently used. The various major tranquilizers, together with their range of daily dosages, are listed in Table 8-3.

7. Department of Health, Education, and Welfare, *Lithium in the Treatment of Mood Disorders* (Washington, D.C.: U.S. Government Printing Office, 1970).

Table 8-3   Major Tranquilizers

DRUGS	TRADE NAME	RANGE OF DAILY DOSAGE (MG.)
Phenothiazines		
Chlorpromazine	Thorazine	100-1500
Triflupromazine	Vesprin	50-200
Thioridazine	Mellaril	100-800
Carphenazine	Proketazine	50-400
Acetophenazine	Tindal	40-120
Thiopropazate	Dartal	30-150
Trifluoperazine	Stelazine	2-40
Butaperazine	Repoise	10-100
Fluphenazine	Prolixin, Permitil	2-20
Piperacetazine	Quide	10-160
Prochlorperazine	Compazine	15-150
Perphenazine	Trilafon	6-64
Butyrophenones		
Haloperidol	Haldol	1-15
Thioxanthenes		
Chlorprothixene	Taractan	75-600
Thiothixene	Navane	6-60

Based on: (1) Kline and Davis, "Psychotropic Drugs," pp. 54-62; and (2) *Physicians' Desk Reference.*

The effect of the major tranquilizers is a lessening of psychotic symptoms, such as anxiety and agitation, delusions, and hallucinations. All the drugs produce about equal improvement, but one or another drug may work better for certain persons.

Side effects are generally the same for all these drugs, though a particular drug may produce more or less of a given side effect. One group of side effects is known as extrapyramidal; these are akathisia, Parkinsonian-like syndrome, and dystonia. Akathisia is motor restlessness or inability to sit still. Parkinsonian-like syndrome mimics Parkinson's disease with its characteristic shuffling gait, tremors, rigidity, and mask-like expression. Dystonia is an infrequent but severe muscular reaction characterized by bizarre, involuntary movements and painful muscle spasms of the extremities, face, and neck. All of the extrapyramidal side effects may be controlled by administration of an anti-Parkinsonian drug—trihexylphenidyl (Artane), benztropine mesylate (Cogentin), or biperiden (Akineton).

Another group of side effects, produced primarily by chlorpromazine (Thorazine), are allergic reactions; these are serious and are indications for discontinuing the drugs. They usually occur early in treatment and include blood dyscrasias, jaundice, and allergic skin rashes. Although a blood dyscrasia might be detected by periodic white blood counts, the first sign is often a sore throat and fever—signs of infection. This can be fatal; fortunately, it is rare. Obstructive jaundice has also been reported, preceded by fever, malaise, and sometimes gastrointestinal upset. It usually clears up in a few weeks. Allergic skin rashes can occur, including contact dermatitis with liquid preparations. Photosensitivity is common, but it is not serious. People taking the drug should be instructed, however, to avoid direct sunlight as they will sunburn easily.

Other common side effects are drowsiness, postural hypotension, dry mouth, appetite and weight increase, blurred vision, menstrual changes, and sexual dysfunction. These are troublesome, but are not in themselves serious. The drowsiness usually lasts only a few days until the person is accustomed to the drug. Postural hypotension, with possible dizziness and fainting on rising, may be counteracted by rising slowly. Since it is most likely to occur after intramuscular administration, patients should lie down for one-half to one hour after an injection.

Besides being alert for side effects and dealing with them, the nurse is responsible for the patient's taking the medication. Sometimes psychotic patients do not want to take medication because they either do not understand or else misinterpret why they are receiving it. The nurse should attempt to explain to the patient why he or she needs certain drugs, but must also be certain the patient swallows them.

SOMATIC THERAPIES

Electroconvulsive therapy. The most commonly used somatic treatment is electroconvulsive therapy (ECT). It was discovered accidentally in 1935 by Meduna, who observed that, in his practice, there were no schizophrenics with epilepsy. He hypothesized that epileptic seizures prevented schizophrenia and that, by inducing seizures, he might therefore alleviate it. He used Metrazol to bring on seizures. (It should be noted that Meduna's basic premise was inaccurate; it has been found that epileptics can become schizophrenic.)

In 1937, Cerletti and Bini began the use of electric shock to induce seizures. The electric shock, delivered to the brain through placing electrodes on both temples, produces immediate unconsciousness and a grand mal seizure. In the early days of its use, a number of patients suffered fractures from the severity of the convulsions. Today, some refinements render it more humane, for example, the use of a short-acting anesthetic and a muscle relaxant, succinylcholine (Anectine).

The primary usefulness of ECT is for psychotic depression, but it is also useful for the manic phase of manic depression and in some schizophrenias. The effect of ECT is remission of symptoms, for example, relief of depression. How the treatment works is not known; the most likely explanation is that it affects the physiology of the brain. The number of treatments given varies according to the physician administering them, but eight to twelve is a usual course. They are given several times a week until the desired number is reached. An unpleasant side effect of ECT is memory loss. The extent of this varies with the individual; usually it becomes worse with more treatments. Patients forget many small, everyday things, which may be very upsetting to them. The memory loss is temporary, lasting six to eight weeks after treatments are finished.

Insulin therapy. In much less common use, but still practiced in some areas, is some form of insulin therapy. Used primarily for hospitalized schizophrenic patients, it has some characteristics in common with ECT, in that it is thought to exert beneficial effects through inducing a hypoglycemic coma. Patients are given insulin, allowed to fall into coma, kept in coma for a measured period of time, then given some sugar product to terminate the coma. Obviously, the procedure requires careful medical monitoring. Insulin coma was a more favored form of treatment before the wide assortment of drugs currently in use was available. It has several disadvantages compared with drugs. It is dangerous—the mortality rate has been reported at 5 percent; and costly in terms of time, money, staff, and the patient's personal comfort. Its detractors have argued that any benefit accruing from the treatment was attributable to the milieu effects of the unit, a necessarily tight-knit group, rather than to the insulin itself.

A nurse in the position of participating in insulin treatment would be well advised to become thoroughly conversant with the stages of coma before accepting the assignment. The danger lies in the possibility of the patient's falling into a deep coma without the condition being anticipated or noted when it happens. This circumstance can lead to irreversible coma and death.

SUMMARY

Although methods of intervention vary considerably, they share a common ultimate goal: to bring about a beneficial change in a person's coping style. Interventions can occur in a variety of settings, and the nurse in a general hospital is in a favorable position to help patients with restrictive coping styles.

The nurse can be either the principal therapist or one of several people supporting an overall treatment regime. In either case, she or he shares in the dilemma of deciding just what constitutes proper treatment for particular people. The nurse needs to understand the kind of influence he or she exerts on patients, and to examine whose interests are being served by that influence.

There are four main treatment approaches. "Talking" therapies involve some form of verbal exchange between patient and therapist, designed to help the patient arrive at some means of evolving new patterns of relating. Chemotherapy is sometimes viewed as adjunctive and at other times is the sole treatment approach. In recent years the use of varying types of drugs in treating different forms of problems has mushroomed. A wide variety of drugs is commonly used, depending upon specific neurological effect desired. A few forms of somatic therapies are used, chiefly ECT for depressive syndromes.

FURTHER READINGS

Brown, Daniel. "Behavior Modification." *Perspectives in Psychiatric Care* 6, no. 5
   (1968): 224-229.
Cavens, Annie, and Williams, Robert. "The Budget Plan (Behavior Modification of
   Long-Term Patients)." *Perspectives in Psychiatric Care* 9, no. 1 (1971): 13-16.
Cockrill, Velda, and Bernal, Martha. "Operant Conditioning of Verbal Behavior in
   a Withdrawn Patient by a Patient-Peer." *Perspectives in Psychiatric Care* 6,
   no. 5 (1968): 230-237.
Cohen, Roberta. "EST & Group Therapy = Improved Care." *American Journal
   of Nursing* 71 (June 1971): 1195-1198.
Edwards, Joann. "If I Touch, Will You Tell?" *ANA Regional Clinical Conferences,*
   1967, pp. 274-280.
Kent, Elizabeth. "A Token Economy Program for Schizophrenic Patients." *Perspectives
   in Psychiatric Care* 8, no. 4 (1970): 174-185.
Kline, Nathan, and Davis, John. "Psychotropic Drugs." *American Journal of Nursing*
   73 (Jan. 1973): 54-62.
Morgan, Arthur. "Minor Tranquilizers, Hypnotics, and Sedatives." *American Journal
   of Nursing* 73 (July 1973): 1220-1222.
Swanson, Mary, and Woolson, Allan. "A New Approach to the Use of Learning Theory
   With Psychiatric Patients." *Perspectives in Psychiatric Care* 10, no. 2 (1972): 55-68.

CHAPTER NINE:

THE NURSE IN THE TREATMENT PROCESS

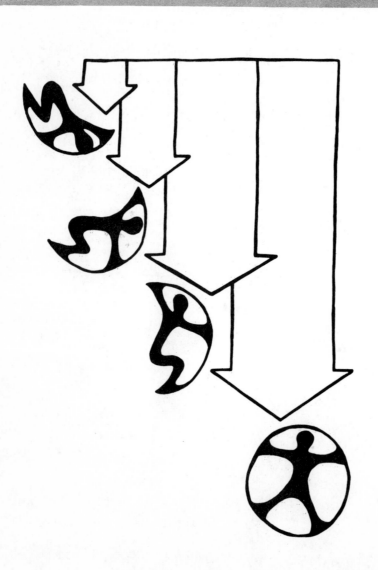

As nurse and patient meet, whether in a general hospital setting, the community, or a psychiatric treatment setting, their initial interactions are based on a set of mutual role expectations. Each individual enters a new situation using the experiences of the past as a backdrop for enacting the drama of the present. This frequently creates problems for both the patient and the nurse. The role of "patient" in the mind of the nurse means someone who is "sick," in many instances physically helpless, and who needs the nurse to "care for" him or her. But psychiatric patients are not physically incapacitated and have few of the treatment regimens common to other patients; they are capable of caring for their physical needs and in no way fit the usual image of "patient." Frequently the nurse, as she or he begins to work with the emotional needs of patients, feels helpless. The thought that all she or he has to offer the person is some form of interpersonal relationship presents a problem. The usual repertoires of role behaviors associated with being a nurse do not include caring for "psychiatric patients."

Similarly, the "patient" is perplexed about how to relate to the nurse. By entering a psychiatric hospital, the person has entered into an implicit agreement, based on commonly held views of "mental illness," that he or she is no longer capable of making decisions or running his or her life. The person entering the hospital knowingly or unknowingly agrees to treatment as it is defined. The nurse, in this situation, is the agent of the hospital.

The definition of "treatment" in a psychiatric setting is somewhat different than in traditional medical settings, and this also creates dilemmas for both patient and nurse. Frequently the person entering a psychiatric hospital tends to emulate a "sick" or helpless role and manipulates the nurse to take care of him or her, even though able to care for himself or herself. If the patient adopts this role and the nurse reciprocates, they may both feel temporarily relieved to have settled the dilemma, but over the long term, this solution compounds the problem. The nurse's "taking

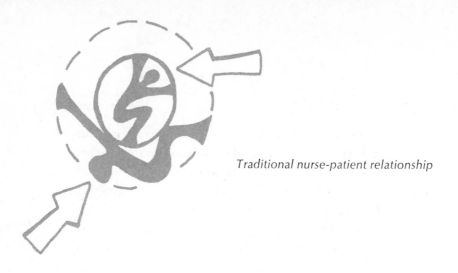

Traditional nurse-patient relationship

over" and caring for the patient confirms the person's already shaky self-esteem and does little to facilitate the development of a more adequate coping style.

Since the traditional role behavior of the "nurse" may not be appropriate in the situation, what other alternatives are open? The nurse plays many other roles in life: daughter, wife, brother, lover, sister, son, friend. Each of these roles evokes a certain behavioral response in the other person, none of which is entirely appropriate given this situation. The patient needs an "other" to whom he or she can relate his or her problems, be encouraged to explore the possible alternatives, and reach more appropriate solutions to these problems than in the past. To accomplish this, the patient needs to know that the nurse is first of all a real person, that she or he is not just playing a role, but sincerely wants to understand the dilemma and explore alternative solutions together. If the patient is to risk disclosing his or her true concerns and problems, he or she must experience the nurse as someone who is trustworthy, who maintains a confidence, and can be respected as a person who sincerely cares about what happens to the patient.

A further problem arises because nurses frequently do not work with one patient alone; they may work with families, groups, in a setting where the patient is involved in other forms of therapy and is seen in a group context. From the many things that are happening, the nurse is constantly faced with having to sort out from numerous stimuli the things to which she or he is going to respond. And how does the nurse adjust the relationship to individual patients within the broader context in which she or he works? In some instances, the nurse provides the supportive role of listener, so that the patient can process some of the things that are going on within his or her particular "therapy" sessions. In other contexts, the nurse plays a role as referee between a number of patients, all of whom are making demands for attention and help. At times the nurse will be placed in the position of having to point out ways in which the patient creates trouble for himself or herself in interrelating with others. In other instances, the nurse is in the position of monitoring the disagreements that commonly arise within group settings, using these conflicts to help the persons involved gain insight into the ways they feed into each other's particular coping problems.

Perhaps one of the most difficult problems for the nurse first entering a psychiatric setting is the absence of the usual forms of work that may have served as a "crutch" in previous interpersonal associations with patients with physical problems. In a medical setting, for example, the main nurse-patient interactions often occur while the nurse is giving some form of care. While the bed is being made, the nurse and a patient may talk of the difficulties he is having with his children. Or patients may talk of their fears and anxieties while being given a bath. The nurse can usually be comfortable talking about even the most intimate subjects while she or he is "busy" giving some form of physical attention to the patient. But what happens when this usual form of work is taken away, and all that remains is "talking with the patient"? One of the common reactions of nurses is to feel that they are not doing "work" if all they do is talk with patients, go for walks, play cards, or knit or sew in a patient group. And indeed, many times these activities are *not* work, in that the nurse has not perceived how they can be used to provide opportunities for exploring new ways of relating.

A nurse who feels that she or he must "do" something in the psychiatric setting and defines that work as "talking about problems" sometimes may so hound the patient to "Tell me what's bothering you" that communication becomes all but impossible. Feeling the pressure to "produce" so that the nurse will feel she or he has accomplished something, the person may retreat into a shell of silence to ponder this dilemma. This in turn makes the nurse even more anxious, and she or he reciprocates with additional demands to "Tell me." The patient will reveal himself or herself, and the problems he or she experiences, when the nurse appears as a real person, one who is flesh and blood but can be relied on as trustworthy.

Having established this basis for the relationship, the nurse plays a vital role in helping the patient sort through his or her situation; plays a supportive and connecting role between the various pieces of the therapeutic process; and frequently is a vital connecting link between the patient and his or her family, the patient and the therapist, and the patient and other patients and personnel on the unit. Through management of this complex set of interrelationships, the nurse can provide positive help to the person who is striving to develop a more satisfying pattern of coping with life.

In this chapter we will consider the intricate matter of relating to individuals in the treatment process. First is the therapeutic use of self; second, the nursing process; and third, the phases of the nurse-patient relationship. Subsequent chapters will consider the nurse's relationships in anticipatory counseling and in crisis intervention, to families and groups, and in the therapeutic setting.

NATURE OF THE NURSE-PATIENT RELATIONSHIP

Patients are people who have been defined as having problems. Their presence in a treatment facility implies some agreement to engage with some "knowledgeable authority" in resolving whatever has been defined as their problem. The nurse in this situation is one of the people clearly regarded as a "knowledgeable authority"—a view which is sometimes not at all the way a beginning nurse sees herself or himself. Let us examine some of the issues involved in how the nurse can use herself or himself as one who can indeed help the patient arrive at more constructive coping patterns.

Basically, the nurse should keep in mind the assumption that, since problems originate in poor interpersonal relationships and are expressed in subsequent interpersonal relationships, they can best be resolved within the context of a relationship. Relationships are seen as the vehicle through which the patient learns the variety of things he or she must learn in order to change. The relationship that the patient forms with the nurse will be one of these key learning experiences. To be helpful, the nurse must be fully involved in the relationship as opposed to being cold, distant, and intellectual. Feelings are important and should not be screened out of relationships with patients. That is, the relationship should not be based on false pretenses or a sense of obligation or duty, but on genuine feelings. The basis for judging the suitability of what is going on in the relationship is always how it moves the patient forward in learning new ways of being in touch with his or her own feelings and expressing them appropriately.

Carl Rogers points out that certain qualities in a therapist are growth-promoting for the patient. These qualities are genuineness, acceptance, and empathy.[1] Genuineness means the nurse is aware of her or his feelings and reactions and is willing to express them in words and behavior. Rogers also calls this quality congruence, meaning that external behavior is congruent with internal reactions. Only through being genuine does the nurse become a real person to patients. The nurse's honesty in expressing her or his feelings enables patients to examine what their true feelings are and thus to begin exploring what troubles them. Genuineness in responding means the nurse shares with patients even those feelings that she or he considers negative, such as anger or boredom. Patients will perceive these feelings on some level anyway, and the nurse's honesty will help in the development of a trusting relationship.

Acceptance means the nurse has a warm regard for patients as persons of worth, regardless of their behavior and feelings. The nurse's acceptance of a patient is the acceptance of him or her as a person and of all his or her other feelings, negative or unpleasant as well as positive.

Empathy is the desire and attempt to understand another person and his or her perception of experience. It implies sensing the meaning and feeling in another's communications, even if he or she does not explicitly state them. While it is not always possible to understand the patient's communications, the nurse's attempts to do so will be meaningful and encourage the person to continue communicating.

Kalisch states that empathy is an essential part of the interpersonal process and forms the basis for the nurse-patient relationship. She clarifies that empathy is for the patient's present, not his past, experience. The pa-

---

1. Carl Rogers, *On Becoming a Person* (Boston: Houghton-Mifflin Company, 1961), pp. 32-34.

tient's feelings change from day to day, and the nurse must tune in to today's experiences. Kalisch further states that the nurse must try to understand the patient's feelings during the interaction, when she or he can be helpful, not after the interaction is finished.[2]

Achieving the qualities of genuineness, acceptance, and empathy is not possible in every nurse-patient relationship, nor even possible completely in any one relationship, but they are goals toward which the nurse works. Their value to the patient is inestimable because, although the motivation for growth comes from within, the nurse can help create the proper psychological climate for that growth to occur.

A word about the differences between social and therapeutic relationships. Social relationships are reciprocal and geared toward serving a wide variety of emotional functions for both parties. The therapeutic relationship, on the other hand, is structured somewhat differently, although there are reciprocal elements. In a therapeutic relationship, one of the people is designated as a recipient of the "treatment" being provided by the other, who is designated as the "therapist." Judgments about what will take place in therapeutic relationships are always based on the welfare of the recipient.

Both social and therapeutic relationships entail involvement and investment. When a nurse engages a patient in a nurse-patient relationship, they must both invest in the relationship and value it if it is to accomplsh anything. Nurses do get legitimate satisfactions in such relationships, or they would not continue to be involved in them. But these satisfactions are a by-product, not the primary goal, and are derived from seeing the person develop new coping approaches. One of the difficulties nurses frequently run into when they are involved and invested in a relationship with a patient is maintaining their objectivity. They must do this so that they can constantly keep in mind the person's movement toward a more open coping style. One of the ways of achieving objectivity is through a review of data derived from the relationship with peers and supervisors.

▪ *The Nurse's Feelings and Reactions.* Self-understanding is basic to effective functioning in psychiatric nursing. The nurse's feelings and reactions influence her or his interactions with patients and may interfere if she or he is not aware of them. For example, one nurse became anxious

---

2. Beatrice Kalisch, "What is Empathy?", *American Journal of Nursing* 73 (Sept. 1973): 1548-1552.

whenever her patient was silent and asked the woman question after question in an attempt to initiate conversation. After a few minutes of questioning, the patient's anxiety increased and she walked away from the nurse. The nurse repeated this pattern of asking persistent questions on a number of occasions, always with the same result, because she was not aware that her behavior was an attempt to relieve her own anxiety. Only with difficulty did she recognize her anxiety, and only then was she able to control her behavior.

Feelings cannot always be controlled, in the sense of directly decreasing or eliminating them. Once a feeling is there, it is there, and it cannot be turned off as one would turn off a water faucet. It is behavior, not feelings, over which one does have direct control. A nurse may, for example, be so angry at a patient that he feels like hitting him The nurse cannot stop the angry feelings, but he can control his behavior and not strike the patient. The nurse can decide, instead, upon some appropriate action, such as leaving the situation until he calms down or telling the patient that such behavior makes him angry.

It is helpful, if at all possible, for the nurse to express the feeling she or he is experiencing, such as, "I'm feeling very angry right now," and then attempt to analyze with the patient what is going on between them to make her or him feel this way. If this approach is used appropriately, the patient may learn how his or her behavior affects others. Sometimes a situation is too emotionally charged to do this exploration with the patient. If this is the case, after such an interaction, the nurse should reflect on what happened and on how his or her feelings affected the interaction. He or she should try to understand the reasons for these feelings. For example, if she felt anxious, why was this so? Did she feel inadequate to help the patient? Was she afraid she would not know what to say, or would say the wrong thing? Through understanding how he or she felt and why, a nurse will be better equipped to direct his or her behavior, and in the next similar situation, be more effective in facilitating mutual exploration.

Eventually, the nurse can decrease the intensity of some feelings by understanding their source. For example, if the nurse's anxiety is the result of lack of knowledge or experience, acquiring more knowledge or experience can decrease the anxiety. Anxiety is the feeling that is most problematic in nurse-patient interactions because it is the most frequent reaction; hence, the nurse must always examine the sources of her or his

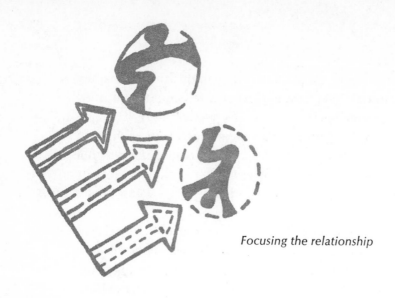

Focusing the relationship

anxiety and seek to resolve them. Most anxiety arises from the ambiguity of a situation. If the nurse clearly sees her or his role as being a listener and a person who assists the patient to explore new patterns of problem-solving, a great deal of anxiety may be eliminated. Focusing the relationship reduces both the nurse's anxiety and the patient's. Not to do so will decrease the individual's effectiveness as a nurse because anxiety prevents her or him from giving full attention to the patient and interferes with functioning to the best or his or her ability.

At times, the nurse's goal is not to decrease her or his feelings, but to accept them as common to all humans. Everyone experiences a variety of feelings, which are neither good nor bad, but simply a part of being human. Everyone, at times, feels anxiety, anger, and depression, and everyone, under sufficient stress, wants to be dependent on others. Nurses' recognition of these basic facts of the human condition will assist them to accept and be comfortable with both their own feelings and those of patients. An ability to be comfortable with their feelings allows nurses to express them in such a way that the patient can examine facets of the interaction that may provide insights into the difficulties he or she has in other settings.

Sometimes the source of the nurse's feelings is something going on between herself or himself and the patient. If the nurse feels, for example, anxious, angry, or depressed, and cannot account for why he or she feels this way, it is possible that the nurse is picking up the patient's feeling. Feelings are communicated from one person to another in subtle ways, perhaps through empathy. Awareness of this process is useful to the nurse in understanding the patient. Sometimes the patient does not manifest his or her feelings outwardly, and the nurse may know what the patient is experiencing only through awareness of her or his own feelings. One nurse, for instance, noticed that she felt irritated and angry each time she talked with a certain patient. She searched within herself and discussed her reactions with her supervisor, but could discern no reason for her anger. She concluded that the patient might be angry, though he did not outwardly appear so, and that his feelings of anger were being empathically communicated to her. This tentative conclusion was valuable to the nurse, because it alerted her to observe the patient for other manifestations of anger.

■ *Therapeutic and Nontherapeutic Responses.* Gendlin, in discussing the client-centered approach to counseling, sets down some guides for the therapist to follow.[3] The therapist focuses on the *feeling* the patient is expressing rather than the content or factual aspect of what he or she is saying. In responding to the patient, then, the nurse reflects the feeling the patient seems to be expressing. This feeling is not usually well-defined, but the nurse does the best she or he can to help clarify what the patient is experiencing. As the nurse and patient continue to talk, the patient's feelings will become clearer, and he or she will then understand the experience better. The important thing is for the nurse to be attuned to the patient rather than making a false construction of the situation. Sometimes the nurse can become entangled in subtle power struggles with patients over trying to make them recognize feelings that are not truly theirs or that they are not, at this point, capable of recognizing.

The nurse must take care, in talking with the patient, to stay with what concerns him or her and not change the subject or pursue a thought for the sake of personal interest or curiosity. Commonly, a tendency to change the subject comes from the nurse's anxiety about the topic the patient is introducing. In trying to understand what the patient is expressing, the nurse will need to try out different ideas, and they will not always

---

3. Eugene Gendlin, "Client-Centered: The Experiential Response," in *Use of Interpretation in Treatment,* ed. Emanuel Hammer (New York: Grune & Stratton, 1968), pp. 208-227.

be right. The nurse observes the patient's response carefully to determine whether she or he is accurately perceiving the meaning. If not, the nurse returns to the patient's original statement and tries again to understand.

As the interview continues, the nurse carefully follows each response the patient makes, whether or not the response is what was expected. Step by step, the nurse helps the patient understand more of what he or she feels. The goal is to help the patient understand his or her experiences better and relate his or her feelings to them. A person with a problem is usually unclear about it. A person who has had problem-solving difficulties usually is not able to understand how he or she gets into these repeated troubles. The nurse can help the person identify these difficulties and explore alternate behavior.

Hays, in a study of more than one hundred verbatim recordings of student-patient interactions, categorized student responses as therapeutic or nontherapeutic, depending upon whether they facilitated or cut off patient communication. Therapeutic responses were further divided into categories of offering self, giving broad openings, encouraging description, using silence, making observations, suggesting collaboration, giving information, reflecting, encouraging evaluation, and seeking consensual validation. The most frequent nontherapeutic responses were asking for explanations, introducing unrelated topics, reassuring, probing, and making stereotyped comments. Other nontherapeutic responses were offering advice, drawing unwarranted conclusions, testing, introducing personal data, and showing disapproval.[4] Many of the responses Hays classifies as therapeutic correspond with Gendlin's approach of helping the patient clarify his or her experience, while what Hays calls nontherapeutic responses direct the interview away from what the patient is trying to express. Each of the types of therapeutic and nontherapeutic responses will be discussed briefly.

THERAPEUTIC RESPONSES

Through *offering herself* or *himself,* the nurse indicates in some way a willingness to be available to the patient. The nurse might indicate this

---

4. Joyce Hays, "Analysis of Nurse-Patient Communication," *Nursing Outlook* 14 (Sept. 1966): 32-35.

verbally, for example, by saying, "I will stay with you until you feel better," or nonverbally by simply remaining with the patient. Being "with the patient" means more than physical presence. It entails communicating in some way that the nurse is on the patient's side, to help him or her seek out solutions to dilemmas.

Giving broad openings allows the patients to direct the interaction according to their needs. For instance, if a patient says, "What do you want to talk about?" the nurse might reply, "Whatever is on your mind." One nurse asked a patient, "How do things look to you now?" This broad opening allowed the patient to express her feelings, and she responded, "Well, I know this job isn't the answer to all my problems, and I really don't have any idea of what I want to do with my life, but it gives me something to do." A word of caution, however, about avoiding certain clichés that tend to become commonplace in some psychiatric settings. The most common cliché is an opening of "How are you feeling?" which is a carry-over from the physical-care settings with which the nurse is most familiar. The important part of initiating a communication is to indicate clearly that one is attempting to get in touch with the person as a person.

Encouraging description is similar to giving broad openings in that the nurse makes a comment to allow the patient to pursue what he or she has brought up. The nurse might say, "Go on," or "Could you tell me more about that?" or a similar statement, as in the following situation:

> *Nurse:* How did your weekend go?
> *Patient:* Terrible.
> *Nurse:* In what way?

The patient then explained why the weekend had not gone well.

Using silence is an essential skill for the nurse. Silent periods often produce anxiety, but they need not do so. Sometimes both patient and nurse need time during an interaction to think, and sometimes the nurse should wait out the silence until the patient brings up whatever is of concern. The nurse can also utilize silence to observe the patient's nonverbal communication, and this approach leads into the next area, *making observations*. Here the nurse comments on what the patient is communicating nonverbally. For instance, the nurse may say to a patient who is chain-smoking, "I notice you are smoking more than usual. Are you feeling nervous today?" Or to another patient, "You look sad when you talk about leaving the hospital." Making observations gives the patient an opening to discuss what he or she is feeling.

In the following interaction, the nurse used several approaches—offering oneself, using silence, encouraging description, giving broad openings:

> *Nurse:* After a morning of making myself available to the patient, I finally spoke to her: "Jan, dinner is here."
>
> *Patient:* (Remained curled up in bed.)
>
> *Nurse:* Would you like to tell me about it? I have about fifteen minutes before I leave.
>
> *Patient:* (Indicated no, but I felt she did not want me to go.)
>
> *Nurse:* After sitting with her about ten minutes, I said, "Could you tell me what is troubling you?"
>
> *Patient:* (After a pause) I'll never be able to work again.

From this the nurse and patient go on to explore her fear that she will never be able to return to her job.

In *suggesting collaboration,* the nurse enlists the patient's help in solving his or her problems. The nurse might say, for example, "Would you like to tell me more about this so we can together sort out what happened?" indicating that problem-solving is a mutual endeavor.

Giving information allows patients to arrive at their own decisions or conclusions. For instance, to a patient who said, "What if I won't take my medicine?", the nurse replied, "Then the voices you have been hearing will probably come back." In the following example, the patient was questioning the nurse about his disease:

> *Nurse:* During a discussion of the patient's illness, I said, "Some epileptics can be controlled. If they take their medicine and regulate their living patterns, they don't have too many problems."
>
> *Patient:* Can epileptics get married?
>
> *Nurse:* I don't see why not. You probably would need to talk to your doctor about the type of epilepsy you have and how this might affect children you might have.
>
> *Patient:* Can I be controlled?
>
> *Nurse:* We don't know enough about what particular type of epilepsy you have, but most types can be controlled or treated. As soon as we know we will tell you more about your particular type.

Reflecting back to the patient what he or she is expressing, especially feelings, helps the patient understand better what he or she is experiencing and also communicates that the nurse understands these feelings. When a young patient with a degenerative disease that kept him confined to a wheelchair said that he wanted to go to college and have a girlfriend like other boys his age, the nurse said. "It must be very sad to have lost these things that you want very badly." In reflecting upon the person's communication, the purpose is to tie together these communications and use them as a means of getting the patient in touch with his or her feelings. As with all forms of communication, it is important to clearly differentiate the patient's feelings from the nurse's. In the example given, one might very easily picture oneself in the patient's situation and think that one would certainly feel sad. But it is important to keep the focus on what the patient is experiencing rather than imputing one's own feelings to the patient, or else clearly stating, "If I were in your position, I would feel sad." This is particularly important in situations in which the patient has difficulty in maintaining his or her ego boundaries.

Encouraging evaluation assists the patient to examine the various facets of a situation as well as his or her ideas and feelings about it. In the following situation, the patient was asking to be discharged:

Patient: I want to get a room somewhere; then I'll be forced to decide something.

Nurse: Do you really think that once you get a room you will be able to decide about a job?

Patient: (No reply.)

Nurse: (After a pause) I'm not quite sure what brought you to the hospital originally.

Patient: I tried to commit suicide.

Nurse: Have things changed so that you don't feel the same way any more?

Patient: Nothing much has changed, but I'm not getting any help in here.

Nurse: We've arranged for you to go out on job interviews, but you don't seem to want to pursue this. What other kinds of help could we be giving?

Patient: Well, I'm not worth much to anyone. Why should I get a job? I only have to pay alimony to my wife and kids, and they don't care for me.

Nurse: I think you could get some help in sorting some of these things out while you stay in the hospital.

NONTHERAPEUTIC RESPONSES

Requesting explanations often takes the form of "why" questions. Since patients frequently do not know the "why" of a situation, asking such questions does not help them explore what occurred. For example, to a patient who said she had not been sleeping well for several weeks, the nurse asked, "Why not?"

Introducing unrelated topics directs the conversation away from the patient's concerns and interest. When a patient told the nurse he had attempted suicide on two occasions, the nurse, being surprised and not knowing what to say, changed the subject by asking, "Did your wife visit last night?"

Offering false reassurance is usually meaningless to the patient. When a patient said she wondered if she would ever get better, the nurse said, "I'm sure you will." The important thing to note about giving reassurance is that it has the effect of cutting off communication rather than facilitating exploration. However, there are certain instances in which the nurse can give reassurance that helps the person structure his or her expectations. For example, the person who has lost a loved one has an intense feeling of loss. It may be helpful to tell such a person that in a week or so the intensity of this feeling will diminish.

Probing, or asking unnecessary questions, may be insensitive to the patient's feelings and needs. One nurse asked a patient question after question ("How long have you been in the hospital?", "Are you from this area?", "Does your family live here?", and so on) until the patient finally said, "You're just like all the rest. All you want is information." On the other hand, probing for the meaning of what the person is saying may serve to facilitate in-depth exploration.

Making stereotyped comments is likewise insensitive and communicates that the nurse is not tuned in to the patient and his or her feelings. To a patient who said he was being discharged the next day, the nurse said, "That's good." The patient may not have thought it was good, but the nurse's stereotyped response kept him from expressing what he felt.

Offering advice serves to reinforce the helplessness of the patient's position. It is the patient who ultimately must decide for herself or himself. One nurse said to a patient, "I think you should have an abortion. You have so many problems already, and another baby would only add to them." Instead, it would have been helpful if the nurse had encouraged the patient to explore her feelings about being pregnant and the alternative options that were available to her. It is important that the nurse withhold value judgments and encourage patients to make decisions that are based upon their own value systems.

Drawing unwarranted conclusions may cut off communication if the nurse's conclusion is incorrect. To a depressed patient, the nurse said, "From what you've said, it seems your depression is because you don't feel needed any more." Instead, the nurse could facilitate the patient's exploration by a statement such as, "Can you identify what it is that makes you feel this way?"

Testing of the patient is not therapeutic. One nurse came late to a meeting with a patient to see what he would do. Patients often test the nurse, but the reverse is not appropriate.

Introducing personal data must be done with thought about its effect upon the patient. While giving information about oneself or one's experiences is sometimes helpful, more often it has no meaning to the patient, who is more concerned about his or her own situation. If the patient asks the nurse personal information, he or she can reply briefly and refocus the conversation on the patient.

Showing disapproval conveys rejection and a lack of understanding of the patient. To an unmarried pregnant patient who said she wanted to give her baby up for adoption, the nurse said, "How could you give up your own child?"

THE NURSING PROCESS

Nursing intervention takes place within the context of the nursing process, that is, the planning, implementing, and evaluating of nursing care. Planning intervention entails collecting data, identifying needs, and determining specific nursing care goals and interventions. Implementation is carrying out the planned intervention. Evaluation entails assessing the effectiveness of the intervention and planning how it might be improved in the future. It is important that the patient and nurse share these activities so that there is mutual agreement about the goals of the nurse-patient relationship.

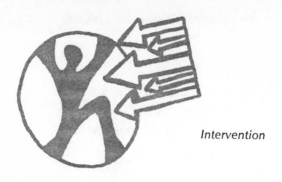

Intervention

To begin planning, the nurse has several sources of data or information about the patient—the patient's own communications, the nurse's observations, the patient's family and friends, observations of other staff, and the chart. The patient's verbal and nonverbal communication is the nurse's primary source of data. Through words and behavior, the patient provides the nurse with data about his or her problems and needs. Occasionally, if the nurse observes and listens to the patient attentively, she or he will note discrepancies between reports of family members and what is recorded on the chart. Such discrepancies should be noted, for they frequently are clues about the way the patient's social network reinforces his or her problems. Observation also provides cues for ways in which the nurse may alter the person's behavioral patterns within the social network. Through empathy and attentive listening and observation, the nurse may gain an idea of the patient's usual coping patterns. It is appropriate for the nurse to check this conceptualization of the patient's difficulties, and from it identify particular problems to work on. A plan of care should be based on mutual agreement between the patient and nurse about what the patient sees as needing to be changed.

A prime requisite for the successful implementation of a plan, which of course requires consistency among other staff members, is a workable format for communication. Although the format for communicating may change from time to time and from place to place, a very workable system is the problem-oriented psychiatric record. When this format is used, staff perceptions of the patients' problems are the organizing focus for formulating treatment goals. (Several of the references given in "Further Readings" pertain to this system.)

As a guide to collecting data, the nurse may organize his or her observations under three categories: appearance, behavior, and conversation. Specific observations possible within each category are numerous, and only a few examples will be given. Regarding appearance: Is the patient neat, slovenly, meticulous? Does he or she attend to personal hygiene and grooming? Does she or he appear anxious, depressed, elated, angry? Regarding behavior: How does the patient spend his or her time? Does he interact with others? Is she restless, agitated, withdrawn? Regarding conversation: Does the patient talk to others? To whom and when? What does she talk about? What does she avoid talking about? Does he manifest delusions, hallucinations, a thinking disorder?

These three areas of appearance, behavior, and conversation will give the nurse some guidelines for observing patient behavior. Although these observations provide a general impression, it is important to place them in perspective. Appearances can be deceiving. For example, persons in rebellion against society adopt particular styles of dressing as indicative of their revolt. Also, it is important to place these observations in a social and cultural context.

Family and friends, if they are sympathetic toward the patient, can also be a valuable source of information about his or her recent and past behavior. They can relate their perception of how the patient has changed and when these changes began. The nurse can also observe the interaction between them and the patient. If the family seems antagonistic toward the patient, the nurse should be aware that their antagonism probably biases their views. The converse is also true; for example, the mother who is oversolicitous of her son has a biased view of his behavior.

Other staff's observations can be combined with those of the nurse to give a more comprehensive picture of the patient. In addition to general observations, other staff can provide specific helpful information, such as a family history or psychological test results. The chart is an extension of the staff and may also be useful to the nurse. For instance, from it the nurse can learn why the patient came or was brought for help, if he or she does not say. Reading the chart is of no particular benefit, however, in initiating a relationship with a patient. In fact, it may interfere. Sometimes nurses, having read the chart, initiate conversations as if they already "knew" the patient, which, from the patient's point of view, is confusing. It results in depersonalization. Knowing the details of a patient's history and behavior does not assist the nurse to relate to him or her as a unique person.

After collecting data, the next step in planning care is to identify needs; from the needs evolve specific goals and interventions. An example will clarify this process:

> A nursing student noticed that Mr. B., a recently admitted patient, spent a great deal of time in his room and did not talk to any of the staff or patients. His family brought him to the hospital because he had quit school and his job and did nothing now but sit around the house. When the student talked to him, he looked at her but did not reply. On the basis of the above data, indicating primarily withdrawn behavior, the student decided Mr. B., although needing to relate to others, feared the closeness involved in relating to others. For several days she sat quietly in his room. Finally he began to talk with her in a limited way. As he became trusting of her, the student gradually encouraged activities that involved others on the unit and thus helped him begin to overcome his fears of relating to others. She phrased her nursing care goal in terms of reducing his fears of relating.

After the plan is decided on and implemented, the intervention must be evaluated. In fact, some evaluation takes place even as the intervention is being carried out. As the nurse is interacting with a patient, she or he observes the effect of the interaction and alters the approach if necessary. The nurse also evaluates the intervention after each interaction, recalling and analyzing what took place.

In the situation of Mr. B. just described, for example, the student carried out her plan and began to spend time with him each day. After three days, she became discouraged because his withdrawn behavior continued, and she talked with her supervisor about changing her approach. The supervisor pointed out that patients as isolated as Mr. B. do not change their behavior quickly and suggested the student continue her approach and observe him for small signs of improvement. As the student did this, she began to notice that Mr. B. was becoming less tense and looking at her and other people more frequently. After three or four weeks, he was talking to her and beginning to relate in small groups.

This example brings out two other aspects of evaluation. One is that the nurse does not change his or her intervention approach without allowing adequate time. To expect rapid or immediate improvement in patients is unrealistic. Behavior changes gradually, and new behaviors will be inconsistent at first. The nurse must allow the patient time to experiment with new behavior. She or he likewise should appreciate small improvements and expect that patients will sometimes fall back into their previous behavior. The other aspect of evaluation brought out in the situation with Mr. B. is that supervision is helpful and sometimes essential in deciding whether to change one's approach and what changes to make. Discussing interactions with the patient with a supervisor will help the nurse view the patient's behavior more objectively. Supervision gives the nurse the opportunity to validate his or her observations and ideas with another person.

■ *Process Recordings and the Nursing Care Plan.*   Process recordings and the nursing care plan are two tools useful to the nurse in planning, implementing, and evaluating care. The process recording is a written record of the nurse-patient interaction. It includes the verbal and nonverbal behavior of both the nurse and the patient. It is also helpful to include at the end of each process recording the nurse's interpretation of the interaction—what she or he felt was its meaning, as well as any observations she or he wishes to record for future reference. The nurse should also think about what his or her feelings were during the interaction and record them as a help in analyzing their significance in the interaction. The process recording is a source of data in planning intervention, as well as a record of the actual intervention and a document to study when evaluating it.

The nursing care plan is an organized way of recording the patient's needs, the nursing care goals and intervention, and an evaluation of the intervention. If nursing care is to be purposeful, it is necessary to have specific goals and interventions and to evaluate the interventions regularly. The nursing care plan will facilitate this process. A written plan requires that the nurse organize his or her thoughts and state specifically what he or she intends to do. It also provides an opportunity for regular evaluation and serves as a written record of the evaluation and the changes resulting from it.

PHASES OF THE NURSE-PATIENT RELATIONSHIP

In analyzing a relationship between a nurse and a patient, one can distinguish different phases with identifiable characteristics. Authors label the phases of a relationship in various ways. In this book, they are called the initiating, working, and terminating phases. Although it is useful for purposes of analysis and discussion to separate a relationship into phases, it is also important to remember that there is no clear-cut division between the phases. Progression from one phase to the next is gradual, and the change may be imperceptible at the time. Also, certain characteristics of one phase may carry over into the next phase. For example, characteristics of the initiating phase may appear from time to time in the working or even in the terminating phase.

■ *Initiating Phase.* During the initiating phase, the nurse and the patient become acquainted with each other and arrive at an agreement about a meeting time. The initiating phase is characterized by the beginning development of trust, by the nurse's observing the patient in order to understand her or his needs, and by obtaining the patient's view of her or his problem. The major goal of this phase is to establish a trusting relationship. This can only be accomplished through an open communication network. The chief problem in achieving such a pattern of communication is the anxiety of both patient and nurse.

Becoming acquainted is an important aspect of the initiating phase. The nurse and the patient must get to know each other as persons. Nurses who are learning to form a relationship with a patient often overlook the patient's need to become acquainted with the nurse. Such nurses seem to want to start a relationship in the middle instead of at the beginning, and they tend to push the patient. A nurse may, for example, ask personal questions she or he would not think of asking in another setting. In so doing, the nurse is responding to his or her own anxiety, not the patient's needs. The nurse needs to remember that the patient needs time to get to know her or him.

Becoming acquainted is the beginning of the larger process of developing trust, which is the foundation of the nurse-patient relationship. Patients who trust the nurse believe she or he is interested in their personal welfare and will accept them as a person, despite their problems. Trust will enable patients to expose their deep thoughts and feelings, even if they are ashamed of them, because they know the nurse will not reject them. Every patient has a need to learn to trust. Persons who are emotionally or mentally disturbed have difficulty trusting other people. Before a patient can begin to work through problems with another person, he or she must have some trust in that person. Some patients have such difficulty with trust that the development of it becomes the goal of the entire nurse-patient relationship, not only of the initiating phase.

How can the nurse nurture a feeling of trust? She or he can be consistent, reliable, and honest with the patient. If a nurse says, for example, that she or he will talk to the patient every day from 11:00 to 11:30 a.m., the nurse does so. If, on a certain day, circumstances require that the time be changed, the nurse explains this. Through the nurse's consistent and reliable behavior, the patient learns that one can depend on her or him to do what is promised. Honesty also supports the development of trust. A patient who asks a question is entitled to an honest answer. The qualities of genuineness, acceptance, and empathy, discussed earlier in this chapter, also contribute to the development of trust.

While trust is developing in the relationship, the patient will test the nurse's interest. Testing takes many forms. The patient may show rejection initially to ascertain whether the nurse will persist, or may withdraw at some point later in the relationship. The patient may express anger or some other feeling to see whether the nurse will still accept her or him. He or she may ask the nurse to do some favor, to see whether the nurse will comply and to test the limits of the relationship. These are a few ways that patients test nurses. If the nurse passes the test, trust will be strengthened. Some patients continue to test the nurse periodically during the relationship, probably because they need a reaffirmation of interest.

The contract. Setting up the contract is a formal way of saying that the nurse and the patient come to an agreement about the days, time, and place of their meetings, the length of time the relationship will continue, and the goals of the relationship. The agreement may be arrived at in any number of ways, and no one way is right for all nurses and all patients. One important component of the agreement is that the patient understand how long the relationship will continue. The patient also needs to know how much time the nurse will spend with him or her each day and what days to expect a meeting. Some patients will be too confused or anxious to remember what the nurse says, and the information should be repeated as often as necessary.

The nurse should decide on a way of setting up the contract that will be comfortable for both participants. Many students who are making their first agreement with a patient go about it in an unnecessarily formal way because they are anxious, and thus increase both their own and the patient's anxiety. It would be preferable for such students to make the agreement one step at a time, giving the patient an opportunity to think about each aspect. Many students find that a comfortable approach is to say, after talking with the patient a few times, that she or he has enjoyed spending this time and would like to see the patient each day that the nurse is in the hospital. After the nurse and the patient have talked about this, the nurse can bring up the details of time and place.

It is advisable to limit the length of time the nurse and patient will spend together each day. Some patients have a tendency to become dependent and will use all the nurse's time if some limits are not set. Excessive dependence is an emotional drain on the nurse and is not in the patient's best interest. What the length of time should be depends upon the patient's need and is a judgment the nurse makes, with the assistance of the supervisor if necessary.

The nurse should expect some anxiety from the patient when the contract is set up, even if it is done in a relaxed and informal manner. The thought of entering into a relationship is threatening to most patients. They fear their shortcomings will be revealed, or that the nurse has certain expectations they will not be able to meet. Also, because their self-esteem is low, they may be unable to believe that someone is interested in them as individuals. Such feelings and ideas cause anxiety, and the patient will need reassurance. The general purpose of the meetings should be explained, but with the qualification that the nurse does not expect any particular behavior from the patient, who may use the time as he or she wishes.

Determining needs. During the initiating phase of the relationship, as the nurse and the patient become acquainted and trust is developing, the nurse has the opportunity to observe the patient and collect data about his or her behavior. From these observations, and through interaction with the patient, a definition of the patient's problems will emerge. As the contract is developed, the patient and nurse should identify together some problem(s) that they agree to work on. It is important that this be a point of mutual agreement that provides a focus for the relationship.

Anxiety. Anxiety in both the nurse and the patient is the major problem encountered in the initiating phase. One source of this anxiety—the patient's fears about entering into a relationship—was mentioned in the discussion of setting up the contract. The nurse, too, will have anxiety on entering into a relationship, especially if this is her or his first relationship with a person seeking psychiatric treatment. Beginning nurses may feel inexperienced and perhaps incapable of helping the patient. Since they are not yet acquainted with the patient, they do not know what behavior to expect, and this very uncertainty is anxiety-producing. They do not have the usual nursing procedures to carry out and may be at a loss for something to say or do. They may feel the supervisor expects them to function in a certain way, and that they will receive a poor evaluation if they do not perform well.

All these issues should be discussed with the supervisor. In this way, the nurse can discover the supervisor's expectations as well as obtain some relief from the anxiety through talking about it. She or he can also examine the cause or causes for the anxiety and thus increase self-understanding. In addition, the supervisor may have some specific ideas or suggestions that will help the nurse. As the relationship becomes focused on working on certain problems, the nurse's anxiety will decrease.

▪ *Working phase.* The working phase begins when some trust has developed and the nurse and the patient begin to work toward the nursing care goals. Travelbee says the introductory phase (as she terms it) ends when the patient and the nurse begin to view each other as unique human beings, which may take a few minutes or a few days.[5]

During the working phase, while the patient and nurse work on the problems identified, the nurse continues to collect data and continuously evaluates the patient's progress.

▪ *Terminating phase.* There are different reasons why termination of the nurse-patient relationship becomes necessary. The nurse's experience in that setting may be ending, the patient is discharged, or the mutually agreed-on goals have been attained. Whatever the reason for termination, it precipitates a feeling reaction in both participants, usually one of sadness and loss. Both persons in the relationship experience what is called separation anxiety at the ending of a meaningful relationship, and both will react in some way.

Patient's reactions. Sene discusses three types of patient reactions to separation—regression, withdrawal, and an attempt to prolong the rela-

5. Joyce Travelbee, *Intervention in Psychiatric Nursing: Process in the One-to-One Relationship* (Philadelphia: F. A. Davis Company, 1969), p. 146.

tionship.[6] In what she characterizes as a regressive reaction, the patient's anxiety results in exhibiting increased symptoms; for example, delusions that were previously given up may reappear. A reappearance of symptoms is upsetting to staff, who may conclude that the patient is not ready for discharge. However, regressions at the time of discharge or separation are usually temporary, and the patient will regain his or her former level of functioning in a few days if given support.

In some cases patients try to deal with their feelings by abruptly withdrawing from the relationship. Typically, they may reject the nurse, refuse to meet, miss meetings, or talk only about superficial topics. If the patient is withdrawing gradually, he or she will talk less about problems and feelings and assert his or her independence more. Withdrawal of emotional investment is necessary if the relationship cannot continue. Gradual withdrawal at the end of a relationship is healthy.

Sometimes a patient will attempt to prolong the relationship by refusing to discuss termination, by bringing up new problems, or by suggesting the nurse write or telephone.

Nurses' reactions. Nurses, too, experience a loss at the termination of a meaningful relationship with a patient, and they, too, react to the impending separation. Sene discusses nurses' reaction—feeling guilty and devaluing their contribution, anger, avoidance, and intensifying the relationship.[7] Nurses, may feel they are abandoning the patient while he or she still needs them, and such a realization arouses guilt feelings. Guilt may also be aroused if nurses feel they have contributed little to the patient's progress. Pessimism about the patient's future and devaluing their own contributions are common reactions. Another reaction is anger, which may be directed at society or the patient's family for making him or her sick, or at the hospital or the nurse's supervisor for not giving more assistance. The nurse may also avoid discussing the subject of termination with the patient or the supervisor, or may attempt to prolong or intensify the relationship, for example, by spending more time with the patient or agreeing to write or telephone later.

Intervention. Preparation for termination begins when the nurse initiates a relationship with a patient. At that time, it is understood that the

---

6. Barbara Sene, "Termination in the Student-Patient Relationship," *Perspectives in Psychiatric Care* 7, no. 1 (1969): 39-45.
7. Ibid.

relationship will continue until the patient or the nurse leaves the setting, and the patient is told the length of the nurse's time there.

As the time for termination draws near, the nurse reminds the patient of this fact and discusses it with her or him. Two or three weeks before termination is usually time enough to bring it up. There needs to be sufficient time for the nurse and the patient to work through their feelings, but introducing the topic too early might result in premature termination.

The first step in dealing with the feelings and reactions of both nurse and patient is to identify what they are. Only then will the nurse be in a position to do anything about them. Many nurses are reluctant to deal with termination because of the pain involved, and they need encouragement from the supervisor to do so.

The nurse's intervention should concentrate on discussing termination with the patient, decreasing his or her dependence, and dealing with any special problems that arise. In discussing the feelings surrounding termination, the patient may be encouraged to express these feelings if the nurse expresses hers or his first. Termination is painful to discuss, and it is unlikely that the patient will spontaneously initiate expressing these feelings. Sene suggests that the nurse and the patient review the relationship and exchange memories of its satisfying and difficult aspects. This is a way of solidifying the patient's gains and pointing out progress.[8]

Near the end of the relationship, the nurse should attempt to decrease the patient's dependence on her or him. This may be done in a number of ways. The nurse might lessen the intensity of the relationship by decreasing the time spent together or, if the patient is to remain in treatment, by including other people in the relationship. The latter approach will help the patient transfer his or her emotional investment to other people. The nurse should discuss with the patient the reason for such actions and the necessity of terminating their relationship. The nurse can also explore with the patient what life will be like after he or she is discharged or the nurse leaves the hospital. Discussing these matters ahead of time will enable the patient to adjust better when the time comes.

If the patient's reaction to termination is to avoid it or to try to intensify the relationship, the nurse needs to talk to the patient about this and help him or her to deal with these feelings. For instance, the nurse

---

8. Ibid.

might mention certain behavior and suggest or ask if the patient is reacting to termination. The patient may be helped to deal with his or her feelings if the nurse also acknowledges that separation is difficult.

To deal with her or his own feelings about termination, the nurse should seek supervisory help. This is a necessity for the inexperienced nurse because these feelings may cause her or him to distort what is going on in the relationship or to use it to meet her or his own needs rather than those of the patient. Talking to the supervisor about the situation will help the nurse clarify his or her feelings about the patient's feelings and reactions and to decide upon a reasonable plan for termination.

SUMMARY

Nurses play a vital role in the overall treatment process. Their most valuable assets are their own personalities, through which they can engage patients in relationships that differ from their past patterns. In the context of these relationships, the patient can examine the difficulties he or she has in relating to people and develop more adequate means of interacting. Self-understanding is important to the nurse as a protection from entering into and reinforcing distorted relationships with patients. The most helpful form of interaction encourages the patient's open exploration of his or her problems with honest feedback as to how the patient comes across to others. Commonly there are three phases to any therapeutic relationship: (1) the initiating phase, in which goals are developed and trust is established; (2) the working phase, in which movement toward achieving those goals takes place; and (3) the terminating phase, in which the benefits accrued in the relationship are consolidated. The terminating phase represents a prototypical separation, which provides an opportunity for the person to prepare for other separations he or she might anticipate in the future.

FURTHER READINGS

Aguilera, Donna. "The Use of Physical Contact (Touch) as a Technique of Nonverbal Communication With Psychiatric Patients." *ANA 1965 Regional Clinical Conferences* 4 (1966): 33-38.

Andrews, Dixie. "A Process-Recording on a Schizophrenic-Hebephrenic Patient." *Perspectives in Psychiatric Care* 1, no. 5 (1963): 11-39.

Babrick, Marie. "Re-Learning Through a One-to-One Relationship." *Perspectives in Psychiatric Care* 2, no. 5 (1964): 23-28.

Bermosk, Loretta. "Interviewing: A Key to Therapeutic Communication in Nursing Practice." *Nursing Clinics of North America* 1 (June 1966): 205-214.

Christoffers, Carol. "An Existential Encounter." *Perspectives in Psychiatric Care* 5, no. 4 (1967): 174-181.

Davis, Barbara C.; Fleming, Mary Jo; McCormick, Maryann and Bealcher, Joyce. "Implementation of Problem Oriented Charting in a Large, Regional Community Hospital." *Journal of Nursing Administration* (Nov.-Dec. 1974): 33-41.

Dillon, Kathryn. "A Patient-Structured Relationship." *Perspectives in Psychiatric Care* 9, no. 4 (1971): 167-172.

Donahue, S. M. "The I-Thou Relationship." *Nursing Outlook* 14 (Aug. 1966): 59-61.

Ehmann, Virginia. "Empathy: Its Origin, Characteristics, and Progress." *Perspectives in Psychiatric Care* 9, no. 2 (1971): 72-80.

Flynn, Gertrude. "The Nurse's Role: Interference or Intervention." *Perspectives in Psychiatric Care* 7, no. 4 (1969): 170-176.

Geach, Barbara. "The Problem-Solving Technique." *Perspectives in Psychiatric Care* 12, no. 1 (1974): 9-12.

Geach, Barbara, and White, James. "Empathic Resonance: Countertransference." *American Journal of Nursing* 74 (July 1974): 1282-1285.

Hagerman, Zerita. "Teaching Beginners to Cope With Extreme Behavior." *American Journal of Nursing* 68 (Sept. 1968): 1927-1929.

Hays, Joyce. "Analysis of Nurse-Patient Communications." *Nursing Outlook* 14 (Sept. 1966): 32-35.

Hays, Joyce, and Myers, Janesy. "Learning in the Nurse-Patient Relationship." *Perspectives in Psychiatric Care* 2, no. 3 (1964): 20-29.

Hobart, John. "The Problem of Silence in a Nurse-Patient Relationship." *Perspectives in Psychiatric Care* 2, no. 5 (1964): 29-34.

Holmes, Marguerite, and Werner, Jean. *Psychiatric Nursing in a Therapeutic Community*, pp. 75-102. New York: The Macmillan Company, 1966.

Joel, Lucille, and Davis, Shirley. "A Proposal for Base Line Data Collection for Psychiatric Care." *Perspectives in Psychiatric Care* 11, no. 2 (1973): 48-58.

Johnson, Betty. "The Blotting Paper Syndrome: A Counter-Transference Phenomenon." *Perspectives in Psychiatric Care* 5, no. 5 (1967): 228-230.

Johnson, Betty, and Myers, Janesy. "Learning in the Nurse-Patient Relationship." *Perspectives in Psychiatric Care* 2, no. 3 (1964): 20-29.

Kachelski, Audrey. "The Nurse-Patient Relationship." *American Journal of Nursing* 61 (May 1961): 76-81.

Kalisch, Beatrice. "What Is Empathy?" *American Journal of Nursing* 73 (Sept. 1973): 1548-1552.

Mansfield, Elaine. "Empathy: Concept and Identified Nursing Behavior." *Nursing Research* 22 (1973): 626-530.

Melat, Shirley. "The Development of Trust." *Perspectives in Psychiatric Care* 3, no. 4 (1965): 29-35.

Mercer, Lianne. "Touch: Comfort or Threat?" *Perspectives in Psychiatric Care* 4, no. 3 (1966): 20-25.

Morris, Karen. "Approach-Avoidance Conflict in the Orientation Phase of Therapy." *ANA Regional Clinical Conferences, 1967,* pp. 289-298. New York: Appleton-Century-Crofts, 1968.

Naugle, Ethel. "The Difference Caring Makes." *American Journal of Nursing* 73 (Nov. 1973): 1890-1891.

Nehren, Jeanette, and Gilliam, Naomi. "Separation Anxiety." *American Journal of Nursing* 65 (Jan. 1965): 109-112.

Parks, Suzanne. "Allowing Physical Distance as a Nursing Approach." *Perspectives in Psychiatric Care* 4, no. 6 (1966): 31-35.

Phillips, Bonnie. "Terminating a Nurse-Patient Relationship." *American Journal of Nursing* 68 (Sept. 1968): 1941-1942.

Phillips, Lorraine. "Language in Disguise: Non-Verbal Communication With Patients." *Perspectives in Psychiatric Care* 4, no. 4 (1966): 18-21.

Rector, Cynthia. "Indices in the Development of a Working Relationship in Nurse-Patient Psychotherapy." *ANA Convention Clinical Sessions 10* (1964): 26-31.

Schaefer, Jeannette. "The Interrelatedness of Decision Making and the Nursing Process." *American Journal of Nursing* 74 (Oct. 1974): 1852-1855.

Schwartz, Morris, and Shockley, Emmy. *The Nurse and the Mental Patient,* pp. 218-281. New York: John Wiley & Sons, Inc., 1956.

Stastny, Joy. "Helping a Patient Learn to Trust." *Perspectives in Psychiatric Care* 3, no. 7 (1965): 16-20.

Steiger, Thelma. "Shadow Child." *American Journal of Nursing* 73 (Dec. 1973): 2080-2086.

Tescher, Barbara. "Distance Maneuvers." *Perspectives in Psychiatric Care* 2, no. 2 (1964): 19-23.

Travelbee, Joyve. *Intervention in Psychiatric Nursing: Process in the One-to-One Relationship.* Philadelphia: F. A. Davis Company, 1969.

Ujhely, Gertrud. "The Uses and Abuses of the So-Called 'Nondirective Technique' in Nursing." *ANA Regional Clinical Conferences, 1967,* pp. 299-303. New York: Appleton-Century-Crofts, 1968.

Van Dervort, Dolores. "Both Hands Clapping." *American Journal of Nursing* 73 (June 1973): 999-1000.

Vidoni, Clotilda. "The Development of Intense Positive Countertransference Feelings in the Therapist Toward a Patient." *American Journal of Nursing* 75 (March 1975): 407-409.

Weed, L. L. "The problem-oriented record as a basic tool." In *Medical Records, Medical Education and Patient Care.* Cleveland Press of Case Western Reserve University, distributed by Year Book Medical Publishers, Inc., 1969.

Woody, Mary and Mallison, Mary. "Problem-Oriented System for Patient-Centered Care." *American Journal of Nursing* 73 (July 1973): 1168-1175.

Zerad, Loretta T. "Empathic Nursing. Realization of a Human Capacity." *Nursing Clinics of North America* 4 (1969): 622-655.

CHAPTER TEN

ANTICIPATORY COUNSELING AND CRISIS INTERVENTION

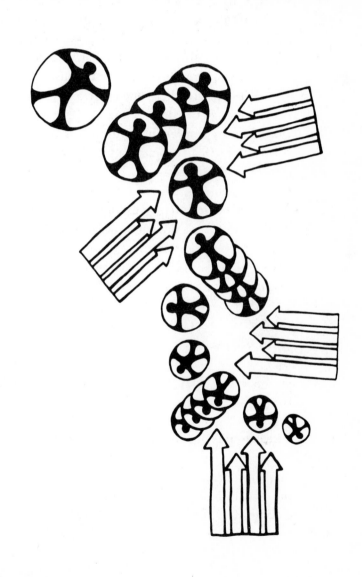

Earlier in this book, we have defined a crisis as a turning point where a person is confronted by a situation in which his or her usual problem-solving mechanisms no longer work. Faced with a problem one temporarily is unable to solve, one may retreat into a maladaptive pattern of problem-solving or may develop an innovative solution. Depending on the response, one may either end up more constricted in one's problem-solving capabilities or, through an innovative approach, develop heightened abilities to deal with problematic situations.

At the point where one is mired in the dilemma—before he or she has been able to figure out any anxiety-reducing moves—one recalls other situations that are similar in nature to the present problem. These prior situations automatically come to mind. Thus, as one attempts to solve a current crisis situation, one is also in a sense reworking prior attempts to resolve similar problems. Because of this facet of crisis work, a person is much more amenable to change, for good or for ill, whenever he or she is experiencing a crisis situation. Because of the increased vulnerability at these points, it is important that those who assist the person be aware of the nature of crisis work and be prepared to assist him or her in reaching new and more satisfying problem resolutions.

Most commonly, people experiencing difficulties do not contact a psychiatric agency for help. Rather they seek help from family members, ministers, friends, fellow workers, family physicians, and sometimes nurses; they look to those immediately available to them for help and frequently do not define their problem as a mental health problem in need of professional psychiatric treatment. Most crisis intervention work is never identified as such but, is described as "helping someone get back on his feet." The columns of Ann Landers and "Dear Abby" represent another form in which the general public gets advice on how to deal with problems that may or may not be defined as crises. One common type of letter concerns the husband who has run off with his young, attractive secretary; the wife, feeling shattered, writes for advice. The usual response of "You're fortu-

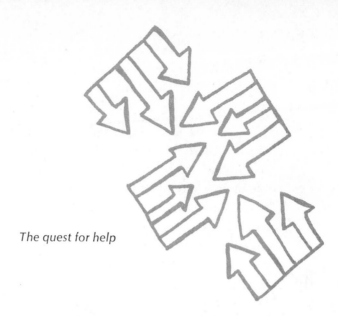

The quest for help

nate to be rid of the louse," while not usually viewed as crisis intervention, certainly is advice about how to solve the problem in such a way that the woman's self-esteem is maintained.

Sometimes, when people reach out to their family and friends for help in confronting a problematic situation, the help they receive increases or magnifies the problem rather than helping them reach new and better resolutions. Take, for example, the pregnant woman who, while not yet in crisis, is bombarded with horror tales of all the dreadful things that have happened to other women—women who have been in labor for twenty-four hours, those who have delivered deformed or retarded children, and the like. In these instances, the help proffered reflects the giver's views and is perhaps part of his or her unresolved dilemmas. Its effect is to generate increased anxiety in the person receiving the information, and its result may be to create a crisis rather than to help the person deal with the situation. In other instances, the magnitude or unusualness of the problem may exhaust the usual network of informal crisis interveners.

Whom, then, does the person turn to in seeking an answer to these seemingly insoluble dilemmas? And how might these situations be used to help the person achieve more positive resolutions than those reached in similar situations in the past?

TYPICAL LIFE CRISES

First, let us examine some of the life crises that all individuals face. We have described crises as being of two types: developmental or maturational, and accidental or situational. There are predictable points in the life cycle where some persons have difficulty making necessary role transitions. The move from childhood to adulthood, represented in the stage of adolescence, is commonly viewed as a crisis both for the adolescent and for his or her parents. Although becoming engaged and moving toward marriage is regarded as a happy event for most couples, in our research into family beginnings, planning the wedding was identified by most couples as a situation of great stress, and in some instances it constitutes a crisis.[1] Parenting, another common role transition, is a period of major role disruption, a time when people redefine themselves and their relationship to one another. Similarly, moving into the world of work, going into a new career pattern, or making readjustments that accompany retirement are periods in the life history of a person when he or she is likely to seek help from others and is more vulnerable to processing and using help.

Accidental crises are also predictable to a degree. All people encounter various losses. Almost everyone experiences some loss of body integrity, through specific disease problems, accidents, or the natural aging process. Loss of body integrity may occur in conjunction with some surgical procedure, such as mastectomy or other amputation. It may also accompany the loss of some capacity, such as that incurred in certain debilitating diseases, for example, muscular dystrophy. As persons age, they experience the loss or diminution of many physical capacities of their youth.

Another form of accidental crisis is the loss of loved ones. The death of a parent or spouse is a disrupting experience that causes one to reexamine the meaning of his or her own mortality. Loss of a loved one also entails a shifting of roles. Death is not the only form of this loss; divorce, separation, or distancing of persons in a marriage over the years, as both go separate ways and there is no longer any psychological closeness, are other forms.

---

1. Helen Grace and Kathleen Knafl, "Family Beginnings: The Dynamics of Role Making," in *Psychiatric Nursing: Perspectives-Issues-Trends,* ed. C. R. Kneisl and H. S. Wilson (St. Louis: C. V. Mosby, 1975).

In other instances, the losses may not be as concrete or tangible as those described above. Loss is involved, for instance, when children grow up and leave home or when one fails to achieve what one expects. It is impossible to know what may be a loss for another person, since each person's situation is different. For some, not having enough money to buy food or not being able to have a house free from rats represents a loss, particularly if one has higher expectations or if such circumstances are seen as something that could have been avoided. Although some may accept these conditions as necessary, the influence of television has made many people expect and aspire to a better way of life. Loss of self-esteem is perhaps one of the most devastating losses.

With this plethora of situations and of people faced with problems and seeking resolutions, the nurse is in a key position to offer assistance.

ANTICIPATORY COUNSELING

Caplan has suggested that it is possible to avoid some crises altogether through the use of anticipatory counseling with people identified as likely to experience certain stresses. Anticipatory counseling functions like a practice session before the main event, in which a person can be guided through identifying troublesome spots and planning how to manage them and can become familiar with the events that will occur. This practice helps enlarge one's problem-solving skills and renders him or her less vulnerable to the anticipated stress. This principle was applied to the Peace Corps program, where it was found that volunteers who had anticipatory counseling adjusted much better than others to the stress of living in foreign, sometimes exotic, surroundings. An interesting point to note is that persons who were prepared to make adjustments to problems of living in foreign countries were nonetheless unprepared for re-entering the United States, and many of them had more adjustment problems at that point than they did while living in a foreign culture.

Anticipatory guidance has been described by Caplan as a form of "emotional inoculation." Through anticipating a hazardous event and preparing oneself for it, one is presumed to be less likely to experience crisis when the event does occur. Since it is relatively easy to identify situations that may constitute a potentially hazardous event, it is possible to work with specific target groups or individuals to attempt to ameliorate the psychological effects that may ensue from maladaptive coping. For example, pregnant women, patients about to undergo surgery, persons about to be married, those planning to retire, and those faced with problems of aging all face one or another kind of stress that could be greatly ameliorated by anticipatory counseling.

AN EXAMPLE: THE UNMARRIED PREGNANT ADOLESCENT

As an example of the application of anticipatory guidance to one target group, let us consider the situation of the unmarried pregnant adolescent. Caplan suggests that ". . . in small group discussions, the specialist draws attention to the details of the impending hazards, and attempts to evoke ahead of time a vivid anticipation of the experience with its associated feelings of anxiety, tension, depression, and deprivation."[2] The process of group counseling in anticipation of an impending hazard may be illustrated through data drawn from group interactions of pregnant unwed adolescents. This group of girls is faced with a number of problems, one of which is that of being pregnant. They are also coping with the stresses of being adolescent, and of not being married while pregnant. Group counseling in this situation has multifaceted goals, one of which is to prepare the girls for the hazards of the birth experience and the ensuing adjustive problems of being a mother.[3]

As previously noted, most crisis situations involve a shift in social roles. The pregnant adolescent girl epitomizes these shifting roles. First, she is an adolescent and so is faced with the developmental tasks of moving from childhood to adulthood. Instead of having a period of transition in which to work through these role shifts, she is catapulted into an adult role, that of "mother." While most adolescents make the necessary transitions within the framework of a peer group culture, the pregnant adolescent girl is estranged in many instances from her peers. She is thus faced with working through the development tasks associated with adolescence,

---

2. Gerald Caplan, *Principles of Preventive Psychiatry* (New York: Basic Books, 1964), p. 84.
3. See Lucille Davis and Helen Grace, "Anticipatory Counseling on Unwed Pregnant Adolescents," in *Nursing Clinics of North America* 6, no. 4 (Dec. 1971): 581-590; Barbara Bryan-Logan and Barbara Dancy, "Unwed Pregnant Adolescents: Their Mothers' Dilemma," *Nursing Clinics of North America* 9, no. 1 (March 1974): 57-68.

while simultaneously coping with the normal stresses of being pregnant, further compounded by the societal stigma attached to being pregnant and unmarried.

Anticipatory counseling for these girls is frequently done in a group context. It focuses on preparing them to deal with the hazards of the birth process as well as on working through some of the role shifts that are involved in moving into motherhood while an adolescent and unmarried. In the first stage of such work, most of the girls' questions are directed toward gaining an understanding of what is happening inside their bodies as the baby develops. Frequently, they have many fantasies and mistaken ideas about their own bodies that need to be clarified. In the early stage of the group's formation, one of the ways for a nurse to establish credibility with the group is to provide factual information in response to the girls' search.

In addition to information, the girls frequently need to discuss, within the context of a supportive group, the difficulties they encounter with parents and peers. In many instances, girls try to keep the information that they are pregnant from their parents as long as possible. During this phase, they have tremendous fears about what will happen to them when their parents find out—they are afraid of being thrown out of the home or of being physically punished. In most instances, parents suspect that their daughters are pregnant well in advance of being told. A nurse working with pregnant adolescents, then, has a role in helping the adolescent work out how she is going to tell her parents and what response she might anticipate. In most instances, parents are upset initially, but in a relatively short period of time they find ways of accepting the daughter in her current state.

In considering the problems of the unwed pregnant adolescent, a number of important cultural differences should be noted. A number of studies indicate that the black culture tends to be more accepting of pregnancy in adolescent girls. This does not imply that illegitimate pregnancies are condoned, as is sometimes thought outside the black community. Rather, the family extends its boundaries to incorporate the adolescent's child; in many instances the grandmother serves as a surrogate mother, enabling the daughter to continue in school or in her normal activities. This may be related both to the inability of adoption serving as an easy solution to the problem of illegitimacy in the black culture and to the high value placed upon the family and the kinship network (another contradiction of a common stereotype of black family life). In any event, the reaction to the pregnancy of an adolescent in the black culture tends to be initial outrage ("How could you do this to me?" and "I always wanted my daughter to have a chance that I didn't") changing to acceptance and support for the girl as she goes through pregnancy. The family tends to rally round and share in planning for the coming child. In white families, in contrast, the traditional response tends to be different. Generally, the approach is to send the girl away and encourage her to give the child up for adoption. More recently, abortion has become another favored alternative.

In both cases, the family becomes actively involved in advancing solutions for the girl to follow. In both cases also, the adolescent is first severely chastised, and then others become actively involved in working out solutions to the dilemma she presents to the social network. The nature of the crisis depends on the cultural variants. If the girl is to keep the child, she must work out solutions about how to manage with a child, while if the child is given up for adoption, dealing with this loss constitutes a problematic situation.

In work with pregnant unwed adolescents, it is important not only to prepare them for the anticipated reaction of their parents, but also to help them deal with their feelings about the facts that their parents are likely to become actively involved in working out solutions and that these in many instances will not be the same as those the girl would choose, given the opportunity. The unwed pregnant adolescent, unlike other unmarried pregnant women who have had a choice in their decision to give birth to a child, are in a relatively powerless position, as they have no financial resources that will allow them to be more independent in their decision-making.

A further factor that complicates issues for the unwed pregnant adolescent is the role of the baby's father in the girl's life at this time. In many instances, the girls think of getting married as a way out of the powerless position in which they find themselves. But to do so means jeopardizing both his and her career and educational aspirations, and in most instances, they would have to live with one set of parents in order to "make it." A sizable proportion of pregnant adolescent girls are closely tied to the baby's father and wish to share the experience of parenthood with him, but counseling programs tend to ignore the "unwed father." Anticipatory counseling, to be of maximum effectiveness, should attempt to include the father, so that he also has help in working through the problems he faces, which in many ways are not dissimilar to those confronting the girl.

Considering these multifaceted relationships, a portion of group interaction time needs to be devoted to encouraging the girls—and, if possible, the boys—to express their feelings and to explore solutions for the problems that confront them.

■ *Preparation for the Birth Experience.* In addition to the psychological needs of these girls, they also need preparation for the hazards of the birth experience. As Caplan describes it, the task is to evoke in the person "a vivid anticipation of the expected situation." One way of achieving this with pregnant adolescent girls is to show them a movie of the labor and delivery process. Doing so usually evokes an accentuated emotional response; generally one of horror and disbelief. Some girls cover their eyes, while others complain of feeling nauseated. Comments frequently made are, "Oh, how awful," and "That's nasty." The group often will discount the film as not really representing what will happen or deny that it has any relevance to themselves. Such maneuvers as talking about their doctors' promises of spinal anesthesia or medications so they will not feel pain are common. Showing the film evokes a preview of the forthcoming crisis experience and thus provides an opportunity for the nurse, in advance of the actual situation, to work toward preparing the girls to cope adequately with the anticipated reality.

Subsequent sessions of the group provide additional information about the actual birth process. After the emotional impact of the film, the girls are much more open about asking questions as to what they may expect, and they are able to process and make use of information the nurse gives in response to their questioning. The nurse who leads such a group can take the girls through the entire sequence of events that they are likely to experience in the birth process: What is happening in their body, ways of coping with the anticipated pain, what they may expect after delivery, both in terms of physical and psychological responses, and what steps they plan to take following the birth of the baby. This prepares them psychologically for some of the emotional hazards that lie ahead.

■ *Preparation for Postnatal Adjustment.* Anticipatory counseling for the unwed pregnant adolescent should not end with the birth of the baby. Following birth of the baby, the girls are then faced with working

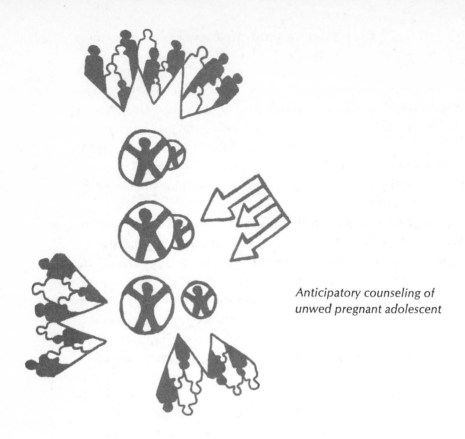

Anticipatory counseling of unwed pregnant adolescent

out in actuality its addition to their life style. While they may have made many plans beforehand, rarely are they prepared to cope fully with the many changes they experience after the baby is born. Many of them report considerable difficulty in negotiating the care of the baby with mothers and boyfriends. As their mothers and grandmothers "take over" the care of the baby, they feel displaced from their mothering role. On the other hand, if they attempt to resume their social life as before, their mothers frequently refuse to baby-sit for any social activities. They thus find themselves cut off from their network of peers. They frequently report great difficulty in attending to school work, and many of them drop out of school because they are unable to manage the multiple demands they face.

Anticipatory counseling should attempt, first of all, to prepare them for this phase of the process, and then should provide group support so they may discuss what they are experiencing. The group should be used as a forum to help them clarify possible resolutions to these multiple problems. The counselor's role in this situation may be to bring up aspects of the issue not faced or thought of by the girls or their boyfriends. The counselor should anticipate the problems the girls will face and facilitate their working out, in the group, some possible resolutions.

A further very sensitive area surrounds the use of birth control measures. Frequently girls are immediately placed on some form of birth control; many times they are given limited information and no choice of the form of birth control prescribed. Both parents and medical professionals tend to unite in a frenzied attempt to prevent repeated pregnancies; the attitude that these girls are promiscuous permeates our common cultural views. The girls, however, do not define themselves in these terms and, in fact, tend to be quite moralistic. Therefore, using contraceptives may indicate to them that they indeed are "bad" girls. Taking "the pill" is equated with accepting a societal definition of themselves as "bad"; therefore, they soon become negligent about taking it regularly. A second factor compounds the problem. Many of them have heard reports of the damage birth control pills can do to their bodies and of potential damage to children they might have in the future. The tendency is to treat the girls as ignorant and not to provide them with adequate information and the freedom of choosing methods of birth control that they see as appropriate. Another related issue is that, with everyone's attention focused on birth control, which has become associated with confirmation of their "badness," the girls avoid coming to terms with their own sexuality. The group can counteract this outcome by providing a forum for anticipating these and other future issues that the girls will inevitably face as time goes on.

THE NURSE'S ROLE IN ANTICIPATORY COUNSELING

Anticipatory counseling and the principles involved have a wide application for nursing. The range of groups a nurse might work with is extensive and includes (1) prenatal groups to prepare parents for the hazards of childbearing, as well as for the role shifts they will need to make as the child enters the social network; (2) parents' groups related to significant transitional points in the life history of the family, such as children going to school or away to college; and (3) groups with common problems, such as retardation, physical illness, or troublesome behavior. The group's intervention can be effective in insulating families against hazardous conditions they are likely to experience. Other areas of preventive work are with certain target groups who face adjustive problems as they make shifts in employment or place of residence, or dramatic readjustments such as those accompanying retirement or a move to a senior citizen's residence or retirement community. The nurse is particularly valuable to persons facing hazardous conditions as a result of physical problems. Patients confronting medical procedures or surgery, or facing major problems of readjustment following certain illnesses are all people whom it would be appropriate for the nurse to assist in preparing for the hazards that lie ahead. Examples of some target groups are persons experiencing heart attacks, amputations, surgery for cancer that may result in alteration of bodily functions, such as colostomies; or patients facing life-threatening situations, such as those who have impaired kidney function and are waiting for a kidney transplant.

Research findings demonstrate that when patients have been given factual information about what to expect in common medical procedures, they experience much less discomfort and are psychologically less disorganized.[4] It is logical to assume that one of the major responsibilities of nurses, no matter what their area of specialization, is to provide patients with a "road map" of what they may expect, and within this context, allow them as much informed control as is reasonable, either in the hospital or as they return home. By providing patients with a framework in which to understand their experiences and to make decisions, the nurse may contribute to both their physical and psychological well-being. This presents a challenge to the nurse to be "in touch" with the patients; too frequently, nurses prepare patients for abstract things rather than common, everyday experiences. Referring back to the model of anticipatory counseling, patients need to have a "vivid anticipation" of the experience that lies ahead, so that they can begin to work through possible solutions to these situations.

To help patients achieve these vivid pictures of what lies ahead, the nurse needs to garner data about what they may expect through questioning and listening carefully to others who have undergone similar experi-

---

4. Jean Johnson, "Effects of Structuring Patients' Expectations and Their Reactions to Threatening Events," *Nursing Research* 21, no. 6 (Nov.-Dec. 1972).

ences. Too often, nurses and doctors rely on textbook explanations of what patients might expect as the aftermath to certain medical or surgical procedures. The language used to describe these experiences is frequently that of the textbook, rather than what they mean to the patient in real everyday living situations. It behooves nurses and all caregiving personnel to listen carefully to their patients' reports and to use the information gained from these patients' real-life experiences as the basis for preparing others for the hazards that lie ahead. Anticipatory counseling in all its forms is an effective tool for nurses to use in working to prevent the maladaptive coping that frequently occurs when people have not been adequately prepared for the crisis situations they face.

CRISIS INTERVENTION

A crisis occurs when a person encounters an obstacle in attaining an important life goal. Barrell, in summarizing the crisis literature, notes:

> . . . the critical attributes of the crisis concept include a person (in a state of relative equilibrium or emotional balance) with a repertoire of problem-solving skills, and a hazardous event or an obstacle to a goal which for the time being cannot be overcome by the usual problem-solving or coping skills. This lack of fit between the event and the skills proves disorganizing and disrupting for the person and his anxiety increases; with the increase in anxiety, the coping powers further decrease. The resulting crisis is clearly the person's reaction and inability to cope, not the event or obstacle.

She notes that a crisis is an *individual matter;* there are no blanket definitions of crisis situations that fit all people. Some persons react to a situation that on the surface seems insignificant, but to them is very meaningful. Their inability to deal with it constitutes a crisis for them. Others may face overwhelming situations that would precipitate a crisis for most people, but they are able to manage without experiencing the situation as disruptive, overwhelming, or demanding of resources they do not possess. It is important, therefore, to be in touch with the individual to ascertain if this person defines himself or herself as being in crisis.[5]

---

5. Lorna Barrell, "Crisis Intervention: Partnership in Problem Solving," *Nursing Clinics of North America* 9, no. 1 (March 1974), p. 6.

The goal of intervention is to restore the person in crisis to at least his or her usual level of functioning. To achieve this goal, the person having the crisis is engaged as an active partner in the problem-solving endeavor, rather than made to play the role of a passive recipient of advice. Crisis work is goal-directed and action-oriented. The person is always viewed within the context of his or her life situation and in reference to significant social relationships.

The first step in the crisis intervention is making an accurate assessment of the problem. This entails authenticating that the person or client is indeed experiencing a crisis, and then focusing on the specific nature of this insurmountable difficulty. Bear in mind that if a person is truly in crisis, his or her anxiety level is mounting and it is difficult for him or her to focus on the specific nature of the problem. It is therefore important for the therapist to structure the situation actively and concretely so that the client may begin to think more rationally and logically. Further, recognizing the person's anxiety and fear of certain doom, it is important in the initial stage to instill hope. The client needs to perceive the therapist as interested in and committed to helping solve his or her problem.

In the initial stage, it is typical for the person to describe a diffuse and unfocused situation in which he or she is helpless and unable to cope. The therapist may demonstrate an ability to assist the person by helping him or her focus on the situation and identify some of the critical factors that make it problematic. In so doing, the therapist helps the person structure and begin to view the problem in a rational framework, something he or she has been unable to do because of the degree of anxiety involved. The following example illustrates the way in which an individual in crisis typically presents herself or himself:

> Susan Connors, a 25-year-old single woman, comes to the mental health center, and as she waits to be seen, she cries. When she is seen, she says to the interviewer: "I'm depressed. I've lost my job and my apartment. I had my own secretarial service but that failed. I woke up when I had that business. I found it's very difficult for a person to run a business individually. I should be okay. I looked at all those people here while I was waiting and I have so much going for me compared to them, but I just can't motivate myself. I wake up in the morning and say, 'Okay, Susan, what are you going to do today?' I should look for a job, but I don't do anything. People have been good to me, but I can't respond back. A friend in the building is letting me stay with her since I got thrown out of my apartment for not paying the rent.

"People tell me this feeling is normal and that I should get over it, but I can't. I should feel good. I just can't get motivated. I should be unpacking my things. My roommate is on vacation this week and I have all the time in the world to unpack, but I haven't done anything. I can't read or watch television because I can't concentrate. I don't know why I came today. I should be looking for a job so I can pay my bills. I know what I have to do, but I'm all screwed up."

Assessment involves identifying specific events immediately preceding the onset of the crisis that the individual perceives as problematic. In this instance, Susan Connors identifies, "I've lost my job and my apartment." She has lost a valued role and her position within significant social groups. Using this as a starting point, the nurse attempts to help Ms. Connors focus more specifically on her problem.

FIRST INTERVIEW

Nurse: What happened that you lost your job?

Susan Connors: Oh, I don't know, things just started falling apart. I had this secretarial service and I just couldn't get good secretaries. They would accept work to do and then do a poor job or wouldn't get finished when it was promised. I'd end up having to redo it, and I couldn't handle all of it. Then the people who had hired secretarial services would holler at me and wouldn't pay me for the work because it wasn't right or it wasn't completed when they wanted it. And I got further and further behind in paying my bills. I lost my apartment because I got behind in my rent. And this is not the way I am as a person.

Nurse: How do you see yourself?

Ms. Connors: Well, I was a very good secretary for this company. I was promoted to executive secretary, and that's pretty good for someone my age. But then the company moved to Atlanta. I didn't want to move because my mother isn't well and my father is dead, and I thought I should be in this area. Some of the people I worked with thought that I should go into business for myself because I was such a good secretary, and I thought that it was a good idea. With my references I was able to set up my office, and when I first started and was handling the work myself it went okay, but then I got these secretaries to help out, and they just didn't do the work. And now it's all done, and what am I going to do? I'm in debt, and I don't know where I'm going to live, and nobody likes you when you're down.

In this interaction, the nurse gets a more specific idea of the loss that Susan Connors has experienced: she has lost her role as a competent individual and now perceives herself as inadequate. Her role has changed from that of executive secretary to that of unemployed "nobody," from her point of view. As Ms. Connors has talked, the nurse is able to formulate some of the alterations in role relationships and expectations that have occurred: She no longer is surrounded by a supportive group of co-workers who commend her on her competence; now she must deal with angry creditors who constantly reinforce the image of incompetence. As the interaction continues, Ms. Connors states: "My family always was pleased with my abilities to handle my job. I was helping put my brother through college and now I can't do that any more."

Having defined the specific dimensions of the problem confronting the individual, the next step involves appraising factors that might influence the resolution of the problem. Aguilera et al. have developed a paradigm illustrating the effect of balancing factors in a stress situation.[6] Using Paradigm 10-1 in analyzing Susan Connors's situation, the following assessment can be made: (1) Ms. Connors has an unrealistic perception of the event. She sees the loss of her business as a reflection of her incompetence as an individual rather than viewing it as a difficult learning experience that does not reflect on her capabilities as a person. (2) She lacks adequate situational supports. She has always viewed herself as the type of individual who "makes it on my own." Instead of receiving support from her family, she has been the one who provides support to them. Her closest friends have transferred to Atlanta, so that she no longer has them as supports, and although a friend is allowing her to stay in her apartment, she finds it difficult to impose further on this friend by talking about her problem. (3) Her coping mechanisms were inadequate in this situation. Ms. Connors responded to crisis by withdrawing, and this was not adequate to resolve this situation; it only compounded her problems.

With such an assessment, the nurse then attempts to assist the individual to gain a greater understanding of factors underlying the crisis.[7]

SECOND INTERVIEW

Nurse: I can understand that you are upset by all the things that have happened to you, but it's not the end of the world.

Susan Connors: It may not seem to you that it is, but to me it's terrible.

---

6. Donna C. Aguilera, Janice M. Messick, and Marlene Farrell, *Crisis Intervention: Theory and Methodology* (St. Louis: C. V. Mosby, 1970), p. 63.
7. Ibid., p. 52.

Paradigm 10-1

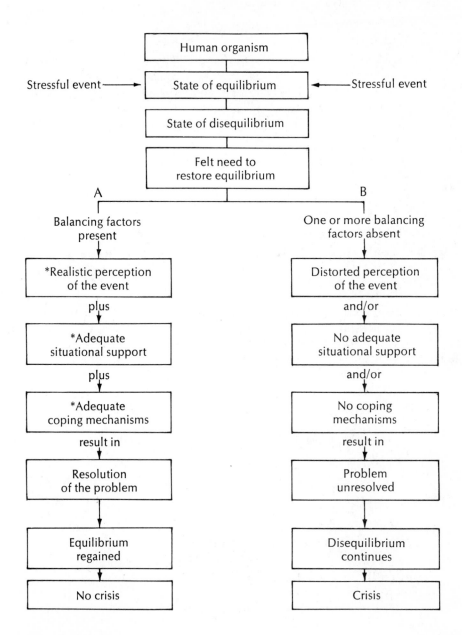

*Balancing factors

Nurse: But just because you've had this experience, it doesn't mean that you aren't still a good secretary.

Ms. Connors: But who would hire me?

Nurse: Have you thought a lot about that?

Ms. Connors: I've looked in the Sunday papers, but I haven't been able to concentrate.

Nurse: I've heard that it is really hard to find good secretaries today, and one with your background could be in demand.

Ms. Connors: But if any company knew the debts I had, they wouldn't hire me.

Nurse: I'm sure if you told them the circumstances they would understand.

Ms. Connors: But it's so embarrassing. I'm not that kind of a person. I've always paid my bills.

In the interactive process, the nurse assists the individual to bring into the open feelings to which she or he may not have access.[8]

Nurse: It must make you feel very angry to find yourself in this predicament.

Susan Connors: Yeah, I feel that I had everything going for me, and now nothing. If I'd been able to go to Atlanta, I'd still have the job I had before and I wouldn't be in this predicament, and the only reason I'm here is to try to help my family out. This is what happens, you strike out all over the place.

Nurse: I can understand your feelings.

Ms. Connors: Other people seem to have such a carefree life, with no responsibilities. I've had to carry people all my life, and now I've failed for everyone. I just don't know what to do. If only those secretaries that I hired had worked like I used to work.

The nurse then explores the coping mechanisms the individual employs.[9]

THIRD INTERVIEW

Nurse: How do you usually respond when you are angry?

Susan Connors: Well, I don't believe much in fighting. Usually I just go off by myself and I get over it. What's the use anyhow? Life is just the way that it is, and maybe if I hadn't been such a fool to think that I could run a business, I wouldn't be in the predicament that I'm in now.

8. Ibid., p. 17.
9. Ibid., p. 17.

Based on the knowledge that Ms. Connors usually retreats under stress, the nurse then attempts to assist her to work out new relationships and reopen her social world.[10]

> *Nurse:* You're telling me that you generally retreat when things get rough, but that doesn't seem to be working too well for you now.
>
> *Susan Connors:* No, it just gets worse and worse; the longer I don't work the more in debt I get. I don't know how long I can stay with this friend if I don't get a job, and it's too embarrassing to go home to my family without being able to contribute something to their support.
>
> *Nurse:* Would it be so bad to go home to your family until you work things out? I'm sure that they would understand.
>
> *Ms. Connors:* Well, I've thought of that, but I don't know. It's hard to go back; my mother is an invalid and she's always thought of my being able to take care of my problems myself.
>
> *Nurse:* I'm sure your mother doesn't care for you only because you've provided for her. Maybe she'd feel good if for once she thought she could be doing something for you.
>
> *Ms. Connors:* I hadn't thought of that before, and my brother really didn't want to continue college anyhow. He wanted to get a job, but it was my idea that he should stay in college. Maybe if I went back there, I would be in a better frame of mind to go out and get another job, and then I wouldn't be going deeper and deeper in debt to my friends. In fact, I guess my family might owe something to me in exchange for all that I've done for them. And if I found another job, then I could develop some new friends. Maybe that might just work out.

Through supporting the individual, the nurse helps the patient to see her problems and possible solutions in a new light. The final phase in crisis intervention involves a resolution of the crisis and anticipatory planning to prepare the individual for encountering subsequent stressful experiences.[11]

SIXTH INTERVIEW

> *Nurse:* How are things working out since you've moved back home?
>
> *Susan Connors:* Quite well. It's been a new experience to find that I'm accepted in the family for myself and not for what I can do. I've spent a lot of time talking to my mother, and she's got a lot of good advice to give me, and I've gotten to know my brother in a new way. He is doing so well in his job; it was probably much better for him that he dropped out of school. He's going to school now in connection with his

---

10. Ibid., p. 17.
11. Ibid., p. 17.

job and he's motivated now to learn, while he wasn't doing much when he was just going to school.

Nurse: Are you able to think things through better?

Ms. Connors: Yes, and I've been out looking for a job. I have about three good possibilities, but I'm going to be sure it's the right kind of job for me.

Nurse: What are you looking for in a job?

Ms. Connors: Well, I don't want to get into the same situation again. I'm looking for a job that I can count on that it won't be taken away. I'm looking for a position where I'm primarily responsible for my own work and where I don't have to supervise others. I've been offered executive secretary positions, and that's probably what I'll take.

Nurse: What happens if things don't pan out there?

Ms. Connors: I've found that there are lots of opportunities for me as a secretary, and I've found a lot of new friends. It really wasn't the end of the world, and if it happens again maybe this will give me confidence in myself. And I've found that my mother and my brother really don't need me to be a martyr for them. They can manage, although it does help if we're all working together.

Not only was Susan Connors helped through a crisis, but she also was pushed into re-evaluating her significant relationships and subsequently developed a new role for herself within the family constellation.

To summarize, crisis intervention follows a problem-solving model. The goal is first of all to help the individual reach an accurate formulation of the nature of his or her problem, then to assess resources and limitations in the situation that affect resolution, and finally to support the individual as he or she advances possible solutions and tests them out in reality.

The focus of crisis intervention must be on understanding the complex web of interrelationships surrounding an individual. Crises disrupt usual relationships. Having experienced a disruption of relationships, the individual then has difficulty in relocating within relevant social groups. Crisis intervention focuses on assisting the individual's problem-solving endeavors to restore balance and perspective. The goal of crisis intervention is to help the individual alter or develop appropriate roles that serve to reaffirms his or her worth within significant groups.

Crisis intervention can be viewed as a means of helping a person resolve an immediate problem. The crisis situation, in making the person much more aware of his or her underlying feelings, may be an opportunity for growth, provided the person receives appropriate assistance to work out

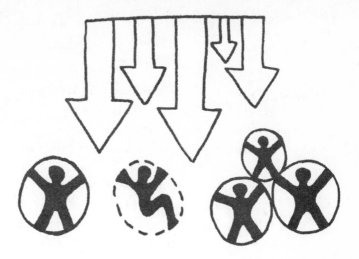

Successful crisis resolution

better solutions to problems than might have been possible in the past. Unlike Susan Connors, who was functioning at a relatively high level before her job loss, many persons come for help after a succession of life crises, each of which has left them less able to cope. Let us consider a contrasting situation.

At intake interview, Julia Mosca discloses that she has been divorced for the past ten years (after being married four years) and lost the custody of her three children to her husband four years ago because of a drinking problem. She has not had a drink for the past three years (with the help of Alcoholics Anonymous), has been very dissatisfied over the child visitation rights she was given, and has engaged a lawyer to help her regain custody of her children. A week ago, she received notice from the court that her petition would be heard the week before Christmas.

Mrs. Mosca has held a job for the past three years and has a two-bedroom apartment in the neighborhood. Her daughter is eleven years old, her sons are twelve and fourteen. It is the fourteen-year-old she focuses on as she asks for help, the most prominent complaint being that he wants to stay with his father. "I can't make him realize that children should always be with their mother. Everybody knows that! But he says he won't come. I need some advice on how to change him." She states that the other two children do not say anything one way or the other, so they will not be any trouble.

She is vitriolic in describing her husband's faults. She complains that he has not followed the visitation ruling reasonably at all, but acknowledges that she has never tried to exert any legal pressure to change that. She reveals that her drinking was a problem before their divorce and complains, "He was always disappointing me. I wanted a strong husband to really take care of us, and he was a mama's boy. He always ran to his mother—spent more time there than at our apartment. He never obeyed my advice, but anything his mother said went! Well, he shouldn't get to keep those kids. He can't manage them the right way. Kids need their own mother!" She also confides that she has been unable to concentrate on work and has had difficulty sleeping during the past week. "If only someone would help me about the kids. When I get them back, I'll bring Tom (the fourteen-year-old) here for counseling."

In assessing this situation, the therapist notes the onset of Mrs. Mosca's difficulties as directly related to the court notification that her petition to regain custody of the children will be heard shortly. Since that time she has been unable to concentrate on her work and has had difficulty sleeping. One notable thing about her situation is common in many crisis situations: the onset of difficulty may be related to what, on the surface, appears to be an event that will bring happiness to the person, rather than one that portends emotional crisis. In making note of the factor (or factors) that seems to be implicated in the onset, the therapist, from the story presented by the client, attempts to formulate the nature of the crisis.

A first thing to note is the person's characteristic coping style. Mrs. Mosca has a long history—at least fourteen years and probably much longer—of difficulty in reaching adequate problem resolutions. After four years of marriage and the birth of three children, she divorced her husband. The reasons given are that her husband was a disappointment, that instead of taking care of them as he should have, he was a mama's boy. This would seem to point to a basically dependent style of coping in which she wished for someone to take care of her and was disappointed when these wishes were not fulfilled. It is likely that Mrs. Mosca has consistently had difficulty in letting those close to her know what she really wants from them. In describing her relationship to her husband, she further comments, "He never obeyed my advice, but anything his mother said went!" It is likely that instead of communicating her wish that her husband would be more demonstrative toward her, she sat at home, seething with anger that her husband would choose his mother instead of her. She would have pitying thoughts about her lot and derogating thoughts about him.

It is further possible to conjecture that all of these angry feelings about her husband's inadequacy as a man may be, at least partially, a projection of doubts about her own adequacy as a person. Her life style seems to indicate a progressive retreat from problems, first in relationship to her husband and later in relationship to her children, as she relies increasingly upon alcohol as a means of coping with her problems.

In further analyzing the story that Mrs. Mosca has presented, it is important to note the point at which difficulties were accentuated. Four years ago, when the children were ten, eight, and seven, she lost custody of them because of her drinking problem. As the children grew up, it is likely that they presented increasing problems for their mother, reflected in her drinking problem. She may have been able to manage adequately when the children were small and dependent on her, but as they become increasingly independent, her position and role as mother became less and less secure. It is further important to note that Mrs. Mosca's problems with drinking have been under control for the last three years, since a year after the children left her. She has been able to go out and get a job and has managed quite well in establishing a more independent role than she had before. In fact, she has become aggressive enough to try to regain custody of her children, and now, when that goal is in sight, she suddenly goes into a crisis.

A further factor that is important to note is her tendency to fixate on the fourteen-year-old boy as the problem. In fact, her stated goal in coming for help is to enlist the therapist's help in changing the fourteen-year-old so that he will want to come and live with her. Later in the interview, however, she states, "If only someone could help about the kids," and promises that she will bring the fourteen-year-old in for counseling when she gets them back. In assessing any crisis situation, it is important to consider that a crisis situation always reactivates old conflicts. In this instance, when she has been coping fairly well, the thought of the children returning has probably reactivated all of the struggles Mrs. Mosca has gone through, first of all in the divorce, and later as she progressed into alcoholism, ultimately losing custody of the children. The return of the children, although something that she wants, also reactivates the old conflicts and fears that led her into alcoholism; she fears that regaining the children might lead to her downfall.

To place this situation within the framework of the crisis model outlined previously in this chapter: Prior to the crisis, Mrs. Mosca had been able to establish a state of equilibrium in which she was working and maintaining herself in an independent position. Return of the children represents a major disruption in this state of equilibrum and arouses all of her old fears and anxieties. She is constantly seeking ways of restoring a state of equilibrium. As she presents herself to the counseling center, she cannot verbalize, nor is she consciously aware of, the underlying basis of her conflict. She focuses on the eldest child who does not want to return to her as the problem, rather than articulating or identifying her fears of being inadequate and once more moving down the path to alcoholism if the children return to her.

Although we have limited data available, it looks as if Mrs. Mosca has little or no situational support in helping her work through the situation; she lives alone, works in a marginal job, and seems to have a limited network of social friendships. Her coping mechanisms have traditionally been those of retreat, although she has modified this to some extent in recent years.

With the possibility of winning a custody fight for the children, she is faced with a situation from which she cannot retreat. One can imagine that she would not have been in a crisis had the judge not awarded her the privilege of a hearing regarding custody of the children. In fact, this would have allowed her to maintain the negative image of her ex-husband that serves as a stabilizing force, and she could continue to play the role of martyr. But now she is faced with re-establishing her role as mother, and this is an unsettling experience. The fourteen-year-old poses the greatest threat. Seeing no solution, Mrs. Mosca reaches out to the mental health center in an attempt to reach a resolution. However, she does not see this in terms of herself; rather the center is to serve the role of bringing her son into line for her, and, in fact, the therapist is cast into the role she feels her husband never played. The mental health center is seen as the force that will help her out of her difficulty by handling her problem, the fourteen-year-old son.

The first step in the intervention process is to support the client's wisdom in coming for help; knowing she has difficulty with her son is a positive insight on her part. The therapist communicates that she is interested in helping Mrs. Mosca with her boy and with the other adjustments she will undoubtedly have to make if the court grants her custody. With that slight but crucial change in emphasis, the major task of the session is to help her identify her anxieties and fears. In the second session, the therapist works with Mrs. Mosca to help her delineate her fears more precisely.

SECOND INTERVIEW

Nurse: Can you tell me a little bit about how you think things might be if you regain custody of your children? Now you live in a two-bedroom apartment and are working. What types of plans have you made for how you might manage?

Mrs. Mosca: I don't know. Things are going along in just a certain way right now. I'd have to get a different place to live, and I don't know if I'd be able to keep my job. A mother should be home and available to her children, and I'd have to get them lined up with school.

Nurse: Can you tell me a little about how things were for you when the children were with you the last time?

Mrs. Mosca: (Pause) I don't like to think about that time. I loved my children, but they were so hard to manage. I just couldn't keep up with everything. They always needed things for school, and they wanted me to help with their homework. They were always wanting to bring their friends in, and they'd start to fight and things would get out of hand. I didn't manage very well.

Nurse: I would imagine that thinking of having the children come back might arouse some mixed feelings in you.

Mrs. Mosca: Well, I really want them back. They should be with their mother, and their father is not doing too well with them. They are with his mother a lot, and that's not a good influence.

Nurse: It sounds like you are giving yourself reasons for why they should be with you, but what about your underlying feelings?

Mrs. Mosca: (Begins to cry) I'm just so scared. I want them back. I want them with me, but I don't want things to be the way they were. I'm so afraid I'll start drinking again and it will start all over again. (Sobbing) I'm just not sure that I can manage.

In this session, Mrs. Mosca begins to explore the underlying fears that surround the return of the children. As she faces this change in her life, she is faced with all the losses of her life and the fears of sustaining further loss through regaining her children. She may regain them only to lose them again because of her inability to cope. It is important at this stage in the crisis intervention process to allow the client to explore her feelings fully and not to rush in with premature reassurances that everything will be all right. As the session progresses, Mrs. Mosca pours out in great detail the difficulties of the previous time when her children were with her, her inabilities to cope with them, and the demands and insults poured on by their father.

At the conclusion of the session, the nurse summarizes, "I can understand how painful this has all been, but let us explore ways in which you might prevent the same sort of thing happening this time if you regain custody of your children." A statement of this nature communicates an understanding of the person's situation, but offers hope that there may be ways of preventing a reoccurrence of the same problems, and that the therapist will help Mrs. Mosca find a way out of her problems.

In the third session the therapist begins by making a summary of the prior two sessions:

THIRD INTERVIEW

Nurse: Now, in the first session you told me about your situation, that you are going to soon have a hearing about regaining custody of your children. At that time you were concerned about your oldest son, Tom, and that he didn't want to come back to you, but that when he returned you would bring him in here for counseling. Then, in the second session we reviewed how it was for you before when you had the children. You were very frightened about getting into some of the same difficulties. Now today, we were going to explore ways in which you might prevent some of these same things from happening. Have you had some thoughts about this the last week?

In crisis intervention work, it is extremely important that the responsibility for reaching more adequate problem resolutions be shared between therapist and client, and that the client's attempts at problem-solving be the basis on which crisis intervention proceeds. It is all too easy for the therapist to rush in with a set of solutions that in no way relate to the way the individual might choose in solving his or her problem. A second point to note in the way the therapist opens the session is that of first summarizing previous sessions, but also clearly stating the goals for the current session. In this way, the client can immediately begin to focus on the work to be accomplished in the session. Mrs. Mosca responds to the therapist's opening statement in the following manner:

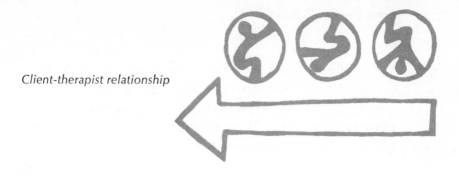

Mrs. Mosca: I have been thinking about it. A funny thing, after all the things I had said here; I really felt better, and I began to think this isn't the end of the world and maybe I could make it after all. Before this, I just haven't been able to think about what I would do. I just tried to keep my thoughts out of my mind and gave myself all the reasons why the children should be with me, without thinking through how I might manage with them back.

But I began to think of how important my job is to me and my friends that I have there. For the first time, I feel like I've been able to do my work, and we have a good time, and I have just decided that I don't want to give up my work if the children come back. They are old enough that they will be in school most of the day, and I think they could manage quite well by themselves. It would just mean so much to me to have my job and my friends, that I think this would help me manage my children. If I just stay home all the time, all I would do would be to worry and think about them and whether I was going to make it all right.

I've been thinking, too, about where I might live. If I'm working and get some child support from the children's father, I should be able to get a bigger apartment. With three children, I need at least three bedrooms. I hadn't dared mention anything to my landlady, because I had heard that she didn't like children in the building, and I didn't know what to do.

Nurse: What did she say about it?

Mrs. Mosca: It just happened that she is going to have a three-bedroom apartment on the ground floor open in a couple of months. Mainly she doesn't like children in apartments where there are other people living under them, because of the noise. But you know, she's gotten to like me. I've been here two years and have never caused any trouble—always paid my rent on time, and she said that if I wanted to, she'd consider letting me have the first floor apartment. That would really be nice because then I would still be with some of the friends I have made, and I'd be close to my work, and the children could play in the park.

While the client may have worked out many solutions for herself, it is important that the therapist encourage the person to explore more than just the surface problems she may have attended to. In this case, the therapist recalls both Mrs. Mosca's concern over her fourteen-year-old son and her prior responses of retreating into alcoholism.

> *Nurse:* The first time you came, you mentioned that Tom wanted to stay with his father. Have you thought any more about how you want to handle this?
>
> *Mrs. Mosca:* Yes, I've talked some more about this with Tom, and I think it might be all right for him to stay with his father. He's growing up, and I can understand how he might want to be close to his father at this time. He said that he'd want to come over to my house on weekends, but he's started high school over where his father lives and he has a lot of friends there, and maybe I just won't make a big point of his having to come to live with me.
>
> *Nurse:* It sounds like that might be a reasonable solution. You mentioned before how you used to feel when the children would get into arguments and you would have to moderate them, and you just couldn't cope, so you began to drink more and more. Have you given some thought to how you might handle this?
>
> *Mrs. Mosca:* Yes, I have. In fact, I brought it up at my AA meeting this week. A couple of women there had had the same type of problem, and they told me that what helped them the most was being able to call one another when they felt this way, and they told me that I could call them and they would try to help me out by listening. That's a real relief, because before I could never talk to anyone about what I was going through. If I mentioned anything to my husband, he would say it was just that I couldn't handle anything, and that if only I was like his mother things would be so much better. That would just make me feel worse, and I didn't have anyone else to turn to who would understand.

Although this example may be somewhat extreme, most persons are adept at seeking their own solutions, particularly when they are freed by being able to explore their underlying fears and anxieties. Once this occurs, all the energies that have been tied up in denying the underlying anxieties can be directed toward problem-solving, and in many instances, people can work out reasonable solutions with little outside assistance. The role of the therapist then becomes that of validating and clarifying as the person goes through his or her problem-solving steps.

As this particular crisis intervention winds to a close, it is important to recapitulate the sessions and then spend some time in planning and preparing the person for the future, discussing the availability of further help should this be necessary. In the case of Mrs. Mosca, it is likely that she will have certain periods when the same fears that have plagued her come to the fore again. She needs some anticipatory work about what will happen if she does not regain custody of the children; while if she does get them back, it is likely that some of the anxiety present in early sessions will be reactivated.

FOURTH INTERVIEW

Nurse: Mrs. Mosca, have you given any thought to what you will do if you don't get the children back? You've made all these plans for how you might manage if you do get them, but what if you shouldn't?

Mrs. Mosca: (Pause) I've thought about this, and then I think that I've not done too bad so far without them. I would like to have them with me more on the weekends than they have been, and maybe I could arrange that. It would be lonely, but I think I might manage.

Nurse: If you actually do regain custody of them, it is likely that you will have some of the same fears as you did at the beginning of these sessions, and as they return, things will come up that might be a problem. Please be sure to call me back if you ever get upset and need someone to talk to. We've identified a number of sources of help for you—your friends at work and the people who live in your apartment building—but if you feel you need someone else, feel free to call me.

Mrs. Mosca: I will. I sure don't want to get back into the mess I was in before, and I really do have a lot of friends I can call on.

This particular case is a good example of how a crisis situation may provide an opportunity for personal growth. Mrs. Mosca, with minimal help from the therapist, continues a progression toward greater independence, in contrast to her earlier patterns of retreating from all problems.

PROBLEMATIC SITUATIONS: AGING, DEATH, AND DYING

Although the principles underlying anticipatory counseling and crisis intervention hold for a wide range of situations, certain areas pose unique problems because of their inevitable outcomes and the general cultural attitudes toward them. Two areas that are felt to be particularly troublesome within this culture are aging, and death and dying; both areas have recently been given more study and attention.

Being old in this culture has few assets to offset the deprivations that accompany it. While many of the liabilities associated with aging are unavoidable, such as loss of physical capabilities and of the companionship of one's peers, other forms of loss are simply the result of common cultural definitions. Old people are frequently poor; they are felt to contribute little to society and are in a devalued position within the family structure also. As they themselves have absorbed the culture's views of older people, and often share in the general high valuation put on youth and the future, a pessimistic outlook on life often develops. If one's total life is lived in anticipating the future and striving to achieve and attain valued goals, when one becomes older, one is lost. Only the present remains, with no further hope for achieving future goals.

This problem is compounded by the loss of friends experienced by older people. This loss of friends produces two problems: first, as significant people die, one has fewer and fewer friends or peers to relate to and therefore is more subject to loneliness. Second, the death of peers serves constantly to remind an older person that he or she, too, will soon face death.

Even if one is not facing imminent death, an elderly person is treated in many instances as though he or she were dead. The elderly person is commonly perceived to be asexual, and any indication of sexual feelings is considered to be disgusting and inappropriate. Even the language used in speaking to elderly persons frequently reflects low regard. "Dirty old man," "Now, dearie, do this," "Be a good girl now," are heard only too often in situations where the elderly are cared for.

With the passage of time, the elderly person frequently becomes the only one who can remember events that had great significance for him or her, but are unimportant to a younger generation devoted to doing their "own thing." Remembering the Wright Brothers' first flight is seldom a topic of conversation, and to have a repertoire of memories that cannot be shared becomes terribly isolating.

To deal with the problems associated with aging in our society, intervention needs to be a multipronged approach that focuses on changing general cultural definitions as well as on enabling individuals to manage successfully the crises of aging. There needs to be public concern about the wisdom of emphasizing young people's "doing" instead of "being," and of encouraging an orientation totally to the future. The practice of excluding the elderly from society either symbolically or actually also requires examination. Nurses working with people of all ages can note the existence of attitudes and practices that will probably not be conducive to their achieving the sense of a life reasonably well used that they will need for a productive and harmonious experience during their elderly years. One of the ways in which this might be accomplished is through encouraging a periodic life review, so that one will arrive at old age having come to terms with life, not leaving this task to a time when one is limited in what one can do to change or rectify areas with which one is unsatisfied.

Nurses working with the elderly may do much to help them confront the problems that accompany aging. First, they may help an older person anticipate changes that accompany aging and, in so doing, clarify what these changes mean and do not mean. For example, the nurse can explain to an aging man that although diminished sexual vigor may be expected, he has not lost his sexual capacities and should be encouraged to continue to express this side of his nature. Older persons need to realize that a loss of acuity in vision, for example, does not mean an inability to think productively. They need to be encouraged to note realistically their losses of physical capacity, so that they can compensate, not simply resign themselves to the inevitability of these losses.

In general, the elderly can be helped to maintain an investment in the areas of their lives that have had meaning for them. If a person who has enjoyed reading now has poor sight, listening to records or having other people read aloud may be a viable alternative. Sharing this type of compensatory activity with the younger generation frequently works out well in families. Reading about the Wright Brothers to an elderly person may evoke a discussion of how it was at that time. The life review shared with a younger generation can enrich the worlds of both the elderly and the one who has the opportunity to listen.

Helping families to look at issues realistically rather than not discussing them is a further way in which nurses can be of help to the elderly. Frequently elderly persons talk about what is to happen when they die, who is to get their favored belongings, and similar topics. The usual response is, "Stop talking like that, you have many years yet," which cuts off any further discussion. It renders both the aging member and the family unable to deal with the ultimate outcome of the aging process, death.

A second, and closely related, area that is a crisis for the whole family is the process of dying, another current area of study. Our cultural views and arrangements concerning dying are undergoing change in many areas. For many years, death replaced sex as a forbidden topic. But the pastoral counselor, the undertaker, hospital personnel, and the public at large have begun to question some of the supports that have maintained a deep-rooted fear of dying and an inability to deal with death as a fact of life.

The way people die and the practices surrounding death are culturally determined. In this technological society, the arena for death has moved from the home to the hospital, and out of the hands of family members into the hands of the health professionals. Even the point at which a person dies has become problematic, with great concern about ethical issues in the use of technological means to preserve body functions; a related problem is the need for good tissues to use in transplants. With the general population concerned with the avoidance of death and with professionals holding the saving of lives as their primary legitimate goal, dying successfully is fraught with problems in our culture. Glaser and Strauss[12] have carefully described the interactions that occur commonly within organizational settings where patients die. They describe the common pattern of collusiveness, in which everyone involved pretends that what is happening really is not. The patient is frequently isolated from family and friends, not only physically, but also psychologically, in that they attempt to deny the situation and rarely talk openly about the expected outcome. The patient then is faced with trying to construct some type of social reality for himself or herself to deal with the ambiguity of this state.

As a result of their studies, Glaser and Strauss make a series of recommendations dealing with the need for those who deal with dying patients to develop an "open awareness" context, one in which there is open communication between patient, family, and professionals about what is going on in the situation. They feel that much of the "protecting" of patients really serves to prevent both professionals and family members from dealing with some emotional issues about what is happening and impedes the dying person's ability to work through a reasonable adjustment to his or her coming death. From the standpoint of crisis intervention, one could

---

12. Barney G. Glaser and Anselm L. Strauss, *Awareness of Dying* (Chicago: Aldine Publishing Co., 1965).

say that professionals and sometimes family have violated the principle of helping the dying person to articulate clearly the nature of the problem, thus extending the crisis rather than modifying it or allowing the person to come to some reasonable resolution.

Other research, such as that of Kubler-Ross,[13] has concentrated on the stages a dying person passes through in relationship to his or her coming death. The stages identified by Kubler-Ross are (1) initial denial, (2) anger, (3) bargaining, (4) depression, and (5) acceptance. The first stage is usually expressed as a state of disbelief that this could happen, followed by anger, that this could happen to oneself. In bargaining, the concentration is on provisional acceptance and an attempt to buy time, while the depression is simply the feeling of hopelessness and despair about the inevitability of death.

Acceptance is the last stage, not reached by all, which entails a feeling of peacefulness about one's fate. The chances of achieving this state are greatly enhanced by having come to terms with the life one has lived. This final phase is usually accompanied by loss of interest in and gradual withdrawal from all outside attachments, including the family. A dying person's family are often upset at this occurrence, since it symbolizes too painfully the impending loss they are helpless to prevent. The help of professionals is frequently a catalyst in enabling dying people to negotiate these stages successfully, and in helping their families to begin work on their grieving.

SUMMARY

Anticipatory counseling leads a person through anticipated periods of stress by exploring, in advance, possible alternatives for action and supporting reasonable problem-solving mechanisms, so that he or she can undergo the stress without being catapulted into a crisis. In this sense, it is an effective preventive approach to insulate the person against possible damaging life experiences.

Anticipatory counseling consists of helping the person imagine all aspects of the stressful experience he or she is going to encounter. Having

---

13. Elizabeth Kubler-Ross, *On Death and Dying* (New York: The Macmillan Co., 1969).

identified the problematic features of the anticipated situation, the person then works out possible approaches toward solving them. With this preparation, the person does not encounter the stressful situation "cold," but is psychologically prepared to handle potential problems in ways that are growth-producing and not stultifying.

Crisis intervention itself occurs at the time the person is actually experiencing a crisis. This form of intervention consists of helping the person marshal the necessary resources, both within himself or herself and within the social network, to master the stressful situation successfully. The first phase of crisis intervention is to reduce the person's anxiety so that he or she can focus on the situation and assess the predicament with some degree of accuracy. Next, a plan of action enabling the person to muster the necessary resources is evolved, followed by an appraisal of his or her handling of the situation, including a review of past performances along similar lines. Anticipation of subsequent crises is a way of consolidating the learnings derived from successful mastery of a crisis situation.

FURTHER READINGS

Berliner, Beverly. "Nursing a Patient in Crisis. *American Journal of Nursing* 70 (Oct. 1970): 2154-2157.

Davis, Lucille, and Grace, Helen. "Anticipatory Counseling of Unwed Pregnant Adolescents." *Nursing Clinics of North America* 6 (Dec. 1971): 581-590.

Hitchcock, Janice. "Crisis Intervention: The Pebble in the Pool." *American Journal of Nursing* 73 (Aug. 1973): 1388-1390.

King, Joan. "The Initial Interview: Basis for Assessment in Crisis Intervention." *Perspectives in Psychiatric Care* 9 (Nov.-Dec. 1971): 247-256.

Kuenzi, Sandra, and Fenton, Mary. "Crisis Intervention in Acute Care Areas." *American Journal of Nursing* 75 (May 1975): 830-834.

Norris, Catherine. "Psychiatric Crises." *Perspectives in Psychiatric Care* 5 (Jan.-Feb. 1967): 20-28.

Robischon, Paulette. "The Challenge of Crisis Theory for Nursing." *Nursing Outlook* 15 (July 1967): 28-32.

CHAPTER ELEVEN

THE FAMILY SYSTEM: NORMALITY, DISTURBANCE, AND INTERVENTION

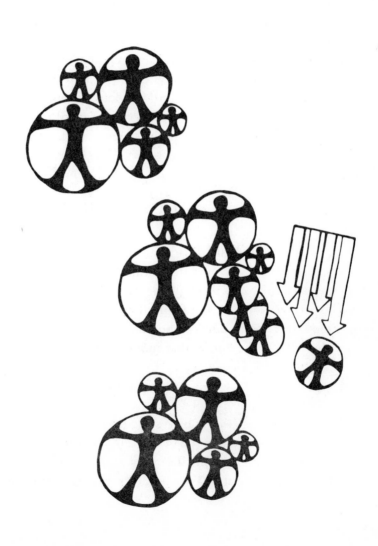

Nurses in all areas of practice relate to families continually, despite the fact that only one member of the family network may be the "patient." Because of this particular relationship to family networks, it is essential that a nurse understand normal patterns of family interaction and be able to appraise constructive patterns of coping with crisis situations. With this as a baseline, the nurse should be able to appraise family systems that are not growth-producing or that are temporarily immobilized in their problem-saving endeavors.

The nurse, because of these relationships to families, is in a unique position to intervene in ways that will help the family resolve their problems and thus allow for more freedom of communication between family members. This chapter first describes normal family processes, then treats disruptive patterns in family systems, and finally, outlines some techniques of intervention.

THE FAMILY AS A SOCIAL SYSTEM

An individual's first relationships are established in the context of the family. The family determines the boundaries of the individual's experimental world through the early years of development. Ideally, these experiences within the family prepare the individual to launch out into the larger world outside the family. What, then, are the processes generated within the family that influence the individual's development?

CONNECTEDNESS AND INDIVIDUAL IDENTITY

First, with the family structure, the individual becomes part of a group. In this context he or she must act out an individual identity while simultaneously defining his or her roles within the family group. Hess and Handel point out: "Two conditions characterize the nuclear family. Its members are connected to one another, and they are also separated from one another."[1] In analyzing families, one of the first factors to assess is the degree of individuality allowed each member. How much is each member allowed to be an individual in his or her own right? Or, in contrast, how much individuality must each member surrender as a condition of being a member of a particular family? For example, in some families, boys are pushed early into playing Little League baseball, whether or not they personally are interested. In situations such as this, the children are encouraged to fulfill their parents' dreams and aspirations rather than being recognized as individuals with differing interests.

An individual can achieve a sense a personal identity only out of an experience of close relationships with others. Erikson, in describing the reactions of a child who has learned to walk, details the process of identity development. In addition to deriving pleasure from having learned a new skill, the child becomes aware of having a new status—"one who can walk"—with whatever connotations it happens to have in his or her culture.[2]

> With the accomplishment of each developmental task the child's self-esteem grows to be a conviction that one is learning effective steps toward a tangible future, and is developing into a defined self within a social reality. The growing child must, at every step, derive a vitalizing sense of actuality from his awareness that his individual way of mastering experience . . . is a successful variant of a group identity, and is in accord with its space-time and life plan.[3]

It is the family that becomes the reference point as the child develops, and it is in this context that the person develops his or her group-rootedness. In the "normal" family, each developmental accomplishment is hailed as another step toward becoming a self-sufficient individual in one's own right. As the individual moves through adolescence, all the identities accumulated in the early stages of development, such as "one who can walk," "one who can talk," or "one who can do school work," become integrated into an overall composite of how one perceives oneself

1. Robert D. Hess and Gerald Handel, "The Family as a Psychosocial Organization," in *The Psychosocial Interior of the Family,* ed. Robert D. Hess and Gerald Handel (Chicago: Aldine Publishing Co., 1967), p. 11.
2. Erik Erikson, *Childhood and Society,* 2nd ed. (New York: W. W. Norton, 1963), p. 235.
3. Ibid., p. 235.

as an individual. Erikson describes this sense of ego-identity as "the accrued confidence that the inner sameness and continuity prepared in the past are matched by the sameness and continuity of one's meaning for others."[4] To separate successfully from the family structure to a world outside, the individual must have the confidence that the identities achieved within the family context are appropriate to a life outside it. Within a broader context, the person needs confidence in his or her capabilities both as a person and as a group member.

In assessing families, one question to ask concerns the degree of connectedness of family members. In a family in which there are extremely loose bonds between family members, or a sense of unrelatedness, the child receives no feedback about the meaning of his or her accomplishmnts. Lacking this appraisal of significant others, the child has difficulty in developing a sense of personal identity. On the other hand, in some families, the parents' sense of worth and competence as individuals is so tenuous that they have difficulties allowing a child to develop as an individual in his or her own right. In these families, an emphasis on "sameness" is an attempt to control this threat. In the "ideal" family structure, the child achieves a sense of belonging that allows him or her to become an individual valued by the family group as well as by himself or herself. As Hess and Handel point out, "the individual's effort to take his own kind of interest in the world, to become his own kind of person, proceed apace with his efforts to find gratifying connections to other family members."[5]

CONGRUENT IMAGES

A second family process surrounds the development of congruent images between family members. Hess and Handel formulate the problem:

> Living together, the individuals in a family each develop an image of what the other members are like. This image comprises the emotional meaning and significance which the other has for the member holding it . . . the image emerges from the holder's past and bears the imprint of his experience, delimiting what versions of others are possible for

---

4. Ibid., p. 261.
5. Hess and Handel, "Family as Psychosocial Organization," p. 13.

him. It says something about him as a person. But it is also a cast into the future, providing the holder with direction in relating to and interacting with the object.[6]

Through the interactive process within the family context, the individual develops a self-image. A person's self-image is the way in which that person perceives himself or herself as an object. An individual's self-image is frequently a composite of the way he or she is perceived by significant others. For example, a boy who is perceived to be a quiet, thoughtful person by others in the family may incorporate this image and, if asked to describe himself as an individual, would most probably say he is quiet and thoughtful. Ideally, an individual's self-image in the family system is built on certain given realities; that is, the child is quiet and thoughtful in actuality, rather than the perception having been misapplied to a child who is boisterous and thoughtless. But rarely can another individual be perceived as he or she truly is; we tend to see others as we wish them to be. Handel and Hess describe socialization as "the parents' effort to get the child to regard himself in substantially the same way they regard him."[7] All individuals confront the dilemma of being both what others wish them to be and the person they perceive themselves to be. But in most instances the divergence between self and others' views is not that great.

In analyzing family systems, then, it is important to evaluate the amount of agreement between how members perceive one another and how individuals perceive themselves. Problems arise when there is too great a discrepancy between "self" and "other" perceptions of individual members. For example, parents may hold an image of their child as being bright, able to achieve in school, and capable of rising to their middle-class aspirations of success in a profession or career. If the child has the potential to be what the parents envision, there may not be too many problems. However, if the child is unable or unwilling to meet these expectations, or has conflicting interests, problems may develop. There is need for consensus about the roles individual members are to play in the family constellation, based on a realistic assessment of the potentialities of individual members.

---

6. Ibid., p. 14.
7. Ibid., p. 15.

FAMILY THEMES

A third significant family process surrounds the "family theme." A family theme, according to Hess and Handel,

> . . . is a pattern of feelings, motives, fantasies, and conventionalized understandings grouped about some focus of concern which has a particular form in the personalities of individual members. The pattern comprises some fundamental view of reality and some way, or ways, of dealing with it. In the family, themes are to be found centered around the family's implicit direction, its notion of "who we are" and "what we do about it."[8]

Typical family themes are built around racial or ethnic origins, religious orientations, or place in the larger community structure. For example, a family of Swedish origin, from a rural area in the West, might have a family theme constructed around stories about grandparents who migrated to America, homesteaded, and faced terrific problems of survival. Despite having to eke out a living on the frontier, they revered education and therefore expected that all children in the family would pursue educational goals. A theme incorporates the story of how a particular family developed and also provides a point of departure for its members. The theme further incorporates a set of expectations held for family members. For example, the family theme presented above communicates multiple messages: "Members of this family work hard, persevere against extreme odds, and value education."

Further, a family theme incorporates a view of behavior considered appropriate. Implicit in the family theme developed above is a view that members work independently toward their goals and maintain stoicism in the face of loss.

Finally, a family theme incorporates a view of the external world that is a measuring standard for the family. For example, the Swedish family theme developed above might incorporate a view of another group, such as the Irish, which is diametrically opposed to their view of themselves. They might characterize the Irish as Catholic, lazy, emotional, and erratic. By maintaining stereotypes of other racial or ethnic groups, a family reaffirms the value of its particular view on life. Children in such a family learn not to associate with the "out group" implied in the family theme.

---

8. Ibid., p. 18.

In analyzing families, one particularly useful way of gaining valuable information is to focus on the family theme. By probing for information about how this particular family perceives its history, it is possible to trace ways in which the family finds its location vis-a-vis the larger social world. As Hess and Handel note, "by determining the salient themes in a family's life, we are able to see more clearly how any individual's fate is shaped, what opportunities he has for interlocking his life with others, and what pressures he must contend with."[9]

BOUNDARIES

A further factor to consider in analyzing a family system is the boundaries established for each individual's experience by virtue of being a family member. The family into which an individual is born sets limits on (1) the amount of differentiation allowed the individual, (2) the intensity or amount of emotional investment of individual members in the family system, (3) the extensity of experiences available to the individual, and (4) the tendency to evaluate experiences in a particular way.[10] In assessing family systems, it is important to ascertain the boundaries established for each of the family members, the expectations held, and the experiences available to the individual.

Finally, the family socializes its members into specific sex roles and thereby prepares individuals to deal with significant biosocial issues of living.[11] In normal families the child can successfully work out her or his identity in relationship to sex role demands.

To summarize, in assessing the growth-producing potential of family systems, the nurse evaluates:

1. The degree of connectedness between family members.

2. Freedom allowed individuals to develop an appropriate self-identity as opposed to fitting into stereotyped roles.

3. The degree of consensus among family members as to their reciprocal roles within the family structure.

4. Family "themes" and their influence upon individual members' perception of themselves and their families.

---

9. Ibid., p. 21.
10. Ibid., p. 21.
11. Ibid., p. 21.

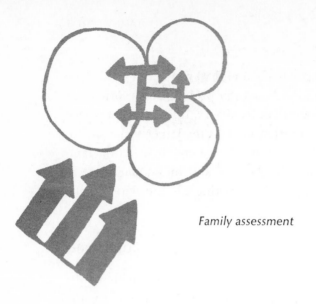

Family assessment

5. Boundaries of individual experiences circumscribed by the family system.

6. Sex role identification patterns within the family.

In assessing a family, the nurse looks at the intricate pattern of role relationships between family members. Each person plays a role, and in viewing a family system, it is important to evaluate the reciprocity between the roles. Let us consider a rather typical family that a public health nurse might encounter.

> The O'Connor family consists of the mother, the father, a ten-year-old son, Shawn; a daughter, Mary, age six; and a newborn baby, Kevin. The public health nurse is making a post-partum visit to see how the newborn baby is faring. She is greeted warmly by Mrs. O'Connor. Since it is a school holiday, Shawn and Mary are home, and Mr. O'Connor is working the evening shift.
>
> As the nurse enters, she sees Mary feeding the baby on the couch. Mrs. O'Connor comments on how interested Mary is in the baby and how she tries to involve the little girl in the care of the baby. Mr. O'Connor is about to go with Shawn to the park lagoon to go fishing. Mrs. O'Connor comments that they usually try to do something special with the children on a holiday. Shawn is excited about a new fishing reel that he received for his birthday a week ago: "It's just what I wanted; my Dad bought it for me." Mr. O'Connor kisses his wife good-bye and suggests she take a little rest while they are gone fishing.

"You know, she just tries to do too much, cooking, cleaning, and taking care of all of us." Mrs. O'Connor beams happily.

The nurse checks the baby and notes that he appears to be well-cared for, clean, and content. Mary watches the nurse carefully: "I'd like to be a nurse when I grow up." Mrs. O'Connor comments on how Mary helps her around the house. Later on, Mary shows the nurse her room. She has a large collection of stuffed animals of which she is very proud.

As the nurse talks with Mrs. O'Connor, she notes the way in which the mother refers to each of the children individually. Shawn is interested in building things and his teacher has noted his adeptness in this area. Mary likes to draw and seems quite artistic, and the baby Kevin seems more active than she can remember either Mary or Shawn being. Mrs. O'Connor apologizes that the house is not quite as clean and orderly as she would like it to be. "We just accumulate a lot of things, and there's always a lot of company coming and going; our families all live nearby."

In this very brief encounter, the nurse can get a fairly good picture of how a family system is operating. First, the family members definitely appear "connected" to one another, through the mother's account of the family's activities and through what the nurse observes—Mary's feeding of the baby, the father's relatedness to Mrs. O'Connor and Shawn. Although each of the members shows a high degree of relatedness, they also demonstrate a considerable degree of individuiality. Mary assumes a number of tasks around the house, but the nurse does not feel that the mother is pushing her into these roles. Each child appears to be viewed realistically by the parents and seen as an individual.

Family members agree on the roles of the other; for example, Shawn and Mary seem settled in roles that are appropriate within this particular family structure. The family theme, while not well-developed in this interaction, may revolve around their being gregarious and welcoming extended family members. "We are a happy family and like to have good times with our friends" may well be the way this family views themselves. The children's boundaries definitely extend outside the boundaries of the home, as evidenced by the mother's statement, "We like to take the children to different places on their days off." Certainly the sex role identification is clear-cut in this family.

In general, one has the impression that all members of this family have clear-cut perceptions of themselves within the family. The mother views her role as that of caring for her children and the house, cooking, cleaning, and other similar house-related tasks. The husband sees his role as that of provider. In this family, one does not get the feeling that people are "bumping into one another" competing for similar roles in the family structure.

Although this is a very traditional family structure, it illustrates the critical factors a nurse might look at in assessing a family system. This does not imply that only a traditional family structure meets the criteria of normality as growth-producing. Indeed, many would argue that such a family does not truly promote the development of the individual family members. But the fact remains, no matter what the prevailing value system, that a family system must provide for the development of each individual member without too much interference from the others.

DISTURBANCES IN FAMILY SYSTEMS

Some families, instead of providing growth-producing experiences for their members, tend to stifle the individuation process. All families develop some type of homeostatic balance.[12] That is, within all family systems, a range of behaviors is allowed for members. Difficulties develop when roles become rigidly circumscribed in ways that do not allow the individual to accomplish necessary developmental tasks. A family system becomes dysfunctional when it cannot adapt to change both within and outside the family structure. Satir summarizes the problem: "Because change must be coped with, a family system which does not have functional ways to assimilate it will have dysfunctional ways. Generally speaking, a system which has rules requiring that the present be seen in terms of the past will be dysfunctional."[13]

LOSS IN THE FAMILY

One of the factors that might contribute to a family's inability to deal with change is an inability to deal with the loss of significant, influential

12. Don Jackson and J. Weakland, "Conjoint Family Therapy: Some Considerations on Theory, Technique and Result," *Psychiatry* 24 (1961): 30-45.
13. Virginia Satir, "The Family as a Treatment Unit," in *Changing Families,* ed. Jay Haley (New York: Grune & Stratton, 1971). Original source *Confinia Psychiatrica* 8 (1965): 37-42.

members, or with loss of position within the larger social structure. Take, for example, a family in which an adolescent son died suddenly in a motor-cycle accident. This son was intelligent, a good student, and a recognized leader. Parental dreams were destroyed by his death. The circumstances of the accident were that the boy was riding a motorcycle given him by his father for his birthday over the mother's protests that "motorcycles aren't safe." Following the death of this son, the parents were unable to grieve their loss adequately or work through their feelings; any discussion of the incident ended in a series of recriminations by one parent against the other.

Instead of resolving their conflicts, the parents gradually began to pressure a younger son to do well in school and, in essence, to fill the dead son's place. The younger son, not able to maintain his own individual identity, begins to act out by engaging in delinquent behavior. Parental recriminations increase, and all their energies become directed toward their now-delinquent son. As a family, they achieve a balance that allows them to maintain personal distance and not deal with the loss of a family member. The family becomes increasingly dysfunctional.

In taking family histories, the nurse should be particularly sensitive in identifying significant family loss, including loss of (1) family members, (2) wage-earning potential, and (3) social status. Sometimes a family has experienced less tangible losses. Loss of the hope of attaining a cherished dream or resignation to never escaping from a life of poverty may be just as devastating as a more well-defined loss. Having identified significant family losses, it then becomes important to discern how these factors have influenced family interaction. How did the family originally cope with the loss? Were they able to grieve adequately and resolve the loss, or are they caught up in a web of unresolved feelings that impede family func-tioning? Frequently, family members get caught up in blaming one another.

SCAPEGOATING

A role frequently played by a disturbed member of a family constella-tion is that of family scapegoat. The family scapegoat acts out the con-flicts of the system. Vogel and Bell describe the process as one in which parents ". . . minimized expressions of affect, particularly hostility, which they strongly felt for each other, and thus made it possible to live with each other. But this equilibrium has many difficulties, the most serious of which was the scapegoating of a child."[14] Thus the scapegoat serves to stabilize the family system. The constellation of roles surrounding the scapegoat, according to Ackerman, includes the "family persecutor," who uses a special prejudice as the vehicle of his or her attack, and the "family healer," who intervenes to neutralize the attack and rescue the victim.[15]

For example, in the family described earlier, the father develops a prejudice against the younger son because he does not excel in intellectual endeavors. He berates the son for being "stupid" and either overtly or covertly contrasts him with his older brother. The mother intervenes as the "family healer" and makes excuses for her son's behavior. The family becomes engaged in a cyclical relationship. For instance, (1) Father reprimands son for not doing well in school. (2) Instead of staying home and doing schoolwork, son goes out with friends and violates his curfew. (3) Mother excuses child's behavior by saying, "He's only a child; you acted out at his age." The total relationship revolves around this cycle, and the parents never resolve their underlying conflicts.

PROBLEMS WITH INTIMACY

Other types of disturbance develop out of the parents' inability to deal with problems of intimacy in their marital relationship. In a family in which there is constant fighting and conflict, it may be hypothesized that this pattern is a defense against closeness in the marital relationship. Each parent may feel inadequate in the marital roles, and to avoid working out these feelings of inadequacy, they fight and so avoid any situation in which they might feel close to one another. Lidz et al. have described such families as schismatic.[16] Conflicts in such families frequently revolve around

---

14. Ezra F. Vogel and Norman W. Bell, "The Emotionally Disturbed Child as the Family Scapegoat," in *A Modern Introduction to the Family,* ed. Ezra F. Vogel and Norman W. Bell (New York: The Free Press, 1960).

15. Nathan Ackerman, "Prejudicial Scapegoating and Neutralizing Forces in the Family Group With Special Reference to the Role 'Family Healer'," *International Journal of Social Psychiatry,* 1964. Reprinted in *Theory and Practice of Family Psychiatry,* ed. John G. Howells (New York: Bruner/Mazel, 1971), pp. 626-634.

16. Theodore Lidz et al., "The Intrafamilial Environment of the Schizophrenic Patient: Marital Schism and Marital Skew," *American Journal of Psychiatry* 114 (1957): 241-248.

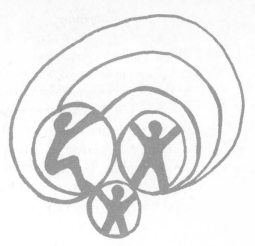

The under-adequate over-adequate family

issues relating to the apparent inadequacy of one partner, combined with the other's appearance as overadequate.[17] The following family illustrates this pattern:

A public health nurse visits a family six weeks following the birth of their third child. She finds the mother crying hysterically. In talking with the nurse, the mother describes the following incident: When the seven-year-old daughter came home for lunch, she dropped her coat on the floor rather than hanging it up. "I don't know what happened; I got so angry I lost control of myself, and I hit her on the head with the baby's bottle until it broke." As the nurse talks further with her, the mother describes her feelings that she has to do everything around the house while her husband is no help; she is becoming increasingly nervous, and she feels she is falling apart. The public health nurse suggests family counseling.

As the family counseling proceeds, the sessions repeatedly revolve around themes of the wife's perceiving the husband as inadequate. "I have to tell him to change his underwear, to brush his teeth, and wash under his armpits. He does nothing around the house but sleep." This theme is picked up and amplified by the fourteen-year-old daughter. The wife and daughter have progressively taken over all decision-making in the family. The husband reciprocates by playing the role of the inadequate man. In one session he states, "I can't do anything right, so why should I try to do anything?" All interactions between husband and wife center around fighting over situations in which the husband has done something wrong in his wife's view.

17. Murray Bowen, "The Use of Family Theory in Clinical Practice," *Comprehensive Psychiatry* 7 (1966): 345-374.

In a marriage such as this, the wife has increasingly assumed the role of the overadequate partner to cover for her real feelings of inadequacy. If she were not constantly complaining about her husband, she might have to deal with her discomfort about feelings of closeness to him. The reciprocal role, played by the husband, is that of the inadequate mate. In another family, the roles might be reversed. By keeping the conflict going, couples such as this can maintain a relationship without working through their difficulties and developing a satisfactory intimate relationship, which would be too great a threat to their personal identities. Children become caught up in their parents' struggles; these families are characterized by the development of factions.

PSEUDOMUTUALITY

A contrasting pattern of family relationships is evidenced in families with the predominating theme of the "happy family," Wynne et al. have described this pattern of relatedness in families as *pseudomutuality*. Pseudomutual patterns are characterized by (1) a persistent sameness of the role structure of the family; (2) an insistence on the desirability and appropriateness of this structure; (3) evidence of intense concern over possible divergence or independence from this role structure; and (4) an absence of spontaneity, novelty, humor, and zest in participating together.[18] Family members are involved mainly in "fitting together" rather than in promoting differentiation of family members. As individuals grow, any affirmation of their sense of personal identity is perceived as possibly destroying the relationship. Family members, as a condition of belonging, must give up their own sense of personal identity.

Such families usually come to the attention of outside persons because of a child's inappropriate behavior outside the family context. The school nurse, for example, may come into contact with families reflecting this pattern of relatedness in making a home visit to look further into the behavior of a withdrawn child. The child, whose behavior is appropriate within the family constellation, appears disturbed in a context where individuation is a necessary component of behavior. When making con-

---

18. Lyman Wynne et al., "Pseudomutuality in the Family Relations of Schizophrenics," *Psychiatry* 21 (1958): 205-220.

tacts with such families, the nurse often cannot understand why a child from this type of family should be disturbed. The family presents itself as a "happy family"—"We always do things together," "We never have any disagreements." The blame for the child's inappropriate behavior is placed upon the teacher. "She's always been a model child; it must be something the teacher is doing."

The primary energies in these families are directed toward maintaining the *status quo*. No conflicts are tolerated. Although such families appear different from the conflictual families described earlier, the basic problem is similar. Family members avoid forming intimate bonds based upon recognition of each other as individuals by investing all their energies in making it appear "as if" they are truly a close, happy family. Behavior becomes ritualized and stereotyped, and in the process individual growth is stifled.

DOUBLE-BIND COMMUNICATION

Other family theorists have focused on communication patterns in family constellations. Bateson et al. describe a pattern of double-bind communication in families of schizophrenics. The necessary ingredients of a double-bind situation, according to these authors' formulations, include the following:

1. Two or more persons, one of whom is the "victim."
2. Repeated experience: the double-bind situation comes to be an habitual expectation.
3. A primary negative injunction, which may have either of two forms: (a) "Do not do so and so, or I will punish you," or (b) "If you do not do so and so, I will punish you."
4. A secondary injunction conflicting with the first at a more abstract level, and, like the first, enforced by punishments or signals which threaten survival.
5. A tertiary negative injunction prohibiting the victim from escaping from the field.[19]

In a double-bind communicative interchange, the individual is faced by a number of contradictory messages, both overt and covert. The indi-

19. Gregory Bateson et al., "Toward a Theory of Schizophrenia," *Behavioral Science* 1, no. 4 (Oct. 1956): p. 252.

vidual can make no appropriate response. Following this line of reasoning, Bateson and his colleagues hypothesize:

> ... the family situation of the schizophrenic has the following general characteristics:
>
> 1. A child whose mother becomes anxious and withdrawn if the child responds to her as a loving mother. . . .
>
> 2. A mother to whom feelings of anxiety and hostility toward the child are not acceptable, and whose way of denying them is to express overt loving behavior to persuade the child to respond to her as a loving mother and to withdraw from him if he does not. . . .
>
> 3. The absence of anyone in the family, such as a strong and insightful father, who can intervene in the relationship between the mother and child and support the child in the face of the contradictions involved.[20]

In this example, the mother of the schizophrenic simultaneously expresses at least two messages: hostility and anxiety at the covert level, and overtly loving behavior. The child does not know which message to respond to. If he or she reciprocates by expressing loving behavior, this stimulates increased anxiety in the mother, accompanied by increased hostility that she in turn must deny. In observing mother-child interactions, the nurse must be alert to double-bind situations. In particular, it is important to be sensitive to mothers who never voice or indicate hostile feelings toward their children. This may be indicative of a mother who must deny and mask all hostile impulses and, in so doing, create a double-bind situation for the child. A child caught up in a double-bind finds it impossible to individuate and become an individual in his or her own right.

To summarize, indications of disturbances in family systems include inability to deal with losses of significant members; prejudicial scapegoating of a member; inability to deal with problems of intimacy, masked by constant conflict or by pseudomutuality; and double-bind communicative interchanges.

PRINCIPLES OF INTERVENTION

The first stage of family intervention is assessment. In most instances, families are seen because one family member has created diffi-

---

20. Ibid., p. 256.

culties either within the family itself or in the larger social networks surrounding it. A starting point in making a family assessment might be to get each family member to give his or her version of the family problem. The following case shows this technique:

> The Taylor family has been referred for family counseling because of the problems of the fourteen-year old son, James. He reportedly was a model child until about a year ago. He then began acting out in school. As a result of his misbehavior, he was excluded from regular school and placed in a school for socially maladjusted children a considerable distance from the home. Currently he leaves home for school in the morning, but frequently does not go there. Instead he spends his days riding around on buses. The truant officer from school is the referral agent. In the first session Helen and William Taylor, the parents, and James are seen. Six other children were not included in the initial family interview.
>
> *Counselor:* Mr. Taylor, would you like to start by telling us something about your family and how you see the problem?
>
> *Mr. Taylor:* Well, I just don't know what's wrong with James. Things have been going so nicely, and I just don't know why he's started cutting up so. You see, I've worked very hard to provide for my family. I came from Mississippi when I was eighteen and went straight to work for the post office. I never had much of a chance for an education, and I've always wanted my kids to have a better life than I did, and James was doing so well in school. He played in the band and was liked by other children, and now he just seems to be throwing it all away.
>
> *Counselor:* How do you see things, Mrs. Taylor?
>
> *Mrs. Taylor:* Pretty much the same way. I've worked hard to be a good mother to my family. We just moved; we bought this six-flat, and I'm working hard to make it go, and then James is bringing me all this grief, and I don't know what to do.
>
> *Counselor:* James, how do you see things?
>
> *James:* (Shifts nervously in chair and twists hands) I don't know. I just feel that I don't belong no more. (Silence)
>
> *Counselor:* Can you tell me some more about that? (No response)

From opening statements such as these, it is possible to ascertain the parents' investment in James as a reflection of their own personal aspirations. Not only is he creating problems, but his behavior is destroying all the things that they have worked hard to achieve. James accurately perceives that they are tied up in their own personal hurts rather than in his pain, and he accurately perceives himself as "feeling left out." In gathering information about the family system, a useful strategy is to guide the family to focus on when their difficulties began. It is especially important to be alert to any family crisis situations that might have precipitated the family's difficulties.

Counselor: (To father) Can you identify when James's problems began?

Mr. Taylor: I just don't know. He was getting along so well in school, and then we moved to our new house. I was busy working overtime, and maybe I didn't spend enough time with him. And then there was the accident. . . .

Counselor: The accident?

Mrs. Taylor: I don't think that has anything to do with James's problems. It's something that's past and we don't think about it.

Counselor: It must be of some importance to you, Mr. Taylor.

Mr. Taylor: Well, you know, boys will be boys. They were just playing around.

Mrs. Taylor: I had told James not to shoot arrows in the house. I guess I wasn't watching, I was so busy working on the garden.

Families will frequently talk about an incident as if the therapist knows what they are talking about. It is important that the therapist seek clarification, as it allows the family to relive the experience rather than getting caught up in guilt or blaming.

Mrs. Taylor: I had always told James that he couldn't shoot arrows in the house. We had just moved into our new house and we have a big basement there. James and some of the neighborhood boys were down there, and they were shooting arrows and I didn't know about it. I sent Denise down to call James for lunch. She went down the steps, and just then James must have shot the arrow, and it hit Denise in the eye. We rushed her to the hospital and they had to take her eye out.

Counselor: After this happened, did you talk about it?

Mrs. Taylor: I stayed with Denise all the while she was in the hospital, and then after it was over I didn't think it would do any good to talk about it. James is a good boy and I know he didn't mean to shoot his sister's eye out.

Counselor: And you've never talked about this as a family?

Mrs. Taylor: What's the use? We can't get her eye back.

Counselor: In the next session it would be valuable to have Denise here, and then maybe we can explore this further.

When a family crisis involves a particular family member, it is important to include him or her in the exploration. In this first session, little attention is focused on the behavior of James that brought the family in for counseling. Rather, the counselor makes the assessment that James's behavior is an outgrowth of some unresolved issues in the family constellation. The next session is a further exploration of the family problem:

> *Counselor:* Denise, in the last session we just started talking about the accident in which you lost your eye. Maybe you would like to tell us something about it.
>
> *Denise:* I just want to forget about it. (Eyes downcast and sad)
>
> *Counselor:* I know it is painful to talk about something like this, but it is important.
>
> *Mrs. Taylor:* I don't like to see my baby so sad. Her artificial eye looks just about real, and I take care of it so she doesn't have to do anything with it. Since this happened, she isn't the same happy girl.
>
> *Counselor:* Did you ever scold James or talk to him about the accident after it occurred?
>
> *Mrs. Taylor:* What's the use? It wouldn't bring her eye back.
>
> *Counselor:* James, can you tell us how you see things?
>
> *James:* Well, it's like it happened (slowly) . . . I didn't mean to do it, and I know I shouldn't have been playing with arrows. We were new in the neighborhood and none of the new boys had a bow and arrow. I was just going to show it to them, and I thought I was pretty important. We got to playing around and I was just going to scare Denise and my finger slipped (begins to cry). And no one ever talked to me about it. If only someone would have punished me or said something. It's like I'm not a part of the family any more.
>
> The session proceeds with the family counselor helping them go through the feelings associated with the accident.

The family system had become immobilized because of inability to deal with a crisis situation. All of the family's energies were tied up in denying that anything had changed. By not talking about the accident, the fourteen-year-old boy was unable to resolve his guilt and was progressively cut off from communication within the family network. His sixteen-year-old sister, Denise, faced with the developmental tasks of adolescence, was similarly hampered. Mrs. Smith, by taking over the care of the artificial eye, was fostering denial in Denise. Further, not teaching Denise how to care for her eye herself precluded her moving toward increasing independence from the family. Mr. and Mrs. Taylor, through the years, had been primarily invested in their separate spheres of work with little communication. They had been unable to talk about their feelings in the situation. At this point the family was immobilized.

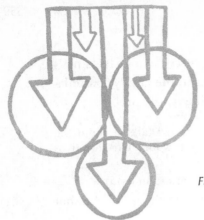

Family intervention

FAMILY INTERVENTIONS

Based on this formulation, intervention then is focused on working with the family to reach a resolution of their difficulties. Strategies employed were centered on opening communication that had become blocked, providing the family with a new understanding of their interrelationships, and developing altered patterns of relatedness.

One approach to opening up the family system is, first of all, for the counselor to present his or her formulation of the problem to the family.

> *Counselor:* James seems to be telling us that not talking about what happened has made him feel that he no longer belongs. It's like he did something and suddenly can't communicate with anyone, and he feels shut out. And he doesn't go to school or behave as a way of "calling for help." It's like he needs to find some way of getting back into the family, but he doesn't know how. The only other alternative he sees is to detach himself completely from the family and his friends.
>
> *Mrs. Taylor:* I thought we were doing the right thing not to talk about it. It's like there was nothing that could be done, and I didn't want James to feel bad.
>
> *Counselor:* It must be very difficult for you to deal with your feelings, and you wanted to protect James and Denise. But James knows how bad you feel and he feels that way too. By not talking about it, James must feel that there is no way for him to be forgiven for what he did.

Although James was the presenting patient, other family members were in pain. Later in the same session, the counselor directed the communication to Denise and the way in which she had adjusted to her eye loss. Mrs. Taylor described in great detail the procedures involved in caring for the artificial eye.

> *Counselor:* Denise doesn't do any of this for herself?
>
> *Mrs. Taylor:* I don't want her to have to think about it.
>
> *Counselor:* Trying to protect Denise keeps her from working through her feelings about the loss of her eye. How do you feel about this, Denise?
>
> *Denise:* It's like everything has changed. One thing I think about and that's that I can never go away from home very far, like I can't go spend the night with my girlfriend or any of the things that I used to do.
>
> *Counselor:* It's like you're totally dependent upon your mother.

After giving the family an overview of the problem, a useful strategy is that of giving the family a task to work on before the next session.

> *Counselor:* Before you come back the next time, Mr. Taylor, I want you to get your whole family together and go through the accident, like we did here today, and for each of you to try to recall the feelings that you had at the time. And Mrs. Taylor, I want you to begin teaching Denise how to care for her eye. Come back in a month and tell me how things are working out for you.

By engineering alterations in patterns of relating, other changes occurred within the family system. At the next session the family reported:

> *Mr. Taylor:* After we got home we got together. It was really strange. I realized we hadn't talked together as a group since this happened. We were able to talk a little about how angry we felt about James messing things up for the family, and Denise talked about how she feels.
>
> *Counselor:* How did it go to teach Denise?
>
> *Mrs. Taylor:* At first she was so squeamish. The first day she sat down and cried, and I cried with her. But then she got so she could touch it. And now she takes care of it all by herself.
>
> *Counselor:* Denise, how are you feeling about it?
>
> *Denise:* For the first time, I went to stay at my girl friend's house, and now it doesn't seem too bad. I don't think most people even notice.
>
> *Counselor:* What about you, James?
>
> *James:* I feel like I'm back in the family. I'm going to go to school so I can get back to my regular school. I can't wait to get back in the band.

In this family the problem was easily resolved. Once the family was given assistance in dealing with a difficult loss, the natural strengths of the family came to the fore and the family members could develop and mature as individuals.

In other families the problems may not be so easily resolved, but the principles remain the same:

1. Identify the family problem.
2. Assist the family to gain an understanding of the problem.
3. Plan interventions to promote change within the system.

SUMMARY

In summary, there are certain processes which occur in a "healthy" family that support both the family as a unit and the individual family member as a person in his or her own right. Ideally, the family establishes boundaries for each member's experiential world, develops patterns of connectedness while fostering the growth of individual identity, and facilitates adequate and accurate self-imagery so that the person perceives himself or herself realistically in relationship to the total family unit. Through family themes it provides the person with an integrated "view of the world" and himself or herself within it.

In viewing family systems, the nurse uses the above dimensions to assess the level of function of the family. Some families, instead of fostering growth, restrict family members. The nurse should be particularly sensitive to the following disturbances in family systems: (1) inability to resolve the loss of a family member, (2) scapegoating, (3) inability to relate on an intimate level with one another, reflected in schismatic or pseudomutual patterns, and (4) double-bind communication.

As with other forms of intervention, the first step consists of assessment and formulation of the family problem. Intervention is aimed at freeing up the family system so that family members need no longer respond to one another in their stereotypical pattern. Strategies are developed to open communication to increase family members' understanding of one another and develop new patterns of relatedness.

FURTHER READINGS

Anderson, Dorothy. "Nursing Therapy With Families." *Perspectives in Psychiatric Care* 7, no. 1 (1969): 21-27.

Barry, M. Patricia. "Feedback Concepts in Family Therapy." *Perspectives in Psychiatric Care* 10, no. 4 (1972): 183-189.

Bulbulyan, Ann. "The Psychiatric Nurse as Family Therapist." *Perspectives in Psychiatric Care* 7, no. 2 (1969): 58-67.

Cornwell, Georgia. "Scapegoating: A Study in Family Dynamics." *American Journal of Nursing* 67 (Sept. 1967): 1862-1867.

Costello, David. "Communication Patterns in Family Systems." *Nursing Clinics of North America* 4 (Dec. 1969): 721-729.

Craven, Ruth, and Sharp, Benita. "The Effects of Illness on Family Functions." *Nursing Forum* 11, no. 2 (1972): 186-193.

De Young, Carol. "Nursing's Contribution in Family Crisis Treatment." *Nursing Outlook* 16 (Feb. 1968): 60-62.

Gerrish, Madalene. "The Family Therapist Is a Nurse." *American Journal of Nursing* 68 (Feb. 1968): 320-323.

Getty, Cathleen, and Shannon, Anna. "Nurses as Co-Therapists in a Family Therapy Setting." *Perspectives in Psychiatric Care* 5, no. 1 (1967): 36-46.

Haller, Linda. "Family Systems Theory in Psychiatric Intervention." *American Journal of Nursing* 74 (March 1974): 462-463.

Hartmann, Kathleen, and Bush, Mary. "Action-Oriented Family Therapy." *American Journal of Nursing* 75 (July 1975): 1184-1187.

Kovacs, Liberty. "A Therapeutic Relationship with a Patient and His Family." *Perspectives in Psychiatric Care* 4, no. 2 (1966): 11-21.

Mereness, Dorothy. "Family Therapy: An Evolving Role for the Psychiatric Nurse." *Perspectives in Psychiatric Care* 6, no. 6 (1968): 256-259.

Miller, Jeanne. "Systems Theory and Family Psychotherapy." *Nursing Clinics of North America* 6 (Sept. 1971): 395-406.

Monea, Helen. "A Family in Trouble (A Case Study of a Family Conjoint Family Therapy)." *Perspectives in Psychiatric Care* 12, no. 4 (1974): 165-170.

Rohde, Ildauro. "The Nurse as Family Therapist." *Nursing Outlook* 16 (May 1968): 49-52.

Salerno, Elizabeth. "A Family in Crisis." *American Journal of Nursing* 73 (Jan. 1973): 100-103.

Smith, Lois, and Mills, Bernadine. "Intervention Techniques and Unhealthy Family Patterns." *Perspectives in Psychiatric Care* 7, no. 3 (1969): 112-119.

Smoyak, Shirley. "Threat: A Recurring Family Dynamic." *Perspectives in Psychiatric Care* 7, no. 6 (1969): 267-274.

Walri, Mary. "Nurse Participation in Family Therapy." *Perspectives in Psychiatric Care* 3, no. 5 (1965): 8-13.

CHAPTER TWELVE

THE GROUP: DYNAMICS, THERAPEUTIC POTENTIAL, AND INTERVENTION

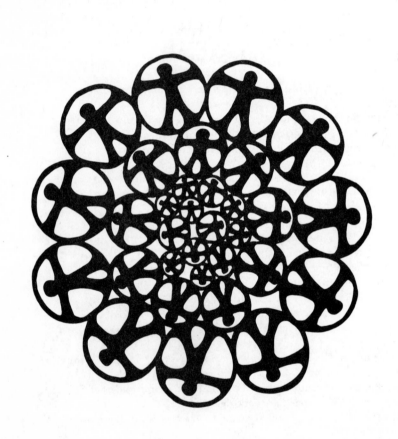

As we have pointed out throughout this book, individuals develop problems of coping in an interactional matrix. Because of this, it becomes important to consider the effects of groups upon the individual. As children we are surrounded by playmates, schoolmates, and teammates. In adulthood, we become involved with a number of diversified groups through work and leisure activities. Personal achievements often are largely contingent on relating to those in relevant social groups.

In light of these observations, psychiatric nursing should, first, include a knowledge of the ways in which groups function and the effect of the group upon the person. Second, since individual problems usually develop within a group context, the therapeutic potential of the group warrants consideration. Third, groups may be used to facilitate personal growth. Groups that are directed toward learning/training to achieve of necessary skills, or remotivation/resocialization for those who have lost the necessary motivation or social capabilities to live successfully outside mental institutions are examples of groups whose major goals are not specifically psychotherapeutic. On the basis of their potential for helping people, the nurse may employ the curative forces within groups to move persons toward more adequate ways of coping with a wide range of social and psychological problems.

THE DYNAMICS OF SMALL GROUPS

If we are to understand how problems develop within groups and subsequently how a group may be used to facilitate problem resolutions, it is important first to be knowledgeable about some general principles of group behavior.

A first question is how to define a group. An individual daily encounters aggregates of people: waiting for a bus, riding an elevator, and other similar situations. These aggregates have only limited influence

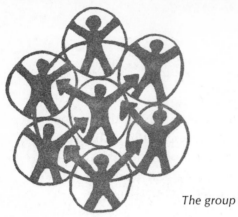

The group rootedness of the person

upon an individual. In contrast to these loosely related associations, individuals participate in groups in which intense interaction occurs, such as work groups, bridge-playing groups, or therapy groups. In these interactions individual behavior is highly contingent on the group. Knowles and Knowles describe groups as having the following stable features: (1) definable membership, (2) group consciousness, (3) a sense of shared purpose, (4) interdependence in satisfaction of needs, (5) interaction, and (6) ability to act in a unitary manner.[1]

A nursing team is an example of a group in which there are assigned members with a shared goal, the care of a specific group of patients. The work satisfaction of an individual member is closely intertwined with the way in which the team functions. A highly developed system of communication develops within the team; in times of crises the team may act as a unitary body. To a certain degree, personal identity merges with that of the larger social group.

Group membership presents a dilemma to the individual. As Cartwright and Lippitt point out:

> ... the individual needs social support for his values and social beliefs; he needs to be accepted as a valued member of some group which he values; failure to maintain such group membership produces anxiety and social disorganization. But on the other hand, group membership

1. Malcolm S. Knowles and Hulda F. Knowles, *Introduction to Group Dynamics*, rev. ed. (New York: Association Press, 1972), pp. 40-41.

and group participation tend to cost the individual his individuality. If he is to receive support from others and, in turn, give support to others, he and they must hold in common some values and beliefs. Deviation from these undermines a possibility of group support and acceptance.[2]

If a person becomes joined in group interaction, his or her subsequent behavior in the group depends to a degree on his or her individual characteristics, but this individuality is molded and shaped by the properties of the group. By committing himself or herself to participate in a group, the person necessarily surrenders some freedom as the price of belonging.

GROUP PROPERTIES

Groups vary in their membership requirements. To understand the conditions of membership in any group and the problems they pose to the individual, it is helpful first to have an overall appreciation of the properties of a group: (1) background, (2) participation pattern, (3) communication, (4) cohesion, (5) atmosphere, (6) standards (or norms), (7) sociometric pattern, (8) structure and organization, and (9) procedures.[3]

■ *Background.*   The pressures that a group exerts upon a person are: to a degree, contingent on its background. A nurse, newly hired on a medical unit, who is assigned to a team with a long history of working together must fit her or his behavior to that of the group.

A first question in analyzing any group is to ascertain its history. How long have they been a group? Why did they initially form a group? What types of persons are group members? What was the basis of their attraction to the group? By ascertaining answers to these questions, one can assess the degree to which the system is open to a new member as well as the pressures to conform that will be exerted upon a new member. A person attempting to join a group with a background markedly dissimilar from his or her own experiences a great deal of anxiety in that it is difficult, if not impossible, to discern his or her place within this social structure.

2. Dorwin P. Cartwright and Donald Lippitt, "Group Dynamics and the Individual," reprinted from *International Journal of Group Psychotherapy* in *Group Development: Selected Readings,* ed. Leland Bradford (Washington, D.C.: National Training Labs, 1961).
3. Knowles and Knowles, *Introduction to Group Dynamics,* pp. 42-52.

- *Participation Patterns.* Each group develops characteristic patterns of participation. In some groups most of the communication is directed from the leader to individual group members, with little interaction among the members themselves. Again using the nursing team as an example, the team leader may see this role as that of giving direct orders to other team members in the initial team meeting for the day; at the end of shift report, she or her expects team members to give a report on their patients. In this type of group, there is little interaction between the members. In other types of teams, the leader may value collaborative planning and enlist active participation of all group members. In the first type of group, involvement of group members may be minimal, while in the second, individual participation is emphasized. An individual joining a group must be able to discern what patterns of participation are expected and gauge his or her behavior accordingly.

- *Communication.* Communication patterns unique to a group develop in the interactive process. Each group develops a language of its own. The development of a language unique to the group serves to limit the communication network only to those who have learned this private language. The nursing team in surgery is a good example. Communication occurs through both verbal and nonverbal symbols. The outreached hand at a certain point in the operative procedure signals the nurse to hand the doctor a scalpel. A newcomer entering this scene would not know what was expected until he or she had an opportunity to observe and be instructed in the meaning of this group's symbols. But once having learned the meaning of the communicative symbols and developed the capacity to respond appropriately, the individual has a feeling of belonging to the group that is personally satisfying.

- *Group Cohesiveness.* As the bonds between group members become established, group cohesiveness develops. It is an outgrowth of similarities between members, attraction to other members of the group, and shared expectations for group membership. The first meeting of any group illustrates the initial process by which group members search for areas of commonality among themselves.

A group of woman nurses meeting together for the first time, for instance, will inevitably present themselves first in terms of their nursing background. They will compare notes on where they went to school and their work experiences, and will attempt to make links on the basis of these commonalities. The next level of interaction will probably involve a discussion related to women's roles held in common by members of the group. Those who are married may talk about their husbands' occupations or their children. Discussion of these roles is more problematic than the earlier discussion of professional roles, for probably not all in the group will be married or have children, and with the upsurge of the women's movement, the commonality of values pertaining to women's roles is questionable. Although there may be different value systems represented in the group, one basic commonality remains—they are all women.

Only after a group has been established over a period of time or has shared experiences that serve to solidify the bonds between members are controversial issues discussed. Politics, religion, and topics of this nature are rarely discussed at a first meeting of a group in which the views of members on these topics are not known. Introduction of a topic prematurely, before group cohesiveness has been developed, is likely to precipitate isolation of the member who introduced the topic before the group had developed to a stage that it was ready to handle controversy.

■ *Atmosphere.*   Each group also develops a characteristic atmosphere. In many instances the group atmosphere varies markedly from the larger organizational context. A nursing team in a hospital frequently has an atmosphere of gaiety that contrasts with the life-and-death matters the team members face in their daily work. A football team, in contrast, frequently has an atmosphere of grim determination and seriousness that is in marked contrast to the mood one would expect in a sport or game. In the first instance, the group provides a means for releasing tension and for group members to gain support from one another, enabling them to cope with the seriousness of their work. In the case of the football team, the team conference is exceedingly important in uniting the team toward the goal of winning. The threat of the outside opponent mobilizes the group to become serious in its attempts to win.

In observing a group, note the atmosphere that prevails and compare it with the overall goals of the group as well as the context of the larger organizational environment. From these observations, it should be possible to hypothesize the meaning of the group to its members. An individual who does not adjust his or her behavior to the general atmosphere of the group may find himself or herself ostracized. The football player who thinks that the game should be played just for fun is likely not to make the team. The nursing team may not welcome a member who will not relax from the on-the-job tension.

▪ *Norms.* Each group develops standards, or norms, for its members. Newcomb et al. describe the process through which group norms become established.

> A *group norm* exists insofar as a set of members share favorable attitudes toward such a regularity—insofar, that it, as they agree and are aware that they agree that the regularity should be regarded as a *rule* that properly applies to the specified persons in the specified situations. The principal characteristics of group norms as distinct from other shared attitudes is that they represent shared acceptance of a rule, which is a prescription for ways of perceiving, thinking, feeling, or acting.[4]

Groups develop their own rules as they interact over time, but they generally are unaware of these unspoken agreements until a member inadvertently violates them. Examples of norms that develop in groups relate to punctuality, attendance, topics that may be discussed, and the emotional affect of group members. As group members interact over time, norms extend to common ways of perceiving events, common beliefs, and common values. A nursing team, again as an example, develops a shared perception of the meaning of the "bleeps" of coronary monitoring devices. A whole series of rules develops about the way in which team members are to respond should there be a disturbance in the expected rhythm. No one need speak a word; each person is expected to play his or her role in the group performance. Other groups similarly develop common beliefs. Nursing team members, for instance, may share the belief that pain-killing medication should last four hours and that a patient who complains after two hours is a "crock," or similar rules of thumb commonly shared in interpreting patient behavior.

As groups exist over time, they develop a set of evaluative norms. Nursing teams, for example, very rapidly develop their own set of "norms" for defining "good" patients. The "good" patient commonly becomes defined as such because his or her behavior lets the nurses reciprocate in such a way that they can perceive themselves to be "good" nurses. A patient who does not complain of pain allows a nurse to feel that she or her

---

4. Theodore Newcomb, Ralph H. Turner, and Philip E. Converse, *Social Psychology: The Study of Human Interaction* (New York: Holt, Rinehart, and Winston, 1965), p. 229.

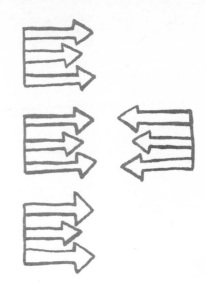

Group alliances

is a "good" nurse. An important facet to observe in groups relates to the
set of implicit agreements that have been reached, which reflect the norms
developed within the group.

■ *Sociometric Patterns.* Over time certain members become increasingly attracted to one another, while others are consistently in juxtaposi-
tion. Alliances usually develop out of perceived commonalities between
certain members. In many instances, the bonds between members become
so strained that when issues are discussed, members interact to preserve
their interrelationships rather than responding to the substantive issues
themselves. In a nursing team, team members may be so intent on demonstrating their agreement with the team leader that they do not explore
relevant issues. A contrasting pattern is one in which members consistently
oppose one another. If a certain member makes a statement, another member predictably disagrees. Again, the logical progression of group discussion does not occur, and the interaction reflects the coalitions and conflicts
between group members. An important factor, then, in assessing group
interaction relates to the sociometric patterns developed within the group.
Which members are attracted toward one another and consistently are
supportive? Which members are in opposition to one another? And what
are the bases of these coalitions and conflicts?

■ *Structure.* Finally, each group develops a unique character with
well-developed structure, functions, and procedures. A newcomer to a

group frequently feels as if he or she is visiting a foreign land until he or she can discern the patterns within this particular group. Members arrive at a set time. Meetings are opened in a standard way, whether it be a formalized structure in which the minutes of the last meeting are read or an informal structure in which the "leader" says, "Does anyone have anything they wish to discuss?" Only a narrow range of topics usually is discussed in groups; in some the rule is to talk only about agenda items, while in sensitivity groups only feelings are to be discussed. As a person moves through the course of a day, she or her interacts with multiple groups, all with their own unique structure and function. The individual must discern accurately a multiplicity of factors if she or he is to function adequately in this complex interactive network.

■ *Stability and Change.* Groups maintain themselves over time by achieving a delicate balance between stability and change. On the one hand, there must be enough cohesion and similarity between group members to maintain the group, but there must also be an optimal level of conflict and competition to generate movement in the group. Groups move through a number of phases over time. Typically, the first phase consists of individually centered contributions. Group members talk about things relevant to their lives outside the group. As people contribute increasing amounts of data about themselves, competition and aggression tend to develop.[5] Using again the case of a group of nurses, an initial discussion may revolve around the group members' professional backgrounds. However, as the group interaction develops over time, competitiveness is likely to arise. For instance, nurses coming from a diploma program will argue the merits of their educational background against those of baccalaureate programs. Usually this type of competitiveness is quite subtle, but as the group continues to interact, it develops to a point of confrontation between group members.[6] Following this phase, the group typically searches for a resolution. In the conflict and confrontation phase, the emphasis is on the differences between group members, while in the resolution phase, discussion shifts to similarities. At this point the group actually begins to function as a group rather than as a number of discrete individuals.

5. D. C. Dunphy, "Phases, Roles, and Myths in Self-Analytic Groups," *Journal of Applied Behavioral Science*, 4 (1968): 195-225.

6. R. D. Mann et al., *Interpersonal Styles and Group Development* (New York: John Wiley & Sons, 1967), p. 172.

Through this process the cohesive bonds between group members are strengthened.

From this point the group can truly become a work group; if the work is therapy, for example, it is possible for the group to provide negative feedback[7] to a member in a way that can be growth-producing. The cohesive bonds have been strengthened so a person is able to process corrective input about his or her behavior without feeling devastated and isolated. If the person feels valued and secure as a group member, he or she can begin to acknowledge how his or her behavior affects that of other members.

A final phase of group interaction is the termination process.[8] This phase helps members integrate the total group experience so that they can successfully incorporate group learnings into their personal behavior. Typically, in the termination phase, the group recapitulates its history. Conflicts are reactivated and resolved. In the final session members usually are constructing a future independent of the group.

In summary, groups have the potential to promote positive changes in people. Knowles and Knowles summarize these potentiating forces:

> A group is an effective agent for change and growth in the individual to the extent that:
>
> a. Those who are to be changed and those who are to exert influence for change have a strong sense of belonging to the same group.
>
> b. The attraction of the group is greater than the discomfort of change.
>
> c. The members of the group share the perception that change is needed.
>
> d. Information relating to the need for change, plans for change, and consequences of change is shared by all relevant people.
>
> e. The group provides an opportunity for the individual to practice changed behavior without threat or punishment.
>
> f. The individual is provided a means for measuring progress toward change goals.[9]

Conversely, persons unable to relate within a group context become increasingly isolated and vulnerable to psychological stress. As they encounter "problems in living," they find themselves with no resources.

---

7. L. P. Bradford, J. R. Gibb, and K. D. Benne, *T-Group Theory and Laboratory Method* (New York: John Wiley & Sons, 1964), p. 16.

8. Mann et al., *Interpersonal Styles and Group Development*, p. 291.

9. Knowles and Knowles, *Introduction to Group Dynamics*, p. 62.

THERAPEUTIC POTENTIAL OF GROUP INTERACTION

Since individual problems commonly are an outgrowth of difficulties in relating to important social groups, resolutions of these "problems in living" similarly must be achieved in the context of group interaction. Yalom categorized the curative factors of group psychotherapy as:

1. Imparting of knowledge
2. Instillation of hope
3. Universality
4. Altruism
5. The corrective recapitulation of the primary family group
6. Development of socializing techniques
7. Imitative behavior
8. Interpersonal behavior
9. Group cohesiveness
10. Catharsis[10]

While these factors are particularly related to group psychotherapy, they may also apply in other kinds of groups, such as educational or re-motivation groups. Certain aspects, such as catharsis, may be emphasized less in these groups, while others, such as imparting of knowledge, may be emphasized more. The particular goal of the group, be it psychotherapy or some other more task-oriented goal, will dictate the factors to be emphasized.

SHARING OF INFORMATION

An important function of group interaction is the sharing of information. In most groups at least 50 percent of all interactions involve asking for and giving information. Information is essential if individuals are to achieve orientation toward one another and if the group is to accomplish its goals. In therapy groups the imparting of information among members is especially important. A powerful curative force in group interaction arises from the sharing of similar experiences. For example, a group of patients who have had colostomies exchange valuable information not only about techniques of physical management but also about common

---

10. Irvin D. Yalom, *The Theory and Practice of Group Psychotherapy* (New York: Basic Books, 1970), p. 5.

psychological adjustment problems. Similarly, a group of discharged psychiatric patients may profit from an exchange of information about their symptoms. A common topic, particularly in groups composed of schizophrenic members, surrounds the meaning of hallucinations. The realization that another person has shared a frightening experience provides support to an individual. Frequently, through an exchange of information of this type, patients achieve an understanding of anxiety-producing situations that precipitate hallucinatory experiences, and thus may find ways of coping more adequately with stress.

INSTILLATION OF HOPE

This sharing of information provides group members with hope. The person realizes that he or she is not alone in facing a frightening experience. He or she may also observe others who have successfully managed to cope with a physical or psychological handicap. The patient who has just had a colostomy, for instance, and feels that he or she will never be able to achieve a normal life is encouraged by interaction with others who have successfully managed this alteration in physical functioning without seriously disrupting their life style.

UNIVERSALITY

The person in group interaction learns that his or her experience is not unique. As Yalom depicts the situation:

> Many patients enter therapy with the foreboding thought that they are unique in their wretchedness, that they alone have certain frightening or unacceptable problems, thoughts, impulses, and fantasies . . . In the therapy group, especially in the early stages, the disconfirmation of their feelings of uniqueness is a powerful source of relief.[11]

To learn that another person feels the same anxieties and fears as oneself makes this particular reaction less threatening. Often times the person fears that he or she is "going crazy." The realization that others share similar feelings allows one to redefine his or her reactions in the framework of normality.

---

11. Ibid., p. 10.

ALTRUISM

The group gives its members the chance to offer help to others in a similar predicament. As Yalom points out, "Psychiatric patients often have long considered themselves as burdens to others, and it is a refreshing, self-esteem-boosting experience to feel that they have become important to others; a morbid self-absorption is temporarily relieved."[12] For example, in a group composed of poor chronic schizophrenic patients, an important curative force within the group may be the building of a supportive network that extends beyond the bounds of the formal group experience. Through maintaining telephone contacts and visiting one another, group members who lack a family network on which they may rely construct a supportive network of group members. This atmosphere of caring provides the opportunity for group members to begin to redefine themselves as important and valuable to other human beings.

RECAPITULATION OF THE PRIMARY FAMILY GROUP

The group provides an opportunity for the individual to repeat in a group context characteristic patterns of interaction first learned within his or her family of origin. In many instances, other group members become cast in the mold of siblings, with the group leader becoming a substitute for parental figures. The curative force in group interaction arises from the possibility of examining these interactions so that the person may gain insight into his or her effect on other people and re-learn more acceptable patterns of behavior.

SOCIALIZATION

Within the context of the group, a person has the opportunity to learn social skills that are important to life. Some rehabilitative groups, for instance, focus on resocialization. Mental patients isolated from the mainstream of life frequently have lost the most basic social skills. Frequently they return to the hospital because they do not "fit in" rather than because of overtly psychotic behavior. Socializing such patients into the accepted

---

12. Ibid., p. 12.

Creative forces of the group

social amenities is an important function of group interaction. Similarly, persons with common physical handicaps may provide an invaluable service to others with similar handicaps by socializing them into behavior acceptable within a broader social context.

IMITATIVE BEHAVIOR

Groups provide a setting in which people can learn through imitating other group members. One technique commonly used is role-playing, in which one member re-enacts behavior characteristic of another group member. Through this experience the person has the opportunity to practice new behaviors and to experience different response sets than those to which he or she has become accustomed. This allows him or her to begin experimenting with new behavior that may be more socially appropriate. These new behaviors in turn generate more positive responses, and the person may thereby begin to achieve a more positive self-identity.

INTERPERSONAL BEHAVIOR

Opportunities for interpersonal learning are myriad in the group experience. The person, by perceiving himself or herself as a member of a cohesive group, may achieve a sense of belonging which he or she has never experienced before. This in turn serves to reinforce and support the growth of self-esteem.

Finally, the group provides an opportunity to ventilate highly cathected thoughts and feelings in a safe and protective environment. The individual has a chance to express the full gamut of emotions in a way not possible in usual social settings. By experiencing a release of emotional expression, the person, through a discussion of the underlying basis for these intense emotions, can achieve a more objective understanding of earlier anxiety-provoking experiences. Psychic energy that has been utilized in repressing these intense emotions thus becomes available to cope with current life situations.

Groups provide a vehicle for helping people. Given the potential curative factors in group interaction, the problem becomes one of developing appropriate interventions so that participants will garner these positive experiences.

INTERVENTION TECHNIQUES

The role of the therapist is of utmost importance in developing and maintaining the group's therapeutic potential. The effective group leader, in Marram's view, "facilitates the benefits of group membership . . . maintains a viable group atmosphere . . . oversees group growth [and] . . . regulates individual growth within the group setting."[13] He or she is responsible first for developing the group and, once it is developed, monitoring group interaction in such a way that the group functions as a curative force for its members. Lieberman characterizes the group leader as a "social engineer."[14] Through the process of selecting patients, instructing them about the purposes of group therapy, carefully structuring the first group sessions, and developing an appropriate communicative network among group members, the therapist can establish a group in which therapeutic work can occur.

---

13. Gwen D. Marram, *The Group Approach in Nursing Practice* (St. Louis: C. V. Mosby, 1973), pp. 131-132.
14. M. A. Lieberman, "The Implications of Total Group Phenomenon: Analysis for Patients and Therapists," *International Journal of Group Psychotherapy* 17 (1967): 71-81.

SELECTION OF GROUP MEMBERS

Perhaps the most significant factor influencing the subsequent development of the group is the process of selecting group members. In assessing clients, the question must be raised as to both the appropriateness of the group as a therapeutic modality for a given person and the suitability of this individual for a particular group. Group therapy is most appropriate for the person who is able to express himself or herself verbally and whose behavior is not grossly deviant from that of other group members.

In selecting members for the group, one primary consideration is the problem of building group cohesiveness. Group members must have enough characteristics in common to be able to share in the initial phase of group development. As Schachter has demonstrated, in a small group, communication is heightened initially as a group attempts to influence the deviant members to conform to group norms. However, if these attempts fail, communication eventually diminishes and the deviant member becomes increasingly isolated.[15] Even before the selection process begins, the therapist ideally conceptualizes the "type" of group he or she hopes to initiate and evaluates potential clients in terms of commonalities that might initially bind a number of discrete individuals into a group. Commonalties may not be found in diagnostic categories but rather in characteristics such as socioeconomic status, race, age, shared problems (for example, alcoholism), or common experiences (such as state hospitalization). The potential group member must envision the group as providing something of value if he or she is to take the risk of becoming a group member.

PREPARATION OF THE PERSON FOR ENTERING THE GROUP

All clients should be interviewed individually by the therapist before beginning group therapy. The purpose of this interview is threefold: (1) to assess treatment needs, (2) to explore with the person his or her feelings about becoming a member of a therapy group, and (3) to outline behaviors expected of the person within the group. All too frequently a

---

15. S. Schacter, "Deviation, Rejection, and Communication," in *Group Dynamics: Research and Theory,* ed. D. Cartright and P. Zander (New York: Harper & Row Publishers, 1968), pp. 165-181.

client is merely told that he or she is to "join a group." If he or she asks why, the response is probably, "To talk about problems," with no further explanation of the meaning of this experience. By translating the expected positive outcomes into understandable language, the therapist can help the person appraise the potential value of group interaction. A typical explanation might include the following type of statements:

> In the group you will meet with other individuals who have problems similar to yours. Through talking with others, you will learn how they manage difficulties similar to yours.
> In the group you may talk about some of your doubts and fears and openly express feelings that you may not be able to share with anyone else, for fear they won't understand or think you are "crazy."
> Through participating in the group, you should be able to gain new understandings of how your behavior effects others and perhaps modify your behavior so that you can get along better.

If a person is going to take the risk of joining a group, the potential value of the experience must outweigh the cost of revealing himself or herself in a group setting. By explaining what the person can hope to gain through participation in the group, the therapist conveys certain expectations: (1) members are expected to communicate their problems within the group context; (2) interaction with other group members is the potential source of help rather than the therapist per se; (3) feelings are to be expressed openly; and (4) alteration in behavior is an expected outcome.

INITIATING THE GROUP

In the first session, the therapist must be actively involved in facilitating the development of the group. The first session arouses considerable anxiety, both in the group members and in the group leader. The basic objective is for group members to find a beginning basis for becoming a group. The therapist's role is twofold; he or she must first assist group members in presenting themselves to the group so that the building of cohesive bonds will become easier. Second, the therapist must develop strategies for diverting communication away from him or her and diffusing it throughout the group. The following interaction typifies some statements by discharged state hospital patients in a first meeting at a community mental health center:

GROUP SESSION 1

Therapist: As I've talked with each of you individually, we have discussed the purposes of meeting in a group—that in the group you can talk about some of the problems you have. All of you have been hospitalized at one time or another, and perhaps you would like to talk about what type of problems you have after coming out of the hospital. I would like for each of you to introduce yourself to the group and tell us something about yourself. Let's start with you, Mrs. A.

Mrs. A.: (Eyes downcast) I'm Mrs. A. I live with my daughter. I've been in the state hospital the last twenty-five years. My problem is that I'd like to get a job. They had me working in a workshop when I was in the hospital and that was nice. But now there's nothing for me to do. I just sit inside all day and sleep.

Mr. B.: That's sort of my problem too. I was working in this factory and I started taking drugs with some of my friends, and then I started seeing things and hearing voices. That's how I ended up in the state hospital. But now I'm better, my nerves are calmer, and I'd like to get a job, but if they know I've been in a state hospital no one will hire me.

Mr. C.: Yeah, man, and then there's the discrimination bit, too. If you're black, you just don't have a chance. The doctor in the hospital told me that sex was my problem. My trouble is that I can't find a woman. I go up to women in the street or in a restaurant and they get angry.

Mrs. D.: My problem is just the opposite—men. My husband isn't nice to me. All I do is sit home all day long. I used to like to go out and have fun, but he won't let me. And I'm afraid to have anything to do with my neighbors. You know how rough the neighborhood can be. I just sat in my apartment so long looking at television that I started to hear the voices, and then they took me away to the hospital.

Miss E.: (Quietly) I'd like to get a job, too. I used to be a good secretary, but now I just stay home and take care of my mother and my aunt, and they get on my nerves. Do you have any typing around here?

In this first session the therapist began by structuring the session so that it was clearly expected that all group members would participate by talking about their "problem." The group leader introduced one element of commonality by mentioning that all have been state hospital patients. The individual members relate their problems as individuals. Their plea is for the therapist to work miracles to solve their problems. The usual response of inexperienced group leaders is, first, to feel overwhelmed by the neediness of the group and then, as a defense against these feelings, immediately attempt to intervene to help the members with their overt problems. In doing this, the group leader blocks the formation of the

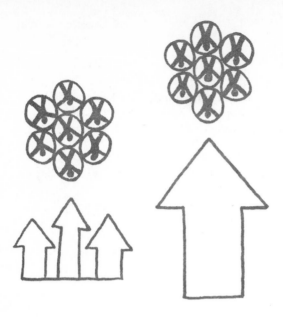

Leadership techniques

group by playing out the role of the "omnipotent" healer. Instead, the first concern should be to mobilize the group to become involved in group problem-solving.

Group members frequently become involved in giving each other suggestions in the first session. Although these suggestions may be no more helpful than those of the leader, they afford a vehicle through which members can initially express an atmosphere of caring. A later phase of the same group meeting described above might sound like this:

GROUP SESSION 2

Mrs. D. (to Mr. B.): What kind of work did you do in the factory?

Mr. B.: I was just an assembly-line worker at a plant that manufactured radios; you had to be very fast and it made me nervous.

Mrs. D.: I hear that they hire discharged mental patients over at the X Baking Company. Have you ever tried over there?

Mrs. A. (to Mr. C.): You say the doctor told you that sex was your problem. Just how do you go about approaching women?

Mr. C.: I just go up to them and say, "Hey baby, let's jive," and they walk away from me.

Mrs. A.: You've got to be more subtle. That would scare a woman off—you can't just go up and talk to them on the street. Have you ever tried getting involved in a church group? You could meet a nice woman there.

Although the initial attempts at helping others to problem-solve may be ineffectual and naive, the process builds an atmosphere in which group members care for one another and the therapist does not play the role of an omnipotent, all-knowing leader.

WORKING PHASE

During the initial stage, the group leader may start to feel that he or she has succeeded in getting a "good group" started. This feeling is frequently shattered when the next stage of group development, conflict and competition, occurs. Members become judgmental toward one another, and the group as a whole turns considerable hostility to the leader.

GROUP SESSION 3

Mrs. A. initiates the session by showing pictures of her grandchildren.

Mrs. E. (a black woman whose skin is very dark): My, they are a pretty color—nice chocolate-brown. They sure are pretty children.

Mr. C.: I think people like me are the most discriminated against. I'm not white and I'm not black. I represent two minority groups, Indians and black.

Mr. B.: You're just a shitty yellow.

Later the discussion progresses to a discussion of God.

Mrs. A.: I think that God is a white man up there in heaven just watching over us.

Mrs. E.: I don't think so. I think he's a light black man with reddish hair.

(The co-leaders of the group were a white man and a light-skinned, red-haired black man.)

GROUP SESSION 4

Mrs. E.: My boyfriend took me to the swellest restaurant last night. It was over in Indiana. We had a big shrimp cocktail and then chicken like you've never seen before, and salad and dessert. Ummm, was it ever good! And you know he tipped the waitress three dollars? It really was an expensive place.

Mr. C.: I don't believe you; you're just making this up to make us feel bad.

In this type of interaction, group members are jockeying for position in the group and are particularly aware of the therapists' responses to their attempts to gain recognition.

Hostility toward the leader (or leaders) develops as members realize that their expectations of a magical cure are not going to be met. Then, as the members' attempts to gain special attention are unsuccessful and each person realizes that he or she is not going to be the favored member in the group, resentment toward the leader increases.

GROUP SESSION 5

Mr. C.: I think that psychiatry is a bunch of hocus pocus. Doctors can't help you anyhow. They just sit here in the group and nod their heads. In the hospital there were all those group meetings. I think they were to entertain the staff. They didn't seem to help us any. If a psychiatrist were any good, he would help me.

Mrs. E.: In the hospital all the nurses did was give me pills, and they held me down when I got disturbed.

Mrs. A.: Yeah, I remember when they took me away to the hospital. I was not that upset until the nurses came after me and they held me down to give me a shot. I tried to run away and they got the biggest man I've ever seen to tie me down, and then they gave me this big needle, and I didn't remember anything until I woke up in this big room at the state hospital.

The attacks on the therapist may at times seem overwhelming and tend to feed into the therapist's feelings of powerlessness. At this stage it is extremely important that the therapist not retaliate or attempt to defend himself or herself, but rather use the experience as an important force in the group's further progress. As Yalom describes the process:

> . . . the therapist who withstands an attack without being either destroyed or destructive in retaliation but instead responds by attempting to understand and work through the sources and effects of the attack demonstrates to the group that aggression need not be lethal and that it can be expressed and understood in the group.[16]

At this stage it is important that the leader intervene in a way that does not indicate taking sides with either party in the conflict, but rather encourages group members to look at the underlying issues.

The third stage, cohesiveness, is one in which there is an atmosphere of mutual trust and disclosure. For example, in the sixth group session the group discussed their experiences in state hospitals.

---

16. Yalom, *Theory and Practice of Group Psychotherapy*, p. 239.

GROUP SESSION 6

Therapist: I would think that a state hospital isn't a very pleasant place, that you would all like to stay out of there.

Mrs. A.: I'd like to stay at home, but it really isn't that bad once you get used to them. At least they've got the bathrooms inside, not like when I was a child in Mississippi. And in winter it's nice and warm there.

Mr. C.: Yeah, and there's that nice fresh home-baked bread there, and you get plenty to eat.

Mr. B.: One thing that's not like outside—in the hospital everybody shares. Here if you want a cigarette, you just can't go up to anyone on the street and ask them for a cigarette, but in the hospital if another guy has a cigarette he'll at least let you smoke half of it. Out here no one cares.

GROUP SESSION 7

Mr. C.: What are hallucinations?

Mrs. A.: Yeah, it sure is scary when you start seeing things.

Mrs. E.: Once I had ordered a chicken dinner to be delivered to my place. The man came to deliver it, and as he stood there in the hall he turned into the devil, and I started yelling, and that's when they took me to the hospital. Could a man turn into a devil?

Later:

Mr. B.: But you can almost feel yourself going. I get more and more tense, and then pretty soon I start hearing those voices.

Through comparing common frightening experiences, group members realize that they are not alone and that others have shared similar problems. A common response of group leaders to a discussion such as the one described above is to divert the conversation to a less anxiety-provoking subject, one in which the therapist feels more competent as an authority. It is important not to do this, but to allow group members to share these experiences so that they can gain new insights into the factors precipitating hallucinatory behavior. As the group develops further, members frequently will bring in experiences they have had, seeking group counsel and advice about them.

GROUP SESSION 8

Mrs. E.: I don't know what to do. You see, I belong to this sanctified church. I go there every morning and night and three times on Sunday. I want to sing in the choir and they have this volunteer group there, but if they knew that I had been in the mental hospital they wouldn't let me be a part of this. When you're a volunteer, you dress in a long white outfit and you go to the hospital and visit people who are sick, and I'd really like to do that.

Mrs. A.: I wouldn't go to any church like that. It seems like things are just turned around—it should be people in the church who would understand about you being sick and all that.

Therapist: How do you know that they wouldn't let you belong if you told them?

Mrs. E.: Oh, I just know. The minister talks about this other lady that was "upset." If you were really sanctified and leading the good life, then you wouldn't have mental problems—according to him.

Mr. B.: Why don't you go to another church?

Mr. C.: I'd never go to a church anyhow; they can't help you.

In these interactions the group leader functions always to try to clarify reality and to encourage the group's problem-solving endeavors.

Ideally, groups vacillate back and forth through these stages. When a period of cohesiveness and group problem-solving has been the pattern, conflicts are activated and the group will go through another competitive cycle. It is important that this be encouraged if the group is to move ahead and the members are to experience the full range of the group's curative processes.

TERMINATING PHASE

Termination is perhaps one of the most significant aspects of group life. In working with groups, it is extremely important to clarify with group members the duration that a group will meet. If this is not planned at the beginning of the group, members ought to be given as much advance notification of the termination date as possible, so that they can accomplish this final phase of group work.

Different members respond to termination in different ways. A particularly maladaptive pattern is for members to terminate themselves by not attending the last group sessions. If this occurs, the group leader should contact the person and encourage him or her to come back to the group or if this is not possible, attempt to work through the separation process on an individual basis. Typically, group members respond with some expression of anger toward the group leader, implying that they are being deserted. Frequently regressive behavior is displayed; it is almost as if group members were trying to show the group leader that they are not improved and therefore cannot possibly terminate the group. Group discussions now commonly are a recapitulation of topics discussed earlier in the history of the group, but the discussion is much briefer and the resolutions much swifter.

A key factor in the termination process is the ability of the group leader to evaluate and express his or her feelings. As Yalom states: "The therapist, no less than the patients, will miss the group. For him, too, it has been a place of anguish, conflict, fear, and also of great beauty; some of life's truest and most poignant moments occur in the small and yet limitless microcosm of the therapy group."[17]

With all the emotions tied up in the termination process having been dealt with, the final session frequently is quasi-ceremonial in nature. Individuals who have appeared regressed throughout the earlier termination phases seem to "pull themselves together." Members frequently talk about plans for the future; ideally, group members can integrate the group experience as something that has been of value, but realize that they will survive and continue to grow outside the context of the group. And the therapist must also cope with the possibility that the members may manage very well without him or her.

SUMMARY

People develop in relationship to a wide range of social groups. These group experiences may be growth-producing or inhibiting. Because of the group-rootedness of human behavior, it is important that nurses understand basic principles underlying group functioning. All groups are characterized by certain properties such as (1) a commonly understood background, (2) unique participation patterns, (3) cohesion between group members, (4) normative standards that govern behavior, (5) characteristic patterns of relatedness between group members, (6) characteristic group atmosphere, (7) communication patterns, (8) particular structure and organization, and (9) a set of procedures, formal or informal. Groups main-

17. Ibid., p. 281.

tain a delicate balance between stability and change. On the one hand, there must be sufficient cohesiveness to hold the group together; on the other, sufficient competition and conflict to move the group forward.

In light of these group properties, groups may exert considerable pressure on individuals to "fit in" to their particular structure. Proper use of these group forces may promote positive changes in people.

Groups may provide the following growth-producing opportunities:

1. Sharing of information.

2. Instillation of hope by learning how others have coped with similar problems.

3. Learning that problems or experiences are common to others and one is therefore not alone.

4. Altruism achieved through reaching out to others in a similar predicament.

5. Reworking of problems whose origins are within the family, which are recapitulated within the group setting.

6. Learning or relearning of social skills.

7. Learning through initiating behavior of others.

8. Interpersonal learnings of how to relate to others.

9. Opportunity to ventilate highly charged feelings.

The group leader has particular responsibility in setting goals for the group and using this curative potential in promoting individual change. The effective group leader carefully selects group members, prepares each person for what will happen in the group, builds group cohesiveness, makes effective use of conflict and competition, and carefully works through the termination phase.

FURTHER READINGS

Baker, Joan, and Estes, Nada. "Anger in Group Therapy." *American Journal of Nursing* 65 (July 1965): 96-100.

Bell, Ruth. "Activity as a Tool in Group Therapy." *Perspectives in Psychiatric Care* 8, no. 2 (1970): 84-91.

Crowdes, Nancy. "Group Therapy for Preadolescent Boys." *American Journal of Nursing* 75 (Jan. 1975): 92-95.

Eddy, Frances, et al. "Group Work on a Long-Term Psychiatric Service . . . as Conducted by Nurses and Aides." *Perspectives in Psychiatric Care* 6, no. 1 (1968): 9-15.

Eisenberg, Joann, and Abbot, Ruth. "The Monopolizing Patient in Group Therapy." *Perspectives in Psychiatric Care* 6, no. 2 (1968): 66-69.

Goodson, Mary. "Group Therapy With Regressed Patients." *Perspectives in Psychiatric Care* 2, no. 4 (1964): 23-31.

Hargreaves, Anne. "The Nurse Group Therapist in a Variety of Settings: Community, Hospital, School, and Prison." *ANA Regional Clinical Conferences* (1967): 281-288.

———. "The Group Culture and Nursing Practice." *American Journal of Nursing* 67 (Sept. 1967): 1840-1843.

———. "Groups in Action." *American Journal of Nursing* 67 (Sept. 1967): 1844-1846.

Jersild, Elaine. "Group Therapy for Patients' Spouses." *American Journal of Nursing* 67 (March 1967): 544-549.

Light, Nada. "The 'Chronic Helper' in Group Therapy." *Perspectives in Psychiatric Care* 12, no. 3 (1974): 129-134.

Loomis, Maxine, and Dodenhoff, Judith. "Working With Informal Patient Groups." *American Journal of Nursing* 70 (Sept. 1970): 1939-1944.

Maurin, Judith. "Regressed Patients in Group Therapy." *Perspectives in Psychiatric Care* 8, no. 3 (1970): 131-135.

Racy, John. "How a Group Grows." *American Journal of Nursing* 69 (Nov. 1969): 2396-2402.

Rogers, Carl. "Facilitating Encounter Groups." *American Journal of Nursing* 71 (Feb. 1971): 275-279.

Rouslin, Sheila. "Relatedness in Group Psychotherapy." *Perspectives in Psychiatric Care* 11, no. 4 (1973): 165-171.

Ward, Judy. "Sounds of Silence." *Perspectives in Psychiatric Care* 12, no. 1 (1974): 13-19.

Werner, Jean. "Relating Group Theory to Nursing Practice." *Perspectives in Psychiatric Care* 8, no. 6 (1970): 248-261.

Yalom, Irvin, and Terrazas, Florence. "Group Therapy for Psychotic Elderly Patients." *American Journal of Nursing* 68 (Aug. 1968): 1690-1694.

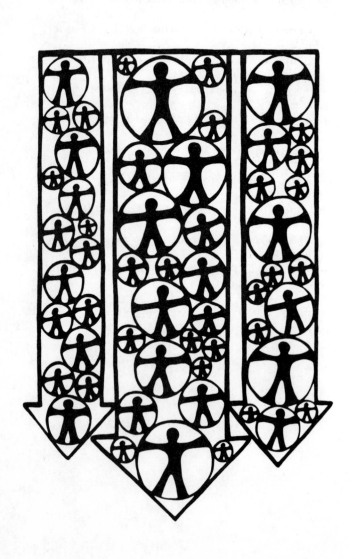

According to the socio-psychological model of mental illness, people develop characteristic responses to coping with problematic situations as they go through life. They tend to become locked into particular coping styles as experience repeatedly reinforces the behaviors that make up their particular style. These styles, while not necessarily satisfying to these persons, do serve to keep their anxiety within manageable limits so that they can maintain themselves at a certain level. However, there are periods when the problems an individual faces are of such magnitude or are connected to such unmanageable feelings that the usual coping maneuvers no longer work. At these points, the person may become so personally disorganized or engage in behavior considered so inappropriate that he or she is hospitalized in an attempt to bring this behavior "back into line."

The point at which a person becomes hospitalized is nearly always a crisis. He or she has reached a point at which the usual coping patterns no longer work, or attempts to cope are inappropriate within a social context. From this standpoint, the person about to be hospitalized is perhaps most amenable to some lasting change in his or her style of coping. Commonly, however, the process of hospitalization is not treated as a crisis; instead, the people involved with getting someone hospitalized tend to be concerned primarily with bringing his or her behavior back within acceptable limits. This usually involves either physical or chemical restraint—placing the person within a secure environment or giving large doses of medication—or both. The emphasis is on getting the person "calmed down." Although this measure may be necessary, often it becomes the main focus of treatment, and the opportunity to treat the situation as a crisis and use the experience for promoting growth is neglected.

The purpose of hospitalization is another problem. It commonly is viewed as a necessary measure when a person's behavior has become unmanageable within a normal social context. From this standpoint, it is used primarily as a means of containing deviant behavior. When the person's behavior becomes "appropriate," he or she is deemed fit to return to

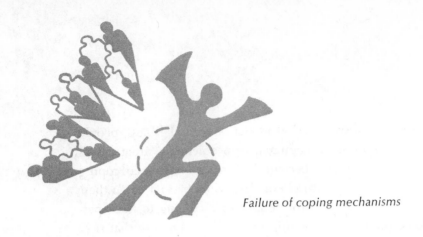

Failure of coping mechanisms

society. From this perspective, then, hospitalization is seen as a necessary step for the protection of society, rather than as a positive vehicle of treatment for persons who have difficulty coping with everyday problems. Because of this point of view, much of the emphasis is on ways in which the patient can learn to manage behavior so that he or she will act appropriately. But if one were to adopt the contrasting view—that hospitalization provides an opportunity for the person to experiment with new styles of coping in a safe environment and with people who may or may not be similar to others he or she has related to previously—hospitalization could be constructed as a therapeutic experience.

Since hospitalization is most commonly viewed from the perspective of social control, the person usually re-enters the community when his or her behavior once more seems appropriate. In far too many instances, this transition from hospital to community is abrupt and disconnected from the overall treatment process. Again referring to the crisis model, it is likely that the process of moving from the hospital back into social groups creates stress that can precipitate a further crisis situation. In the hospital, the person may have experimented with new forms of coping, but with a different set of people from those with whom he or she interacts every day and on a much more intimate basis than in the hospital experience. Further, the person who has been hospitalized for psychiatric reasons also often meets problems arising from the stigma attached to this experience. From this perspective, it is clear that on-going support to facilitate the re-entry process would benefit most former patients.

This chapter, then, first examines the hospitalization experience as a crisis and explores its inherent therapeutic potential. Second, it looks at the social network of the hospital in terms of its therapeutic potential. Psychiatric nursing is directed toward structuring an environment in which people can experiment with new coping styles in a safe environment, one in which they can receive feedback about the effects of their behavior on others and, in turn, can openly communicate their feelings about how others affect them. In this environment, the person has the opportunity to try out new styles of coping that may prove more personally satisfying than those he or she has used previously. Next, the process of re-entering the community and the need for on-going support during readjustment are explored. The chapter concludes with some general principles for relating to people, which may be helpful in responding to the kinds of behavior commonly encountered as people progress through various stages of disorganization and reintegration.

HOSPITALIZATION AS A CRISIS EXPERIENCE

When someone is hospitalized, whether for a psychiatric emergency or for a physical problem, it frequently precipitates a crisis, both for the patient and for significant others. In a psychiatric emergency, the person's inability to cope with particular situations may precipitate the behavior that results in his or her being admitted to the hospital for psychiatric treatment. In medical emergencies, the person's physical condition, which may potentially threaten life, can create a crisis. Hospitalization is a crisis not only for the patient, but also for his or her family. Role relationships are disrupted; the family system goes into disequilibrium. Not only are the patient and his or her family dealing with the realities of the immediate present, but often they are thinking of the future; they may fear that the person hospitalized will not return, that the illness will be fatal, or that the person will suffer permanent damage, either physical or psychological. In any event, at a time of hospitalization, marked alterations in relationships occur, causing people to re-examine and redefine their relatedness to one another.

Bearing this in mind, it then becomes important to consider the process of admitting a person to the hospital in the framework of crisis intervention. As has been pointed out, a person in crisis experiences a high level of disorganization. The first task in crisis intervention is to structure the experience in such a way that the person can begin to bring his or her anxiety level back within manageable levels, so that he or she can deal with the situation. A second factor in crisis intervention is to build rapport with the person and instill a feeling of hope, that he or she will receive help and that the situation is not hopeless. With this framework in mind, consider the usual hospital admission scene.

THE EMERGENCY ROOM EXPERIENCE

Frequently the person who is to be admitted to the hospital comes through the emergency room. Usually accompanied by family or friends, or in some instances the police, he or she first encounters an emergency room clerk who fires questions about the nature of the problem and the specific circumstances of the request for hospital help. In many instances, the person is asked for identification, insurance numbers, mother's maiden name, parents' places of birth, and other detailed information. In a state of crisis, the person frequently does not have this information readily at command. Attempting to manage and cope with the overwhelming anxieties of the moment, the person must direct all his or her energies toward maintaining himself or herself. Faced with this barrage of questions and unable to answer them, the person may go into a panic state. This additional frustration provides the person with further evidence that his or her world is falling apart.

In considering the process of being hospitalized as part of a crisis experience, it is important to consider the impact of various procedures at the time of admission. The nurse, who frequently is in the emergency room, could do much to use even the initial phase of the admission process as a form of crisis intervention. Instead of bombarding the person with questions that may or may not be pertinent, the skilled nurse may use the admission interview to help the person structure the current experience and thereby pull it into an organizing framework. By using the intake interview in this way, the nurse can accomplish two tasks at once; while eliciting the necessary information, she or he can direct the questions in a logical rational way, thus using the interview to help the person make sense out of the experience.

For example, consider the case of Mary Lou Stevens, a 32-year-old schoolteacher who is brought to the emergency room by her husband following a suicide attempt in which she has cut her wrist with a razor blade. The cut itself is not serious, but Mrs. Stevens is in a state of panic over what she has done. She is sobbing hysterically, while her husband tries to calm her down. Upon entering the emergency room, Mr. and Mrs. Stevens are ushered to a private room, rather than having to sit in the waiting room. The nurse, Ms. Adams, immediately comes into the room, makes sure that Mrs. Stevens is comfortable on the examining table, and sits down to take the necessary information. At all points in the admission process, Mr. and Mrs. Stevens are interviewed jointly; this is especially important to cut down on the amount of distortion that may occur between the couple in such a time of crisis. Also, much of what might have led up to the crisis, as well as the aftermath, involves them as a couple rather than as two separate individuals.

> *Ms. Adams:* Can you tell me what happened?
>
> *Mr. Stevens:* I came home from my office and found her in the bathroom holding her wrist, and blood all over the place. I don't know why she would do such a thing.
>
> *Ms. Adams:* Mrs. Stevens, could you tell me what happened?
>
> *Mrs. Stevens:* (Sobbing hysterically) I don't know. Everything had just gotten to me. Today I got my ratings at school and I got a "Satisfactory." That's not very good, and just everything had gotten to me. My husband hadn't remembered our anniversary, and it just seems that nothing is turning out for us the way it should. I came home and there was nobody there, and I just thought that the only solution was to end it all, and then he came home and stopped me.

As the nurse talks, she is putting a tight compression bandage over Mrs. Stevens's wrist until the doctor comes to suture the cut. In so doing, she provides another type of structure to the situation and offers reassurance through the physical care she is providing. This in itself provides reassurance and evidence that the patient can place trust in the competence of those who will take care of her.

> *Ms. Adams:* You must have been really feeling bad about a lot of things. Can you tell me a little about where you teach?
>
> *Mrs. Stevens:* I work in a school for crippled children. I've worked there for three years, and I'm still on probation. I need to get good ratings if I'm going to get permanent certification, and I just haven't

been doing as well as I might. I just can't manage those kids, and I get so involved with their problems. I just can't manage.

Ms. Adams: Can you tell me a little about yourself—where you live, how many children you have, some of those sorts of things.

Mrs. Stevens: We live in Maytown—5012 South Fifteenth—we've lived there for the last ten years, ever since we got married. We've never had any children, and you can't adopt any now. If only I had a child, maybe my life would have some meaning, but the way it is now. . . .

Mr. Stevens: We went through an awful lot trying to see if we could have a child. It's my fault. The doctors say that I'm sterile, and we've gone to adoption agency after adoption agency. Last week they finally told us that we wouldn't be able to get a child they had thought we might get. They told us to give up trying.

Ms. Adams: I can imagine how disappointing this must be to both of you. (Pause) I need to get a little more information about you. I assume you have some insurance from your work at the school; could you give me your account number? And could you tell me a little about your work, Mr. Stevens, what you do and where you work?

Mr. Stevens: I'm an engineer. I work for Magnavox designing components for TV's.

Ms. Adams: Does either of you have families living nearby?

Mrs. Stevens: I'm from California; my parents are out there. I have two sisters and they both live there. I came to Chicago twelve years ago to go to school. I met my husband while I was attending the university, and we got married when we graduated. We've lived here ever since.

Mr. Stevens: My family lives here. My parents came here from Poland when they were young. I've always lived in the city, and all my family are here. We're very close to one another, not like Mary Lou's family who hardly ever see each other. I've worked very hard to get where I've gotten. My father ran a bakery. He still does, and my parents live in the old neighborhood. We've got so much—a nice house, plenty of money—we can live a good life. I don't know why you would want to do something like this.

Mrs. Stevens: I feel like I should be happy, but somehow I'm not. I see you so close to your family, and I don't really have anyone. It all seemed so hopeless and I felt so all alone.

At this point Mrs. Stevens's hysterical behavior has subsided; the doctor comes in to begin suturing her wrist, and the nurse comforts her and reassures her during the process.

After the immediate emergency is cared for, it is important that the person and the family members participate in decision-making about the next steps.

Ms. Adams: Now you have a couple of alternatives. You may wish to be hospitalized; that would give your wrist time to heal, and also you could start looking at some of the problems that have contributed to your getting to this point. You might decide you want to go home, and then see someone here on an out-patient basis, but it looks like it is important for you to have someone to talk to about some of the things that you seem to be troubled about. Would you like to be hospitalized, or would you prefer going home?

Mr. Stevens: I would think it would be better if she were in the hospital. There would be someone around to talk to until she gets over this phase that she's in. And I'd be afraid that something might happen, that her wrist might start bleeding, or that I wouldn't know how to manage. And I'd like to see her be happier; maybe she could work out some of her problems by staying here.

Ms. Adams: What do you think about it, Mrs. Stevens?

Mrs. Stevens: I really don't like hospitals all that well. I've never been a patient before . . . would I have to go to the psychiatric ward where all those crazy people are?

Ms. Adams: We do have a psychiatric ward, and, yes, there are some people there with some rather severe problems. It's a small unit—only twenty patients—and there are two beds in a room, so you would have a roommate. We do try to place people in rooms where they have roommates with problems of about the same severity; and those who are severely disturbed are placed in private rooms. We have a large nursing staff there, and a lot of people to talk to so that you could start looking at your problems in a different way.

Mrs. Stevens: I really need that. I've been just getting nowhere. The more I sit home and think about things, the more impossible they become. And maybe if I could talk to some others, I would start getting some new perspectives on life. I don't want to go through life feeling so miserable. I guess I should be admitted.

In this initial contact in the emergency rom, the first phase of crisis intervention begins. First, the nurse provides some structuring of the experience so that the person's anxiety can return to normal limits. Throughout the course of the interaction, hope is instilled. Although this person obviously has done something to herself that is dramatic and life-threatening, the nurse, through careful structuring of the initial interview, puts the behavior into a perspective that is understandable for both the woman and her husband. The expectation that help will be forthcoming and that she will be able to gain new insights into herself and her style of coping are clearly implicit in this initial intake interview. Even allowing her to participate in making the decision about whether she will be hos-

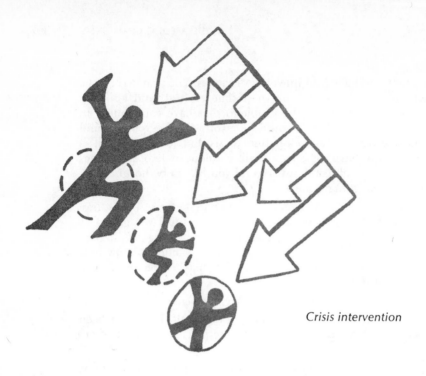

Crisis intervention

pitalized transmits a message that she is considered to be capable of making decisions about her life. If she had been hospitalized without being involved is the decision-making, this would be likely to reinforce her negative self-image as someone who cannot manage. The nurse has provided her with accurate information about the type of unit, explaining that she might expect others to be more disturbed than she, but that the setting would be structured to provide safety and contact with those who might help; and with this information, Mrs. Stevens is able to make the decision to be hospitalized. She is not likely to be startled by the unexpected when she finally arrives on the ward.

Although this example shows a typical "psychiatric" patient, the principles apply to persons coming to the hospital for any emergency. It is safe to assume that all are in a state of crisis, that their lives and relationships to significant others are disrupted, that they feel helpless, and that the situation is in the control of someone else. The hospital, for many people, represents a life-threatening place. Memories of others who have died in hospitals, stories of failures or mistakes by doctors and other hospital personnel—all these combine to make people fearful. This is compounded by not knowing what is going on in their bodies. As has been pointed out earlier, as the person's anxiety rises, the feeling of impending doom is likely to grow. All too commonly, medical personnel whisk in and out while the admitting clerk asks the most personal questions in much the same manner as a robot. The goal is to get the information; and it may seem that it is being garnered about an object, rather than a human being. A series of people "do things" to the patient, but rarely do they explain what they are doing and what for. Many times, another emergency is brought in; people hustle about; and not infrequently the people waiting for care are silent witnesses to the death of another person in a room nearby. All this does little to reassure the waiting patients.

The nurse is one person who, in the midst of this activity, could provide the reassurance and support so desperately needed. But all too frequently the nurse, too, becomes caught up in the demands of technical aspects of her or his role, failing to note the importance of the experience for the patient, not only in terms of physical health but also mental well-being. Certainly the person's physical safety takes priority; but in most instances it is possible to attend simultaneously to both physical and psychological needs. In any event, hospitalization in any form constitutes a stressful situation, and in many cases precipitates a crisis.

ADMISSION TO THE TREATMENT UNIT

The second important phase of hospitalization is the admission of the person to the treatment unit. Here the person is confronted by unfamiliar surroundings, staff and other patients who are all strangers, a lack of familiarity with what to expect as a hospital patient, and fears about the total effects of this hospitalization. While this is true of all persons admitted to a hospital, the problem is frequently worse for psychiatric patients, who have less preparation, via the media, for playing their role as "patient" than do people who enter medical units for a physical disease. And although being a patient for medical reasons is acceptable in our society, hospitalization for "mental" reasons is frequently perceived as unacceptable; the person is said to have a "nervous breakdown," which usually implies some weakness of character or lack of strength. In fact, as Goffman[1]

---

1. Irving Goffman, *Asylums* (New York: Doubleday Anchor Books, 1961).

has pointed out, the process of becoming a psychiatric patient frequently resembles a degradation rite.

As a condition of being hospitalized, the psychiatric patient usually is forced to assume a role of one who is helpless and unable to care for himself or herself. The admission procedures mandatory in many hospitals reaffirm this—the patient is stripped of all clothing, and personal belongings are searched for lethal weapons or drugs, particularly if there is some indication that he or she might be suicidal. This "rite of admission," while not in all instances this extreme, strips the person of his or her identity. In the process, the person becomes a "psychiatric patient."

As has been pointed out throughout this book, people enact roles that are reciprocated by significant others. The physically ill person, for instance, enters the hospital and assumes the "sick" role. This is reciprocated easily by hospital personnel, including nurses, who can then play the roles of "healer," "helper," or "caregiver." But all these roles imply a certain degree of helplessness on the part of the patient to which the others can respond, usually by providing physical care. The physical incapacity of the patient allows the caregiver to provide help, and the roles are thus mutually rewarding, both to the patient who needs care and to the nurse who feels competent in providing it.

But this situation becomes complicated in the case of the psychiatric patient, for the person is not physically incapacitated and is usually capable of taking care of his or her personal needs. Most frequently, the role of the psychiatric nurse is to protect the person from harming others or himself or herself. Instead of being the helper, the accustomed self-image, the nurse becomes the restrainer, or the person who must intervene to prevent certain actions by the patient. Unlike nurses who work with physically ill patients and get personal gratification from patients who are grateful for their help, nurses in the psychiatric unit, who frequently must restrain or interfere with what the patient wishes to do, get an opposite reaction: they are cursed, spit upon, hit, and otherwise castigated for interfering with what the patient wished to do.

Another familiar role for a psychiatric nurse is that of listener to the patients' problems. Again, this is not a role that finds much reinforcement in other areas of nursing practice. From the day nursing students enter a hospital unit, and throughout their careers, nurses are accustomed to being physically active and doing things. Although they talk to patients as they do their work, they are accustomed to a constant stream of activity. The psychiatric unit is a sudden change of pace; here the emphasis is on listening, talking, and doing things with patients. Frequently the activities of the psychiatric unit do not fit into nurses' usual definition of "work," and they can see no tangible product as a result of their efforts. While nurses on a more traditional unit can at least count the number of beds they have made, baths they have given, and the medications they have passed out, the nurses on the psychiatric unit have few guidelines to validate their work. Similarly, they have few guidelines as to when their work has been helpful; changes in patients are often slow and not easily started. Considerable ambiguity surrounds the role of "nurse."

A similar aura of vagueness surrounds the role of "patient." A person enters the hospital, usually after some dramatic event in which he or she has "lost control" in one way or another. Hospitalization is the final evidence of personal incompetence. Most people, while capable of playing the role of patient, have little preparation for playing the role of *psychiatric* patient; the popular concept of this behavior is usually the stereotypical version of the "madman," and the examples one might draw on as a pattern for behavior are extreme. If one is neither physically ill nor a "madman," what, then, is the role of the psychiatric patient?

Bearing these factors in mind, and considering that the person who is being admitted to a psychiatric unit is in crisis, it is extremely important to structure his or her introduction to the psychiatric unit to reduce the ambiguity in the situation and help bring the person's anxiety within normal bounds. Let us again imagine Mrs. Stevens as she is admitted to the psychiatric unit of the hospital. Ms. Adams accompanies her to the unit and introduces her to the head nurse, Ms. Wagner.

> *Ms. Adams:* This is Mrs. Stevens. She is to be admitted to your unit. She was feeling depressed and cut her wrists, and together we have decided that it would be best for her to spend a few days in the hospital.

By clearly communicating the substance of earlier interactions in the emergency room, Ms. Adams is making the transition from one phase of the process to the next. The nurse can make this kind of statement whether it was she who participated with the Stevenses in the decision or some other person, such as an admitting physician. By making this statement in front of the patient, the nurse is attempting to reduce Mrs. Stevens's suspicions that the nurses would talk about her, which would be, to her, evidence of the terrible thing she had done.

> *Ms. Wagner:* I will show you to your room. Thank you, Ms. Adams. I'll take care of the records. (As Ms. Wagner walks down the hall with Mrs. Stevens, she points out the layout of the unit.) There's too much to learn for people to remember everything at once. But let's at least get you started with the physical layout and some of the people you'll be living with. Here is the nursing station; you can always find someone here who can answer any questions you might have. If you need something, either turn the light on in your room or come out here to ask for what you want. Here's the dining room; all patients come here and eat their meals together. There are snacks in the refrigerator, and you can help yourself to anything that is here. One of the rules is that you must help in keeping things cleaned up. This is the lounge area; there's a television here, and we often have different activities here such as our group meetings.
>
> Entering one of the rooms, Ms. Wagner introduces Mrs. Stevens to her roommate, Jean Peters.

Although the steps in introducing Mrs. Stevens to the unit seem self-evident, becoming oriented to the environment is very important for someone who is having difficulty managing her or his life. By pointing out the obvious facets of the unit, the nurse is also implicitly pointing out some of the norms that prevail. First, she communicates the expectation that if the patient has questions or needs something, she may seek out a nurse at any time. Knowing about the area in which people eat, the availability of snacks, and the personal responsibility to one another in keeping the eating area clean tells the patient something more about the kind of place this is. Certain things are expected of patients, such as eating together and sharing responsibilities.

The availability of snacks may symbolically communicate the giving atmosphere of the ward. The lounge area again symbolizes a place where certain types of interaction take place: watching TV, activities, group meetings. This implies that patients are expected to be involved with others on the unit and not remain isolated. In a short span of time, Mrs. Stevens is given a considerable amount of information that helps her to structure a new and undefined situation. The psychiatric ward, which seemed so formidable, rapidly becomes a place of some familiarity.

■ *The Initial Interview.* Ms. Peters has left the room so that Ms. Wagner and Mrs. Stevens can continue the admission process. Both sit

down in the comfortable lounge chairs in the room. In this relaxed atmosphere, the orientation process continues, but now the nurse becomes oriented to Mrs. Stevens's problem.

> *Ms. Wagner:* Ms. Adams mentioned that you had been feeling de-
> pressed and that you had cut your wrists. Would you like to tell me a
> little about that?
>
> *Mrs. Stevens:* I feel so terrible. It's just that everything seemed to be
> going wrong. I got my evaluation at my school. I teach multiple-
> handicapped children, and it's such hard work. I feel so sorry for those
> children, and I guess I just get too involved, and then I don't seem to
> maintain control of my classroom. I got just a satisfactory rating. If I
> don't get a better rating than that, I won't be certified and I won't be
> able to remain in teaching, and I feel so sorry for those children. I came
> home and I felt so useless, like I can't manage anything.
>
> And my husband doesn't seem to be around much any more. He
> just seems to take me for granted. And I couldn't think of any other
> solution. I went to the bathroom and took a razor blade and slashed my
> wrists. I fainted on the bathroom floor and my husband came home and
> discovered me there, and he brought me here. He's disgusted with me,
> and I guess he has a point. I don't know what he's going to tell his
> folks! I don't know why I did this. I've never done anything like this
> before. Do you think I'm crazy?
>
> *Ms. Wagner:* It must be very frightening to you to have done this, but
> we all get into situations where we don't know what to do. It seems like
> there aren't any answers, and sometimes we do things at those times
> that don't make much sense later. That doesn't mean that you're crazy.
> What do you think you might get out of being in the hospital? What
> would you like to have happen to you that would make life a little
> more manageable?
>
> *Mrs. Stevens:* I don't know. I guess one of the things is that I wish I
> could speak up a little more about what is bothering me. At school,
> these other teachers push me around, and sometimes I get blamed for
> things that I'm not really responsible for. And I don't ever speak up.
> I'm just boiling inside, but then I don't know what would happen to
> me if I said anything. This one teacher is always talking about how I
> can't maintain discipline in my room. I see her pulling the children's
> ears and doing all sorts of things to them. It's true I don't do much to
> make the children behave. Every time they do something bad, I think
> of what it would be like to be crippled, and I suppose I do indulge
> them a little more.
>
> *Ms. Wagner:* Are you able to talk to your husband about some of the
> problems you have at school? Does he understand?
>
> *Mrs. Stevens:* I've given up talking about school to him. We've tried to
> have children of our own for about ten years. The doctor says it's be-

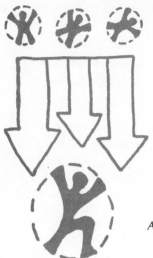

Assessment of coping styles

cause he's sterile. So every time I talk about the kids at school, he thinks I'm too involved with them, and then it all goes back to him feeling guilty about not being able to give me a child of my own. So for about the last five years, we've just sort of reached an agreement not to talk about any of this. And he's got all his worries with his work. I spend a lot of time listening to his problems.

Ms. Wagner: Perhaps one of the things you want to work on while you are in the hospital is to practice talking about how you feel, rather than just burying all these feelings inside of you.

Mrs. Stevens: That is something I would like to be able to do.

In this introductory interview, it is important to get some perspective on the person's characteristic coping style so that an intervention plan can be developed to provide experiences designed to give practice with alternative patterns of coping. In this case, it is important to note the characteristic pattern of burying feelings and not talking about them. In this instance, it is important to build an overall plan that includes experiences to encourage Mrs. Stevens to begin to express herself and to assess the reasonableness with which she does this. Not infrequently, this can be accomplished in the milieu, in specific group experiences, and through family counseling.

The initial interview also can provide the person with some orientation as to how she or he might use the hospital experience to help with the problems she or he is facing. In this case, Ms. Wagner goes on to explain to Mrs. Stevens how the unit operates, and in so doing she provides a "map" for ways in which Mrs. Stevens might begin to relate to other patients and staff.

> *Ms. Wagner:* Would you like to know about how things go around here? And how you might get some experience in expressing your feelings a little better?
>
> *Mrs. Stevens:* I'd like that. I've never been in a place like this before, and I'd feel uncomfortable not knowing what to say or do.
>
> *Ms. Wagner:* Things may be different around here from what you have been accustomed to in the past; for example, we really put a lot of emphasis upon your trying to develop some different patterns of relating to people from those you've used before that haven't really worked too well. You'll find us asking you a lot how you feel about certain things. Sometimes this can be a little irritating, but we do it to try to get you to become a little more familiar with some of the feelings that you try to hide. Now I know it can be uncomfortable to talk about some of your problems to people you don't know, but just remember that everyone here is pretty much in the same boat. We're all trying to find way of becoming more in tune with one another.
>
> There are a number of ways we try to encourage this. First, everyone comes to the dining room to eat, and then there are certain group activities that we try to plan together. Each evening we have an end-of-the-day report, when everyone is expected to tell how their day has gone, and sometimes others comment about how a person's behavior may have affected them. We also have unit meetings every day, where we talk about some of the problems that we have in living together as a group. Then, in addition to this, we have some group therapy experiences where you meet with a small group for the sole purpose of exploring your problems within this setting. And then usually we have some meetings with your family—in this case, with your husband and you, to see if you might find better ways of communicating with one another. You'll find that it seems like hard work at times, to be constantly working at looking at your feelings.
>
> *Mrs. Stevens:* It sounds like it, but if only I could get so I don't feel so depressed and so that I could manage better.

In this type of interaction, the intent is again to spell out the expectations set for the person so that the ambiguity of roles in this situation may be lessened. Ms. Wagner in this interaction clearly places much of the responsibility upon Mrs. Stevens to become actively involved in the group activities. She also outlines some of the things that Mrs. Stevens is to expect and thus further attempts to structure the situation and allay anxiety. The work expected to be accomplished is clearly outlined, based on the person's initial identification of what she would like to see happen in her life. The idea of a partnership between "patients" and staff is communicated clearly in this initial introduction of the unit. The person must be an active participant in the treatment, while the role of staff is to be active partners in the problem-solving endeavor. Although the process of admitting a person to the hospital is frequently viewed as a routine procedure, it is an optimal time to interact significantly with a person in crisis.

THE MILIEU AS AN AGENT OF CHANGE

The role of the milieu in the overall treatment plan has been a subject of considerable controversy in the psychiatric field. One side holds that the milieu is only an adjunct to other treatment processes, while the other maintains that the community of the hospital unit in and of itself provides the major form of treatment.

In this country, milieu therapy was first introduced by the Menninger clinic, and was adapted from an approach developed in Germany in the 1920s. As Almond describes this orientation:

> Milieu therapy required a more specific prescription for each patient. Patients were treated with individual psychotherapy, and the therapist, on the basis of his treatment data, prescribed to the ward staff the manner of social interaction he felt would provide the patient with the most useful therapeutic experience.[2]

In this form of therapy, the ward was viewed as adjunctive to the therapist's work with patients; certain attitudes were to be adopted toward patients so that the staff would reinforce the particular type of therapy being adopted by the therapist.

The problem with this approach is the difficulty that staff may have in adopting a particular attitudinal set while dealing with large numbers of patients at the same time. Nursing staff deal with patients in groups, rather than on an individual basis. To have to deal with each of them from a different attitudinal set is almost impossible, besides being somewhat

---

2. Richard Almond, *The Healing Community: Dynamics of the Therapeutic Milieu* (New York: Jason Aronson, 1974), p. xii.

contrived. Another problem is that an important facet of the treatment process is to give persons who have difficulty with coping the experience of relating to "real" people, who lead them into more productive patterns of problem resolution. But prescribing attitudes implies that staff members will play roles rather than interact as "real" people. The masking of staff identities tends to reinforce and encourage the same process in patients.

A third criticism, frequently voiced by patients who are faced with a staff instructed to interact with them in a particular way, is that they very quickly pick up stereotypic behavior and standardized responses to their behavior, and they respond in turn by mocking the staff. A fourth problem with this approach is that attitudes prescribed (such as "Be firm," "Provide support") tend to be so global that they do little in providing concrete guides for patient-staff interaction.

Although there are these difficulties in adopting a milieu therapy approach, there are also some important positive features in this approach. The most important is that it maintains consistency among the different parts of the patient's therapeutic experience within the hospital. If the therapist is working toward one treatment goal, staff should not be working toward competing or conflicting goals. For example, if a therapist is working toward helping a woman become more independent and more of her "own" person in relationship to her husband, her experience in the hospital unit should similarly be directed toward helping her to greater independence.

Second, the milieu approach directs those involved in the healing process to provide experiences that are supportive to other parts of the overall treatment program. For example, if a therapist is working intensively in helping a man achieve insight into his problems, his experience in the milieu should be structured to create an atmosphere that supports this aim. In this instance, staff would not steadily pressure the "patient" to be involved with the group and look intensively at their behavior in the unit. Rather, the unit would be a place where this man can reflect upon what has transpired in the therapy session and continue work without being disrupted by competing demands from the hospital milieu. For this person, the hospital should be viewed as a "resting" place, where he experiences the sincere concern of staff and finds the support necessary to explore intensely painful and highly cathected experiences that influence his current patterns of relating and of resolving problems.

A third issue in coordinating an overall treatment program is to have an early consensus between the therapist, the unit staff, and the person involved about the long-range goals of hospitalization. Is the goal for the person to return home? Or is it desirable that this person break away from involvement in a social network that may be implicated in his or her problems of coping? These overall goals should be explicit and agreed upon by all participants in the treatment process. All too frequently, the three principals involved—therapist, staff, and patient—are working toward three different ends, and the patient gets caught in impossible conflicts that in most instances reinforce the problems he or she had before hospitalization.

THE THERAPEUTIC COMMUNITY

The other major attitude toward the milieu as a part of the treatment process views it as a "therapeutic community" or, as Almond terms it, a "healing community." In this approach, there is an implicit movement away from the medical model of "milieu therapy," in which the physician prescribes particular approaches to patients as part of an overall treatment plan, to one in which the emphasis is placed on group treatment and decision-making shared by patients and staff. In the "community" approach, the group experience becomes the major form of therapy, while other forms are adjunctive.

Maxwell Jones is considered to be the originator of the therapeutic community approach, which developed shortly after World War II.[3] Jones's description of the therapeutic community and those of others have certain features in common. First, the predominant emphasis is on group activities. Patient government meetings, community meetings, group psychotherapy, psychodrama, family group meetings, recreational and social groups are all commonly mentioned as part of a therapeutic community. These meetings are important in establishing the "patient culture." Almond describes the aspects of this culture as including:

> A stress on pragmatism; facing real life problems in the community and in patients' lives; a here-and-now emphasis on present manifestations rather than on origins of problems; informal sociability and

3. Maxwell Jones, *The Therapeutic Community* (New York: Basic Books, 1953).

friendliness, rather than arbitrary edicts from "on high" or sympathy and commiseration; immediate responses to patient behavior and ward problems.[4]

The emphasis in therapeutic communities is on the creation of a caring environment.

The nursing staff are centrally involved in creating such a healing environment, though whether they share this task with other disciplines is a point of controversy. Practice varies from institutions in which nurses are solely responsible for the milieu to others in which the milieu is the joint responsibility of all disciplines and the patients. But it is usually the nursing staff who are on the unit on a 24-hour-a-day basis, rather than just for particular group activities. Nursing staff either explicitly or implicitly assume responsibility for the managerial aspects of the ward; it is they who are concerned about seeing that the patients receive their food and medication and that housekeeping functions are maintained, and they monitor the living relationships of those on the unit.

Although this strategic position provides nurses an opportunity to have far-reaching impact upon patients' lives, it also presents a dilemma. Those who become "patients" in a psychiatric unit have longstanding coping mechanisms that have served to defend them in their relationships with others. Scher postulates that "the manipulative skill many patients have at creating situations where it is easier for others to do things for them than to insist that they do things for themselves; and the high value many nurses ascribe to their practical activity and helpfulness to others" combine to create a situation in which it is difficult to convince staff that patients should carry out certain work activities within the psychiatrc unit.[5]

■ *Changes in Hospital Attitudes.* Before exploring in greater depth ways in which the milieu may be an effective agent in teaching people more satisfactory ways of dealing with problems, a few cautions appear to be in order. In reviewing differing trends in hospital treatment of psychiatric patients, dramatic swings in treatment ideologies are apparent. As psychiatric hospitals developed as custodial institutions, patients were

---

4. Almond, *The Healing Community*, p. xiv.
5. John Cumming and Elaine Cumming, *Ego and Milieu* (Chicago: Aldine-Atherton, 1972), p. 217, in reference to Jordan M. Scher, "Schizophrenia and Task Orientation: The Structured Ward Setting." *ANA Archives of Neurology and Psychiatry* 78 (1957): 531-538.

often used as a labor pool within the hospital. They did manual labor on the farms that provided food for the hospital, manned the laundries, and did the cleaning. Often they became servants in the house of the superintendent. They were viewed as lifetime residents of the psychiatric hospital and served in a pseudo-slave capacity. Rarely did they quarrel with this arrangement. First of all, they did not dare, for fear of retribution; and second, work was preferable to spending long hours on the ward with no activities. As they remained in the hospital over long periods of time, their attachment to families or other significant social networks became totally severed and they had no other options. In this case, work therapy, as it was sometimes called, did not have the goal of moving the person outside the hospital, but was a way of obtaining a cheap labor force that incidentally provided certain rewards for the patient.

As treatment, rather than custody, became the goal in mental hospitals, the traditional forms of work programs faded from the scene. In fact, the swing was almost to the other extreme. Patients were not expected to do anything while residents in a psychiatric unit. They were to spend full time concentrating on trying to understand the basis of their problems and work them through, mainly in therapy sessions. While this move corrected some of the abuses of the earlier system, it created new problems.

First of all, the person who comes to a psychiatric hospital is not physically disabled. The loss of all responsibility for his or her personal care did much to rob patients of any feeling of self-worth; to become a psychiatric patient meant that one became totally dependent upon others to supply basic needs, such as food, laundry, and housekeeping. With this framework, the person, although not physically ill, was treated as though he or she was not capable of managing the simplest aspects of life. Responsibility was thus removed from the person and assumed by staff. This dilemma is compounded by the fact that most psychiatric units are located within general hospital settings. All hospital services are provided to psychiatric units just as they are to units with a physical care orientation. Meals are delivered, housekeeping takes care of room maintenance, and the same rules governing other areas of the hospital prevail on the psychiatric unit.

For these reasons, many questions have been raised as to the appropriateness of hospitals as treatment locales for those with problems in their approaches to coping with life. The most radical of alternative proposals is the establishment of communes isolated from urban settings, particu-

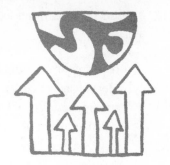

Dependency of the psychiatric patient

larly from hospital-like buildings, where persons can work freely on resolving their problems through interactions with one another and without the constraints placed upon them by other social settings. Although this is a radical approach, its point is that every aspect of life within the psychiatric unit needs to be examined for its potential in providing positive learning experiences for those who have had difficulty in other settings. One problem is that nurses have become enculturated into an orientation toward hospitals that assumes that certain features are unchangeable or unmodifiable and does not allow for an exploration of the therapeutic potential of ward living.

INTRODUCTION INTO THE TREATMENT UNIT

With these issues clearly in mind, let us examine some of the facets of milieu that might be structured to provide exercises in more effective problem-solving for those who enter psychiatric hospitals. Consider again the case of Mrs. Stevens. In her life outside, she has experienced feelings of increasing helplessness and inability to cope. A bad evaluation of her performance as a teacher and her inability to talk to her husband about some of her feelings were perhaps involved in her dramatic suicide attempt. As she enters the psychiatric hospital, she feels more and more out of control of herself; her husband, who has brought her to the hospital, and those who see her there have taken additional responsibilities away from her by recommending that she be hospitalized. She feels increasingly helpless and stripped of her normal role functions as housekeeper and teacher. Now she is also confronted with being a "patient." Often such feelings are compounded each step of the way into the hospital milieu: clothes are checked for any lethal drugs or weapons, and a set of instructions to govern life on the ward is given. The general message is to "fit in." But the price of "fitting in" is surrendering one's individuality and competence.

What, then, are some of the ways a hospital might be structured so that the experience, instead of adding to the person's feelings of incompetence, might enhance his or her self-image and help develop new ways of coping, both of which are goals in most treatment plans for patients?

Mrs. Stevens, after being checked into the hospital in the afternoon, spent a couple of hours unpacking her things and getting settled in her room. She and her roommate, Jean Peters, have had a discussion about why they are in the hospital. Jean has been in the hospital for two weeks; after breaking up with her boyfriend, she became confused and disorganized, and her sister came to her apartment and brought her to the hospital. As the dinner hour approached, Jean encouraged Mary Lou Stevens to come out to the lounge area with her to meet the rest of the patient group. Everyone was interested in why she was in the hospital, and as she explained to some of the patients, they in turn told her something of their problems. In the process she begins to feel that maybe what she did was not all that terrible; that there were others here who had done things that were also somewhat "crazy." In talking about it, she begins to feel relieved. Mary Lou does have some concerns, though, about three or four of the patients who seem so irrational and obviously mentally disturbed. She tries to avoid association with these people, thinking how horrible it would be if she became like that. As the dinner hour approaches Jean asks Mary Lou if she would like to help her on her work assignment, which is to set the table for dinner for the entire group. Mary Lou gladly agrees and they proceed to this task. Setting the table is something that is familiar and easy to manage, and helping out makes the process of fitting in easier.

However, things rarely proceed in the way this scene describes. The early hours of admission usually are accompanied by a steady progression of people in and out of the patient's room. An intern or medical student comes in to take a history, the psychiatric resident comes in and asks questions about why the person is here, the attending doctor pays a visit, a number of technicians come in for various reasons, to draw blood, to take a chest X-ray, and so on, and the nursing staff all pay a visit. Instead of having time to begin to integrate the things that have happened in the course of a hectic day, the person is bombarded with further anxiety-provoking stimuli.

Another thing to note about the experience of Mrs. Stevens: Instead of being forced out into the patient group, she is introduced naturally by her roommate without staff intruding into this process. Again, this serves to reinforce one's independence and ability to manage; while being led by the staff out to the patient unit and introduced reinforces the person's image of helplessness. However, introduction cannot be left to chance. It can be a unit norm that patients will participate in orientation in this way. By naturally experiencing the interaction within the group and telling one's story about how he or she came to be in the hospital, the person gains further control of the situation. Hearing other people's problems places one's own in a broader perspective that again reduces feelings of guilt over having engaged in some behavior that violated significant social norms.

WARD LIVING

A further factor to note is the responsibility that patients hold for some of the work of the unit. In many psychiatric units, meals are delivered to individuals on trays; they do not share a communal eating experience. Or else they are fed in cafeteria style, with someone dishing out their food as they pass by. In either case, the message conveyed is that one is helpless and dependent. The experience of eating together can be a time for relaxed sharing with one another and thus can play a significant part in building relationships within the patient group. It can also be used to instill a sense of responsibility for certain tasks in patients who are struggling with feelings of helplessness and incompetence. Interactions surrounding food, its preparation, or its consumption also bring out people's natural ways of coping with situations; the activities surrounding eating could be used effectively if staff were able to see communal dining as a naturally occurring group experience within the life of the ward. For instance, those whose characteristic pattern of coping is to try to push others out of the way and gratify their individual desires would probably demonstrate greedy behavior in a communal dining situation. Those who tend to be passive and withdrawn (such as Mrs. Stevens) would tend to allow themselves to be pushed out of the way by these more aggressive members. A staff person observing this concrete, tangible piece of interaction could intervene in a way that would be effective as a learning experience related to how people act and react to one another's behavior.

Following dinner, the community group (patients and staff) view a film in the recreational area of the ward. This film, *Death Wish*, was selected by the patient government officers. In the story, an executive's wife and family are killed, and he responds by taking the law into his own hands. Going out on the streets, he sets himself up for various assaults, such as robbery, but just at the point of attack, the business executive shoots down his assailant. The movie is a strong commentary on a number of highly charged emotional issues. During the course of the film, the viewing group become involved in a number of conversations. Mary Lou Stevens is talking with another woman, Karen Anderson; their conversation relates to how much the husband must have cared for his wife and family to become so involved in trying to seek retribution for their loss. Another group is preoccupied with how cruel and unjust it was for him heartlessly to shoot down his attackers: "How could he be sure that they were really going to do harm? Maybe they just wanted a cigarette." Another group is occupied in talking about the problem of violence in our society and how inadequate the police system is in giving protection. In all of these side conversations, an outside observer or staff person might be struck with how the topics of discussion in the various groups reflect the problems they themselves are dealing with.

A movie like *Death Wish* would not be chosen by staff as appropriate for patient viewing because of its highly charged emotional impact. Yet, in this situation, what is depicted in the movie probably reflects a wide range of human emotion representing many of the issues with which "patients" in this setting might be struggling. The usual pattern is for staff to search for a movie that is bland and nonemotional; these films kill time, but usually are not something that the patient population is interested in. Allowing a patient group to make choices even about the movies they wish to see poses risks; a disturbed patient with very tenuous ego controls could be highly stimulated by a movie such as the one described. On the other hand, involvement in watching a movie of this type allows the patients, with the participation of staff, to work through a wide range of emotional issues through viewing the film rather than through direct confrontation with one another. Again, the point is that patients in a psychiatric unit are not helpless children who need staff to determine what is good for them; the staff responsibility is rather to relate to "patients" as responsible adults and to play their roles as those who facilitate patient exploration of emotional themes. One way to do this is through the viewing of films or TV programs that deal with controversial themes about human experiences.

Another factor in this situation is the film's place in the ward schedule. After seeing such a film, patients may not be ready to go to bed immediately. Since psychiatric units are part of an overall hospital structure in which shifts change at 11:00 p.m., the usual norm is for the evening shift of nurses to be sure that everyone is in bed before the night shift comes on. Working under such a system of constraints, the usual pattern is for nursing staff to attempt to whisk the patients off to bed after the evening film, without considering their need to unwind from a charged emotional experience. To relax, patients need an evening staff and the opportunity to talk to one another or to go to their rooms to read or watch TV. And maybe this cannot be accomplished by 11:00 p.m. or even by midnight.

Hospitals frequently assume that all persons who are patients will follow a pattern of going to bed at 10:00 p.m. and rising at 7:00 a.m., completely ignoring a number of facts. First, there are many people who do not follow these "rules of living" for one reason or another. All people have different "biological clocks." Some people work nights and sleep days. Others are not bound by any schedule and sleep whenever they feel like it. Still others may choose to go to bed at 8:00 p.m. Yet when they come into a hospital, all are fitted into a standard mold. Night nurses tend to become irritated when people do not sleep; they do not see their role as one of talking to people, but rather doing something to see that they sleep. Usually they accomplish this by giving sleeping potions. This ignores another pertinent issue, which is that people often do considerable "soul-searching" and introspection about their problems when they cannot sleep. In the silence of the night, they are freed from the usual group pressures that surround them during the day. In the hospital many sleepless patients, instead of seeking a pill to numb their feelings, could profit from being able to sit and talk and explore their problems with a member of the nursing staff.

Again let us consider Mrs. Stevens. In the course of twelve hours, she has gone from being a schoolteacher to being a person who has attempted suicide to becoming an inpatient in a psychiatric unit. She has made major role transitions that have serious implications for the way in which she views herself. In the quiet of the night, she is understandably unable to sleep and seeks out the night nurse to reflect on the things that have happened to her in the course of the day. The night nurse, instead of insisting that she return to bed, accompanies her to the dining area and makes some hot chocolate, and they sit down together to talk. After a half hour in which Mrs. Stevens reviews the happenings of the day with the nurse, she returns to her bed and falls asleep.

■ *Patient Responsibility.*   In a therapeutic environment, the person is given as much power and responsibility as possible. Breakfast is routinely served at 8:00 a.m., but instead of the nurses getting everyone up and ready for breakfast, the responsibility is on patients to do as they choose. If they are not up for breakfast, then they must fend for themselves in getting something to eat. Similarly, responsibility is placed on the patients for the care of their rooms and personal belongings. This presents a particular problem to nurses who are oriented toward seeing a compulsively neat ward environment. An unmade bed is tantamount to disaster in the eyes of some nurses; the image of the supervisor checking behind them to see that they have done their work still haunts many nurses trained in a different system of providing patient care.

Things like going to bed, getting up in the morning, straightening one's room, and taking care of one's personal belongings frequently become the basis of power struggles between the patient and the nurse. Many argue that a person cannot be prepared for life outside the hospital if he or she does not assume certain responsibilities and "shape up" while in the hospital. It is as if getting someone to make the bed and take care of personal belongings were tantamount to success in making him or her "well"; conversely, if this cannot be accomplished, it is evidence that the person is never going to "make it." This attitude ignores the fact that many supposedly "normal" persons are not particularly good housekeepers and have trouble getting up in the morning, and so could be considered irresponsible in this frame of reference.

The important thing is for nursing staff not to get caught up in a series of power struggles that substitute for a sound base of communication between the patient and the nurse. The hospital environment should provide the opportunity for the person to explore with others the ways in which they deal with life and, from this, develop some alternatives.

PATIENT GOVERNMENT

Most therapeutic communities have a number of group activities, the most common of which is some form of patient government. Patient government may take many forms, but in most instances patients and staff meet together, frequently once a day but at least twice a week, to decide on matters that have to do with day-to-day issues on the ward. Cumming and Cumming give certain principles of ward government: "First, the patient government should make and enforce the majority of the ward rules; second, it should organize and execute the majority of the routine ward tasks; finally, no staff member should solve a problem if it can possibly be delegated to the patient group."[6] Based on these principles, patient and staff together should agree upon the rules that are to govern them. Going back to our example of the problems of keeping rooms clean, people getting up, and similar issues, it is important that the entire group be involved in the decision-making process, first to make the rules by which they agree to live, and second, to be involved in the enforcement procedures if these rules are violated.

If patient government is to work, staff must carefully foster a climate in which these interchanges take place. What frequently happens is that staff members violate the structure by making decisions unilaterally without involving the group. To make a patient government system work, staff must consciously refrain from certain decision-making prerogatives and defer to the group. This is sometimes difficult to achieve, particularly with some of the traditional norms of medical settings. In the medical model, it is assumed that those who are the "professionals" in the setting are the ones who have particular expertise in treating the patient's disease. In psychiatric settings the situation is somewhat different. Although the professionals have particular expertise in the area, the patients' problems are not due to a particular disease process, but rather to difficulties in the way

---

6. Cumming and Cumming, *Ego and Milieu*, p. 123.

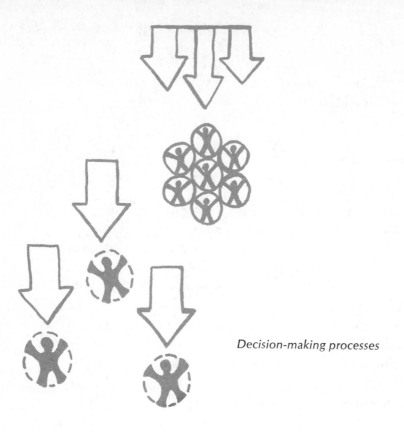

Decision-making processes

in which they relate to others. The treatment process, then, must be focused on disentangling them from their interpersonal difficulties. The only way this can be accomplished is through experiences within the hospital environment.

Therefore, staff in a psychiatric setting are in a different relationship to their clients than staff in other medical settings. Here the emphasis is on fostering the group's relatedness to one another and helping them achieve more satisfying approaches to problem-solving and a more effective exercise of the power they hold. Also, in many instances, "patients" do know what is best for them. The area of expertise of the staff is to foster the patients' decision-making processes so that they will arrive at the most rational decisions possible.

Take, for example, the hassles about people keeping the ward neat and maintaining their rooms. The patient group first needs to decide what standards of cleanliness they wish to have established for their ward. Maybe they will agree that keeping the ward clean is not too big a thing with them. At the other extreme, they may insist that the unit be thoroughly cleaned each day. If these are the decisions they make, they must live with the consequences. If the first alternative is chosen, they have little right to complain about the sloppy habits of some of their group. On the other hand, if they have agreed that the unit should be meticulously clean, then they have to develop a system to accomplish this end—perhaps assigning particular tasks to persons on the unit or developing a rotational system for doing the work. In any event, if they make this decision, then they must be responsible as a group for its enforcement. If a person does not perform according to the standards established, the group must deal with this and reach some rapprochement between the patient who does not follow the rules and the group who established them.

PATIENT-STAFF GROUP DECISION-MAKING

This emphasis on the patients' role in decision-making does not imply that staff sit silently by without having any part in the decision-making. Rather, it means that whatever input staff has to make should be made within the context of the patient-staff group and should not bypass the group structure. Most staff would find it difficult to live with a patient group decision that the the unit could be as messy as they wished it to be. Concern for the health of the group, a view that a messy ward reflects on their competence, and similar issues would be involved. But instead of arbitrarily imposing a set of rules and regulations, staff should express their concerns in the group decision-making context. Usually some compromise will be achieved, but the important thing for the staff to bear in mind is the necessity of abiding by the group's decision. If this is violated, any attempts at patient-government arrangements become something of a farce; it becomes further evidence of the powerlessness of the patient group and the power of the staff. And if for some reason staff have to make decisions contrary to the group, these decisions and the underlying reasons must be made explicit within the context of the patient-staff group.

In most patient government situations, an important part of the activity of the patient-staff group relates to decisions about whether patients should be given certain privileges, such as passes, or whether they are ready to be discharged. The decision-making in these areas is problematic in that staff feel they are responsible for protecting both the person and society and therefore must be very cautious. Legal complications frequently confuse the situation further. What usually happens is that the patient-staff group will discuss whether a particular patient is ready to go on a pass. The person's behavior on the ward will be reviewed, and the patient will be asked what he or she plans to do and whether he or she feels ready to go on a pass. Sometimes, however, this decision-making gets caught up in other issues. For instance, the patient group may be angry at staff for some reason and may hastily decide that a certain patient can go on pass, even though there is considerable evidence against it. Making such decisions is, in some instances, the only way patients can get back at staff. Staff then is faced with a dilemma. A common response is for them to have a separate meeting to make the "real" decision about whether or not a patient can go on pass. Should the staff meeting decide contrary to what the patient group has decided, the situation is set up for a continuing power struggle.

The preferable approach is for staff to discuss the issues that confront them in the open forum of the patient-staff meeting. Their perceptions of the person's readiness (or unreadiness) for certain activities are valid observations that should be stated openly. If there are legal or other constraints, they likewise should be stated. Even though staff may state their reservations, it may be that the patient-staff group will reach a decision different from that which staff wish them to make. And in some instances it is necessary to deny certain requests even though the group may have voted their approval. Again, it is extremely important that these decisions be stated openly and the reasons given, so that everyone has a clear perception of the way in which the decision-making process operates. If this does not occur, the patients have no way of getting clear readings of how the system operates, how decisions are made, or their place within this overall structure.

There are rules that are a necessary part of group living. The important point is that everyone know what these rules are, have the opportunity to engage in decision-making about modifying or updating them, and be clearly involved in discussing the consequences of rule violation. Rarely is this clarity achieved, but it is a goal to be worked toward if the climate of the unit is to foster more adequate problem-solving endeavors.

CHANGING PATTERNS OF COPING

In the case of Mary Lou Stevens, one of her consistent coping styles was to withdraw from any conflict situation, not expressing her anger or other feelings, and then to feel depressed. Let us look at how interaction within the therapeutic community setting might be helpful in developing altered patterns of coping. Mrs. Stevens characteristically is a very orderly person; her life has been rather carefully structured around home and work activities. She has always considered herself to be a good manager, and her home is kept meticulously clean. Her roommate, Jean Peters, is the complete opposite; her life style is in direct contrast with Mary Lou Stevens's. While Mrs. Stevens likes to go to bed at 10:00 p.m. and get up at 7:00 a.m., Ms. Peters would like to stay up all night playing her radio and then sleep all day. She does not care if her bed is ever made, throws things around the room, and is generally disorderly. Mrs. Stevens, in contrast, is very upset by seeing things in a mess.

Mary Lou Stevens's first approach to dealing with this problem is to clean up the room for both of them. While Jean Peters is out on a field trip, she spends the whole time cleaning the room, thinking that her roommate will be pleased when she comes back to find everything neat and orderly. Instead, Ms. Peters complains loudly about anyone touching any of her things and says she cannot find her favorite sweater. In a rage attack, she throws all her belongings around the room, and it is in worse shape than before Mrs. Stevens cleaned it up. Mary Lou Stevens responds by going to an isolated corner of the dayroom and silently crying—this is further evidence that she is "no good" and cannot manage anything right. Ms. Wagner, the nurse, finds her in this condition. She sits down beside her quietly and gently asks if she would like to tell what is troubling her. Mrs. Stevens briefly goes through the story but ends up with a series of self-recriminations. The nurse asks what she said to Jean Peters, and the response is, "Well, I didn't feel that there was anything to say. She was just throwing things around and the only thing for me to do was to get out of there."

> *Ms. Wagner:* You say that was the only thing to do. I can think of some other things you might have done. Can you identify any other alternatives?
>
> *Mrs. Stevens:* I was only trying to do something that would please her.

Ms. Wagner: Did you try to tell her this—that you hadn't meant to do anything that would upset her?

Mrs. Stevens: Well, there wasn't really any chance. I get so frightened of a person who is angry that I just want to get away.

Ms. Wagner: What about your feelings in this situation? You put a lot of work into cleaning up the room. It must have been distressing for you to see it all torn up.

Mrs. Stevens: I just felt bad; it's so like all of my life goes. I try so hard to do things right, but I just can't seem to get them to come out right.

Ms. Wagner: It's as if you somehow think this is all your fault. Don't you have any rights to feelings of your own?

Mrs. Stevens: What good would it do? Oh, I feel a little angry sometimes, but there's no point in getting into a fight.

Ms. Wagner: So instead you retreat and sit here alone crying. What do you think would have happened if you had told Jean that it made you angry to see her throwing things around?

Mrs. Stevens: Well, she would have just been angrier at me, and I really was wrong in touching her things.

Ms. Wagner: But it is your room, too, and your husband is coming to visit you. I would be very upset and angry to have this happen to me.

Mrs. Stevens: Well, I have to admit that I am a little angry, but what's the use? It wouldn't accomplish anything.

Ms. Wagner: Maybe we should discuss this in the meeting tomorrow so that you can get the views of some of the other people here.

In the meeting the following day, this incident did become a topic of discussion. As the situation was discussed, other patients expressed their anger at Jean Peters for the way in which she totally disregarded other people's feelings, while Mary Lou Stevens received a great deal of support from them even though she did not ask for it. She consistently presented the situation as one in which she had done something wrong, but within the group there was considerable support that she had not intended to do anything deliberately to upset Jean Peters, and that Jean really should be more considerate of others and abide by the rules that specified that each person was to keep his or her room clean.

While this was just the first of many instances, the relationship between Mary Lou Stevens and Jean Peters became one in which both were encouraged to develop new ways of coping with their situations. Mrs. Stevens was encouraged to become more forthright in first recognizing her feelings and then expressing them. Ms. Peters was able to begin to see the way in which she, out of anxiety about not being accepted, ran roughshod over others. The relationship established between the two women became a means for learning new ways of relating that were more personally satisfying.

The hospital setting is one in which the person can learn new patterns of relating that will carry over into his or her relationships outside the hospital. For the person to accomplish these necessary learnings, every aspect of the hospital experience must be examined for its therapeutic potential. The nurse, within the hospital setting, is the person who can monitor the situation and try to use naturally occurring incidents as vehicles for helping patients explore new patterns of coping and of relating to others.

PREPARATION FOR RE-ENTERING THE COMMUNITY

Perhaps one of the most crucial aspects of the hospitalization experience is its end—the person's discharge and reintegration into social networks outside the hospital. The significance of this important facet is frequently overlooked or discounted. The person is judged ready for discharge with little consideration or planning for the ways in which he or she will resume life outside the hospital. Anticipatory counseling has been mentioned as a valuable technique to help people prepare for certain problematic situations; by going through the problem-solving process in advance, they are "emotionally inoculated." The same principles can be applied to patients about to be discharged from a psychiatric setting.

Consider the problems that they will have to deal with. When a person is hospitalized, there usually is a shifting of roles in the family, and the hospitalized person is, in a sense, displaced. The family makes an adjustment so that they can "do without" the extruded family member. For instance, Mary Lou Stevens's husband probably managed to do the housework and cooking himself, or has enlisted a family member to help him, or has hired someone to fill this gap. Mrs. Stevens, on coming out of the hospital, cannot just automatically resume her place within the family, but must negotiate with those who have shifted their roles in her absence.

The person also is faced with re-entering a community. Frequently the fact that a neighbor has been hospitalized in a psychiatric setting be-

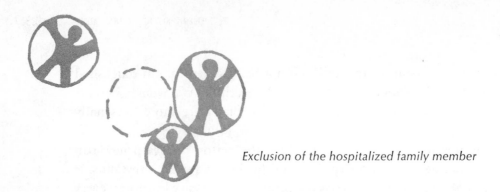

Exclusion of the hospitalized family member

comes a favorite topic for neighborhood gossip. Neighbors advance explanations for someone's having a "nervous breakdown": perhaps there is something wrong with the marriage, or, "I always knew she was a little peculiar, working like she does and no children." The person coming out of a psychiatric hospital then re-enters a neghborhood system where she or he is looked on as somewhat strange. The common stereotype of mental patients is that they are not to be trusted and are unpredictable in their behavior. The relationships between neighbors and the person coming out of a psychiatric hospitalization are likely to be strained, and the person feels he or she must be overly careful lest others think there is still some problem.

A third common problem area is re-entering one's work position. Many of the themes common in the neighborhood setting are repeated, but there is an additional factor—whether the person discharged from psychiatric treatment will be able to manage the work. For example, if Mrs. Stevens goes back to teaching, she is sure to face either over or covert questioning as to her capability to handle her job. Her performance will be scrutinized even more than before her hospitalization. She will be in a position of having to prove her competence rather than having it assumed.

Some persons leaving a hospital do not return to their families, communities, or jobs, but instead must seek out a totally new living situation for themselves. In these instances the work that needs to be accomplished before leaving the hospital concerns where the person is to live, what type of job he or she is going to seek, and in many instances, help in finding a job while still in the hospital.

In any event, before leaving the hospital, people should be encouraged to review every aspects of their plans for re-entering social networks or for establishing alternate ones. The problems that they will encounter should be anticipated, and how they are to deal with them should be worked through before they face the actual situation. In many instances, family members meet with the therapist to work out family arrangements before the person is discharged. Also, the person is encouraged to make contacts with his or her employer before leaving the hospital, in order to have the necessary support.

Leaving the hospital is another potential crisis experience for which one can be prepared. As with all crises, it may be an opportunity for new learning or it may pose a threat to the learnings achieved while in the hospital. People may come out feeling they have some mastery over situations that were overwhelming before entering the hospital, or they may again fall victim to their inadequate abilities to manage the life situations they face. The crucial variable is the assistance they have received in learning new ways of resolving problems, and the anticipatory guidance they have received to prepare them for coping with the problems they face on leaving the hospital.

Hospitalization can be an experience that temporarily protects one from harming oneself or others, or it can provide one with an opportunity to learn new patterns of relatedness that will change one's total life. What transpires during the course of a person's hospitalization depends mainly on the orientation of psychiatric staff and the potential they find within the hospital setting for helping the person with necessary new learnings. Some psychiatric staff see themselves only as custodians, with the primary responsibility of protecting patients. Others see themselves as catalysts in helping patients achieve new learnings about themselves and others. Hospitalization can be a turning point in helping a person develop more flexible problem-solving styles, or it can be a constricting, restricting experience that leaves him or her more vulnerable in subsequent crises.

PRINCIPLES OF RELATING

People who are in the process of becoming familiar with markedly unusual ranges of behavior commonly feel at a loss as to how to respond.

Such behavior can be anxiety-provoking to the nurse who wants to do her or his best to help people, but cannot understand behavior that does not seem to follow the usual rules and may even be bizarre or frightening. Although there are no rules for predicting the appropriate response to each situation, there are some principles underlying all relationships that are particularly applicable in these instances. As the nurse gains experience in relating to a wide range of people, she or he may want to expand on these principles.

COMMUNICATION

A basic principle of communication is that all behavior—commonplace or bizarre—has meaning. Discovering the meaning of particular symptoms or behaviors allows one to plan responses that have a greater chance of being helpful to the patient. Striving for such understanding is a major thread throughout all interaction between staff and patients; as the understanding increases, it serves as strong base for intervention. Take, once again, the case of Mary Lou Stevens, the suicidal schoolteacher who retreated, weeping, to the corner of the dayroom in the face of difficulty with her roommate. The nurse needed to have some understanding of that behavior as a manifestation of Mrs. Stevens's particular coping pattern before engaging in any corrective interaction with her.

In a more extreme case of a severely depressed person who has much more psychomotor retardation, the nurse also would need an accurate notion of the meaning of the stilted, slow-down, uninterested-appearing behavior. Communication in this circumstance is difficult, and nurses are apt to feel put off and useless. It is helpful when the nurse understands that the patient is unable to register input, to think, act, or even remember at a reasonable rate. This person lacks both the confidence and the energy to initiate interaction and cannot maintain an investment in people. With this understanding in mind, the nurse will take the initiative in the relationship, allowing for slowness and a relative lack of activity. The nurse will probably depend on sharing silence and solitude with such a patient, knowing that a low-keyed presence and perseverance will cut through his or her feelings of isolation and unworthiness. The nurse will be communicating acceptance and faith that the depression will lift.

■ *Acting Out.* Another good example of the nurse's need for understanding occurs in situations in which the patient is commonly described as "acting out." "Acting out" is a term used indiscriminately, unfortunately, for situations in which patients are getting into trouble or behaving in a way that makes everyone irritated and disapproving. There are some advantages in considering the real meaning of the concept. For behavior to be appropriately called "acting out," it should consist of rather impulsive behavior that expresses some piece of a conflict the person is not aware of. The person knows that he or she is behaving in a certain way, but that he or she does not recognize what this behavior communicates or what motivates it. It is of key importance that the people concerned with the person, whatever else they may choose to do about the acting-out behavior, also seek to understand its source and meaning. Such understanding is essential in helping the person arrive at a reasonably improved way of handling the conflict.

Take, for example, Jean Peters, Mrs. Stevens's roommate. Much of her flamboyant physical expression of whatever comes into her mind could be labeled "acting out." Ms. Peters, who considers herself an enlightened "free spirit" in contrast to her dull, dowdy family, does not recognize how much her behavior is tied to these family relationships. She is expressing an intense power struggle with her parents, further complicated by her unrecognized wish to be loved by them, a factor that interferes with her ability to make a complete break from them. In addition to simply setting limits for Jean, the nursing staff, being aware of the meaning of her particular behavior, must plan how they might help her work toward greater autonomy. This will involve helping her gain some understanding of her true abilities and how she can use them to gain the positive attention she so desperately seeks. They might also be aware of any opportunities to help her with a realistic assessment of her relationship to her parents.

■ *Countering Patients' False Belief Systems.* Another principle of communication is the general futility of telling people something that runs counter to the belief system that supports their current coping style. Such information is useless, since it is not accepted as fact, and frequently adds to the feelings of frustration and misunderstanding between nurse and patient. If the nurse is particularly strong in maintaining a stance in spite of the patient's opposition, it may simply push the patient to defend himself or herself more effectively against the nurse and the anxiety this stance provokes, or to demonstrate more dramatically the "truth" of his or her position. One application of this principle is in responding to delusions and hallucinations. If a person knows he is a "terrible sinner," then telling him he is not will not alter his conviction, and he may be pushed to prove just how bad he is. This, though, does not imply that the opposite course —agreement with his belief or agreement that the voices he hears are real —is preferable.

Patients (schizophrenic patients in particular) who are disorganized are especially likely to have problems with ego boundaries. In other words, they have difficulty in differentiating themselves from people and things in their environment. Any behavior that seems to confirm the reality of the person's distorted thinking implies that the nurse, too, shares it; this adds to his or her ego boundary problems. When for some reason it becomes necessary to interact around the issue of the delusions or hallucinations, other people—patients or staff—can acknowledge that while they themselves do not hold the belief or hear the voices, they do appreciate that the patient does and is understandably concerned with them. They may want to add that they are interested in helping the patient understand more about the hallucinations so that he or she can gain more control over them and be less troubled. In this way, the experience is identified as the patient's, not anyone else's, and he or she also is presented with a way of achieving some mastery over it.

The failure of efforts to reassure patients, to increase their self-esteem, or to get them to value themselves more, frequently can be explained on the basis of this same principle of communication. Most people who have evolved a restricted, rigid, or otherwise unsatisfactory coping style have suffered many assaults to their esteem; they lack trust in relationships with others and confidence in themselves. In nearly all cases, the nurse would want to nurture that person's self-esteem and confidence carefully, but although it seems logical, labeling certain attributes or abilities of the person as positive, or praising some accomplishment does not really work. The reason for this is that praise or positive remarks will seem foreign to the patient, who will then decide that the nurse either does not know him or her very well or is somewhat inept in making judgments. If a great deal of guilt is involved in the patient's dynamics, he or she may feel even guiltier because praise reaffirm his or her feelings of being a "fraud." The nurse would be better advised to simply help the person become competent, structuring situations to make his or her own competence obvious. A safer approach is a statement such as, "I'm glad you were able to figure out that piece of the pattern, Mrs. Brown. There are two other people who had a lot of trouble with it. Maybe one of these mornings you may care to help them."

■ *Feedback.* Most relationships depend heavily on the participants' getting feedback from one another. This is how they gauge that their messages are being understood and are influencing the other person. In some of the more disturbed behavior situations, however, nurses cannot rely on feedback the way they ordinarily would. Schizophrenic persons who are fearful of relationships because they cannot depend upon being safe in them may be very guarded in responding to the nurse. It is probable that such persons are taking in and attaching meaning to everything that is being said, but they give no outward indication. In ordinary social situations, most people would change the content of their interactions until they evoked some feedback response from the other, or they would abandon the attempt and interact with someone else. This reaction is not particularly helpful in a treatment situation, and it must be assumed that patients are responding, even though they give no outward indication. With the development of a trusting relationship—which may require the nurse to weather many silences, be undemanding, and demonstrate complete trustworthiness—patients will be able to extend themselves a little more openly, and feedback will cease to be such a problem.

Otto Will describes certain characteristics that are desirable in those who would work with schizophrenic patients. Such persons must recognize their own anxiety and want to explore its sources, not be excessively disturbed by the manifestations of anxiety in others, and analyze the motives underlying their own behavior, even though this may produce discomfort. They should be compassionate but not feel compelled to convert the patient to their views or to "cure" him or her; they should identify with the patient, but not to the point that they take on his or her feelings of despair and hopelessness. Finally, they should not use the patient to fill their own needs, for example, for human relationships or for power over others.[7]

---

7. Otto Allen Will, Jr., "Schizophrenic Patient, Psychotherapist, Consultant," *Contemporary Psychoanalysis* 1 (Spring 1965): 113-114.

As a nurse interacts with patients and gains knowledge about their typical ways of behaving, she or he can develop some shortcuts for discerning the level of anxiety that patients are experiencing at any given time and sometimes the nature of what causes the anxiety. The patient's symptoms frequently serve as indexes of anxiety, so that if a particular patient's hallucinations are more frequent or more exaggerated at certain times, the nurse would do well to inquire to discover what is precipitating the anxious response. This same principle is helpful in working with patients who have compulsive behavior patterns. Usually compulsive behavior becomes more prominent when patients are anxious. Noting the points at which the behavior increases is helpful when the nurse is attempting to assist the patient to gain more knowledge about the meaning of these patterns and achieve mastery or control over them.

SITUATIONAL BOUNDARIES

In any situation, the allowable behavior is somewhat circumscribed by the boundaries or parameters of the particular situation itself. For instance, the situation in which patients decided to have a messy unit and forego concerns with cleaning itself exerted certain limits about what would be possible. Matters of sanitation and safety, if not esthetics, would definitely provide parameters. If each person in a situation can be considered an actor, the possible roles of that actor are likewise limited by the boundaries of the situation. Thus, within this situation, Jean Peters can be only so "messy." Violation of role behaviors indicates a need for limit setting, but these limits should be set by the boundaries of the situation, not the personal preferences of people with power. Many staffs' difficulties about limit setting stem from lack of agreement about the boundaries that are being transgressed and, therefore, the limits that need to be stressed. When people are not in complete agreement, there is no consistency and therefore no predictable limits. Since lack of predictability is usually a problem for people in a psychiatric setting, it is especially important that the limits be consistent, clear, and objective, that is, clearly related to what the situation requires.

There are other people who tend to create situations with a high degree of unpredictability so that they can keep things in such an uproar that they maintain their own basic isolation and lack of connectedness. These people are particularly prone to break the unit's rules. They frequently get themselves into a position in which they are labeled in a way that distorts how they are seen. For instance, Jean Peters is generally considered unpleasant by her peers and intransigent and unmotivated by the staff, since she does not seem to take any of the rules seriously and puts staff in a position to be assertive about her complying with them. Of course in this kind of a unit, limit-setting flows naturally from the milieu since it is a shared responsibility, while it also flows naturally from the situational requirements, a point not easily seen in more authoritatively structured settings.

PHYSICAL NEEDS

A final principle relates to physical aspects of care. Although much of our discussion has centered on the need for nurses in psychiatric settings to adopt modes of relating to people other than those used previously, they need not forget their prior skills altogether. Patients with difficulty coping may have both physical manifestations of their problems and other physical illnesses. It is not unheard of for patients to go into cardiac decompensation because no one paid attention to their complaints, attributing them to anxiety or some psychological problem. It is particularly important to monitor patients' physical functions and see that they follow proper hygiene. Very depressed patients, for instance, may have edematous extremities or circulatory problems because of their inactivity. They may also be constipated and either not notice or not say anything about it. People who are in a manic state need similar attention. Seeing that patients get enough to eat and proper rest is a legitimate concern. Noticing any injuries or physical malfunctions is necessary, since patients in such a state frequently do not complain about them. Sometimes compulsive ritualistic behavior can interfere with normal physical functioning, as in the classic instance of a person washing his hands until they are bleeding and raw. In any event, the nurse currently working in a psychiatric unit should not cease using her or his previously learned principles of good health.

SUMMARY

The experience of being hospitalized usually involves a crisis, both for the individual and for his or her family. It therefore affords an opportunity for personal growth or for further restrictive coping. By structuring the situation to reduce anxiety, familiarizing individuals with what they might expect, and orienting them to the new hospital environment, staff can make the experience of entering the hospital the beginning of the reintegrative process.

Proper organization of the milieu can further move the person toward more adaptive problem-solving maneuvers. Carefully planning the introduction of the patient into the treatment milieu, providing opportunities for preserving and maintaining self-esteem through participation in ward activities and decision-making, helping with problem-solving activities and anticipatory planning for a return to life outside the hospital are all essential parts of the treatment process.

A therapeutic community involves equalization of status and responsibility between those being treated and those who are doing the treating. When this occurs, the interlude of hospitalization may be used to maximal effectiveness, as it not only allows patients a respite from their usual role responsibilities so they can concentrate on their difficulties at hand, but also provides a new arena to practice alternative forms of relating. In all hospitalization, for whatever cause, the person is removed from his or her usual supports and identities and is faced with a stressful situation in which new learning may readily take place. The nurse is in a key position to make the hospitalization experience truly therapeutic in helping the person achieve new learnings.

FURTHER READINGS

Berliner, Arthur. "The Two Milieus in Milieu Therapy." *Perspectives in Psychiatric Care* 5, no. 6 (1967): 266-271.

Calnen, Terrence. "Whose Agent? A Re-evaluation of the Role of the Psychiatric Nurse in the Therapeutic Community." *Perspectives in Psychiatric Care* 10, no. 5 (1972): 210-219.

Dixson, Barbara. "Dealing With Passive Aggressive Behavior." *Nursing Forum* 8, no. 3 (1969): 276-285.

Emde, Robert. "Limiting Regression in the Therapeutic Community." *American Journal of Nursing* 67 (May 1967): 1010-1015.

Fagin, Claire. "Psychotherapeutic Nursing." *American Journal of Nursing* 67 (February 1967): 298-304.

Gardner, Kathryn. "Patient Groups in a Therapeutic Community." *American Journal of Nursing* 71 (March 1971): 528-531.

Holmes, Marguerite, and Werner, June. "The Use of Limit Setting as a Therapeutic Process." In *Psychiatric Nursing in a Therapeutic Community*, pp. 43-62. New York: The Macmillan Company, 1966.

Huey, Florence. "In a Therapeutic Community." *American Journal of Nursing* 71 (May 1971): 926-933.

Kincheloe, Marsha. "Democratization in the Therapeutic Community." *Perspectives in Psychiatric Care* 11, no. 2 (1973): 75-79.

Leone, Dolores, and Zahowek, Rothlyn. "Aloneness in a Therapeutic Community." *Perspectives in Psychiatric Care* 12, no. 2 (1974): 60-63.

Loomis, Maxine. "Nursing Management of Acting-Out Behavior." *Perspectives in Psychiatric Care* 8, no. 4 (1969): 168-173.

Robitaille, Normand. "The Organization of a Patient Council." *Perspectives in Psychiatric Care* 3, no. 3 (1965): 23-25.

Saper, Beatrice. "Patients as Partners in the Team Approach." *American Journal of Nursing* 74 (Oct. 1974): 1844-1847.

Schwartz, Morris, and Shockley, Emmy. *The Nurse and the Mental Patient*. New York: John Wiley & Sons, 1956.

Tudor, Gwen. "A Sociopsychiatric Nursing Approach to Intervention in a Problem of Mutual Withdrawal on a Mental Hospital Ward." (reprint) *Perspectives in Psychiatric Care* 8 (Jan.-Feb. 1970): 11-35.

Ujhely, Gertrud. "Nursing Intervention With the Acutely Ill Psychiatric Patient." *Nursing Forum* 8, no. 3 (1969): 311-325.

CHAPTER FOURTEEN

ETHICAL
ISSUES

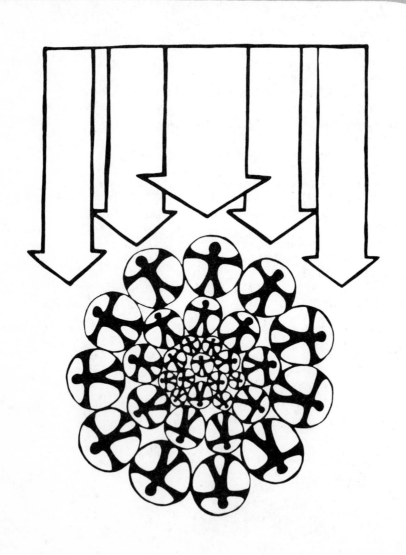

Ethical issues inevitably arise in any field in which the primary goal is to perform some function or service involving people's behavior. Psychiatric nursing is very much affected by dilemmas concerning ethical issues. These dilemmas involve the nature of behavior generally, whether it be "mental health" or "mental illness," and the interface of behavior within a social network. At certain points, conflicts can arise between the interests of a particular person and his or her larger social groupings; in this instance, the dilemma is whose interests shall take precedence, the person's or the social group's. These issues in turn affect the direction and nature of interventions. Szasz feels that our traditional notions of mental illness are poorly conceived because of this dilemma. He succinctly states the position:

> It is customary to define psychiatry as a medical specialty concerned with the study, diagnosis, and treatment of mental illness. This is a worthless and misleading definition. Mental illness is a myth. Psychiatrists are not concerned with mental illnesses and their treatment. In actual practice they deal with personal, social, and ethical problems in living.[1]

Nurses are involved ostensibly in the identification and treatment of mental problems, but in actuality these mental problems consist of personal, social, and ethical difficulties. Although psychiatric nursing has changed greatly in recent years, the nurse still operates predominantly within a medically oriented system concerned with the identification of disease and treatment of specific problems. In most psychiatric settings, the nurse needs to be at least conversant with major diagnostic categories, common etiological explanations, and more usual treatment approaches. This medical background, however, is not of particular help in dealing

---

1. Thomas S. Szasz, *The Myth of Mental Illness: Foundations of a Theory of Human Conduct,* 2nd ed. (New York: Harper, Row, 1973), p. 262.

with the social, personal, and ethical problems represented in the "patient's" dilemma. In the past, dealing with these problems was the domain of those outside the medical profession, for example, social workers and priests. However, patients identified as having "mental problems" come into the medical system, in which the predominant values are oriented toward a medical model of practice.

Throughout this book we have faced the dilemma of how nurses can best be prepared to function effectively in bridging the chasm between this medical orientation and other aspects of the patient's situation. We feel that the traditional medical model of psychiatric illness is inadequate and that the treatment approaches that derive from it frequently do not succeed in touching the areas of a patient's life that would make a difference. This is not to say that physicians do not succeed in helping people, but that when they do, they have probably abandoned a pure medical model for a more encompassing social-psychological approach. We have presented this broader model throughout this book, first to familiarize nurses with the orientation of the medical model, and then to make bridges to an alternative social-psychological model of behavior and intervention. We would much prefer to view "mental illness" problems, from whatever source (psychological, social, or biological), from the broader perspective of societal rule-breaking and its responses and repercussions through the social network. From this perspective, psychiatric nursing practice should be directed toward intervention in these broader social networks.

It is our belief that psychiatric nurses must increasingly be directed toward this broader societal perspective; in the interim, however, they face the problem of transition between it and the medical model. Throughout the book we have attempted to lay a foundation that would prepare nurses for this aspect of their role. No matter what framework is employed, each nurse must weight the moral and ethical dilemmas and make decisions as to the nature of her or his work with people. To assist the nurse in identifying significant issues, this final chapter raises a number of pertinent questions: What should be treated? Who decides? Who defines the nature of the treatment? Who should be the treaters? How shall treatment be financed?

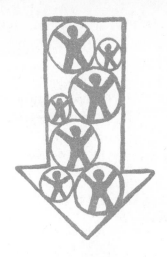

Mental illness in a societal framework

WHAT SHOULD BE TREATED?

With the popularizing of psychiatry, a surface inspection would seem to indicate that everyone is in need of psychotherapy in one form or another. Hardly a day goes by that there is not a newspaper or magazine article or a television presentation on some mental health problem. The bored housewife, anxious businessman, hyperactive child, rebellious teen-ager, and forgetful grandparent are all considered to be candidates for psychotherapeutic help.

Those formally labeled as mentally ill, while constituting 50 percent of the total population of hospitals, are but a small proportion of the population considered to be in need of some type of psychiatric help. That large numbers of people lead psychologically constricted and miserable lives cannot be denied, but what should be done about it?

Many professionals are troubled by this question. They feel that the problems of the people about whom they are consulted, or who consult them directly, are the natural outgrowths of the social conditions surrounding them. Their idea of their appropriate role goes beyond helping people "adjust" to the stresses of their particular positions and includes helping individuals make whatever changes they can in the networks surrounding them. For instance, they may feel that the bored housewife could be encouraged to change her coping style so that she does not need to feel constrained to remain home, but will make many changes with the people who surround her and, indeed, become quite a different person in a different social situation. The anxious businessman might well quit his job and seek to find a more satisfying niche in the social order.

The problem for practitioners develops when there is no satisfying place in a social system which the "patient" can negotiate for himself or herself and the needed changes seem to be in the structure itself. To promote organizational change entails activity commonly regarded as more "political" than that with which most practitioners are comfortable. If we say, for instance, that the situation of minority people predisposes them to depression, then what is needed is a change in the position of the minority person. Assisting in such changes requires commitment and involvement in the political and legal arrangements of society. The question of whether such commitment is appropriate at all—and, if it is, how much involvement there should be—is a matter of current controversy. Frequently ignored in the debate is the equally viable argument that the psychotherapist who works solely with the individual in his or her struggles to "adjust" also is implicitly supporting a political position: that of maintaining the status quo.

WHO SHOULD BE TREATED?

It may be argued that the foregoing issues are clouded and that surely situations arise in which the behavior of an individual person is so extreme that he or she must be treated. Once again, while most people would agree that this is true, the decision about who is to be treated is not so simple as it seems. The complexity usually involves questions of individual rights and how decisions for treatment are made.

In cases related to hospitalization, for example, psychiatric professionals tend to evoke the rule of thumb that if a person is potentially dangerous (to himself or herself or others), he or she should be hospitalized.

From their perspective, hospitalization is an humanitarian gesture. Patients frequently do not share this view. The question is one of the moral right of hospitals or psychiatric professionals to decide that a person needs to be confined to a hospital. Recent legal decisions also have supported the right to confine people as long as there is tangible evidence of treatment. From a legal point of view, protection of society through the enforcement of laws is necessary to maintain the social order. In the example of the "mental patient" who needs to be confined, the medical and legal systems join. The patient is legally confined, but the problem is treated as a medical one that is the cause for his or her acts. The patient is regarded as not capable of making decisions about necessary treatment, so that others must make them, including the decisions about if and when he or she is to be released from confinement. The person who is evaluated as suicidal is a case in point. It is generally maintained that the wish to commit suicide is evidence of mental imbalance and that this person must be protected from himself or herself and not allowed to follow through. The consensus is that as the person's problems are solved, he or she no longer will feel this way and will be grateful for having been saved.

Szasz represents the opposing view. He argues strongly that the client (not "patient") is the one who should decide about whether he or she is to be treated, hospitalized, or whatever. Implicit in this stand is the one's responsibility for oneself. This view holds that if one violates some law, one is responsible for his or her behavior and its consequences and cannot be excused as "mentally ill."

As Szasz points out, psychiatry has increased in scope so that problems that used to be treated as moral or legal have become mixed in with psychiatric treatment. A psychiatric professional, he argues, is not prepared to deal with these moral or legal dilemmas. But what frequently happens is that the psychiatric professional does deal with these issues, but they are not identified as such; rather all the issues are considered together as part of the person's problems. When this happens, the treatment situation becomes clouded. Halleck[2] points out that psychiatric treatment is a political activity and that the values of the psychiatric professional tend to set the standard for defining the values considered proper for the person defined as "patient."

---

2. Halleck, Seymour, *The Politics of Therapy* (New York: Science House, Inc., 1971).

Recognizing these problems, Szasz argues strongly for the necessity of a contract between patient and psychiatric professional as essential in defining the parameters of treatment. It is the client who decides whether he or she wishes psychiatric treatment, not the family, employer, school, or some other agent of society defining him or her as in need of treatment. Once the person has been identified by these social agents, he or she is likely to be directed to a psychiatric professional. But the psychiatric professional is then an agent of whoever has referred the person, rather than an agent of the client. Frequently the definitions of the person's problem made by these social groups become the basis for assuming that he or she does have a particular problem. For example, the child who is defined as "troublesome" in the classroom is automatically judged to have a problem in need of treatment, without other factors being considered. The word of certain authority figures, such as a teacher, is frequently taken as more authentic than the person's own account of the situation. The psychiatric professional is seen as the agent of change who will work with the patient to make his or her behavior more acceptable to the social group, whether the patient wants this or not. The power placed in the hands of psychiatric professionals is great, and many are seduced by this rather "god-like" position to go about changing people in the manner prescribed by society.

Given this arrangement, does a person have any right to decide whether he or she wishes to be changed? Perhaps the norm-breaking individual does not wish to change his or her behavior—if not, what should be done? Now many will argue that one cannot let this person decide what he or she wishes to change. Indeed, one of the problems attributed to a person who is identified as "mentally ill" is that he or she is not capable of making rational judgments. How could this person possibly decide whether he or she wishes to receive psychiatric treatment?

Children present particular problems from the standpoints of both legality and maturity. Usually parents are regarded as responsible for them and have the power to make decisions for them. It is fairly easy to see that a five-year-old is not able to perceive many reality situations that will affect his or her future. On the other hand, in situations such as child-abuse, the parents are not particularly good at making these decisions. The problems of how to make the best decisions for children have not been addressed, primarily because of legal problems. One proposal has been to establish a "child advocate" position, so that someone would function as an adult but would act in the interests of the child. This advocate, in essence, would not be part of either the legal or the family system, but would bring maturity and specialized knowledge to bear upon the decision-making process.

Informed consent is another frequently raised issue. Since many psychiatric patients have limited legal voice, they are particularly vulnerable to being exploited in matters of experimentation and treatment by methods whose potential for ill effects is not explained. This treatment is due mainly to the tendency to regard mental patients as incapable of making decisions. A whole range of treatments is involved (lobotomies, electroshock, and medication regimes, for example), in which the professional assumes that the long-range advantages outweigh the patient's protestations that he or she does not want this type of treatment. The reciprocal of this issue is the staff's responsibility for the results of their decisions on the people they treat. Consent for various procedures is generally obtained from family members, who often feel at the mercy of the psychiatric professionals and will agree all too readily to the proposed prescriptions. Convincing other family members that the person should have a particular treatment instead of negotiating this issue with the patient only contributes to his or her basic problem of powerlessness.

WHO SHALL TREAT?

Considerable controversy also surrounds the issue of who is qualified to treat either actual or potential "mental patients." Again the issue is tied up in the definitions of "mental illness." For those who hold to the medical model, "mental illness" is considered a disease, which is to be treated only by those with specialized knowledge about its diagnosis and treatment. Others may be involved in the treatment process, but only in a limited way. The psychologist's role is to provide the psychodiagnostic testing, while the social worker is to deal with the family and make necessary job contacts in preparation for the patient's leaving the hospital, and the nurse is to function in the hospital setting, following the doctor's orders for treatment. The patient is seen as having a disease, and a specific treatment procedure is developed to manage it. In this strict medical model, the primary arena of service by any member of the team, except for the psychiatrist, is the hospital setting. The persons treated are only those who enter the medical system voluntarily or through the actions of other people on their behalf.

If one takes the alternate model—"mental illness" embedded within a social network—the issue of who should treat becomes more controversial. Here the intervention will be into social network problems, to free the person from the problems that have developed for him or her within the realm of interpersonal relations. Who should intervene then becomes tied to the issue of who has access to the social networks in which the problems exist. The people with most ready access to social networks are those who are a part of them, and for this reason some segments of the community mental health movement have argued strongly for the development of a core of indigenous community mental health workers, with ready access to the social structures involved. These endeavors have taken many forms, such as training of housewives, bartenders, funeral directors, and a wide range of similar people to be "front line" mental health workers. Working in this framework, psychiatric professionals take responsibility for training these nonprofessionals, provide consultation to them, and give treatment—individual, group, or family—to those who need more than the emergency interventions of the community workers.

Although this appears to be a rational and feasible approach, there are a number of difficulties. First, psychiatrists have not been socialized into such a view of the problem, and the skills of working with nonprofessionals are not built into their professional background. They similarly are uncomfortable in working outside their private office or the hospital setting. Few have the capacity to go into a community and relate to its problems on a meaningful level. Many come from a different socioeconomic group from the people they serve and so have difficulty comprehending the problems of those who live in unfamiliar circumstances. They have little practice in going into a home situation and have difficulty overcoming the "social distance" issues in a community setting.

Community psychology programs have perhaps done more than other disciplines to prepare professionals to function specifically in community settings. Most clinical psychology programs have a built-in option of concentrating in this area of study at the doctoral level. Social workers, while their background is somewhat different, are similarly familiar with community work, although traditionally those specializing in psychiatric practice

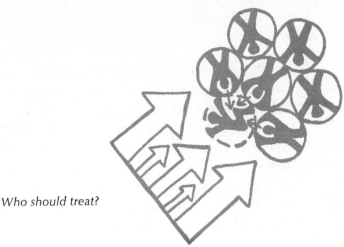

Who should treat?

are oriented toward casework, that is, a one-to-one relationship with the patient. Nurses in general have little orientation to community work of a preventive or curative nature. Although all baccalaureate programs include community experience, they tend to be limited to physical care dimensions rather than mental health considerations. By and large, psychiatric professionals entering the community are on foreign turf. But it is still very difficult for a person who has devoted a number of years to becoming a psychiatric professional to take the stance that he or she really does not know how to engage in community work. The situation is further complicated by the indigenous workers who, in many instances, are perceived to be the experts.

A number of complicated status issues emerge. If indigenous community workers with no formal education can be successful treaters, why should the psychiatric professionals devote years to formal education? A common response to this problem is for the professionals to become overly invested in training the indigenous workers, in effect, transforming them from nonprofessionals to professionals. In the process, they, too, are socialized so that they become distanced from their own social networks. As professional values are imposed on these community workers, most are encouraged to "better themselves," and frequently they become involved in formal educational processes that make them professionals in the same system.

Theoretically, it seems feasible that the point of intervention should be to people at the time of crisis, within the network of social relationships, but the question remains as to how this can be achieved. While it is beyond the scope of this book to address this broad issue, it is important to consider the unique role the nurse can have in relationship to people at points of stress. Whoever is to intervene must be accessible to those who are having problems, and the interventions need to be real and tangible, not abstract and theoretical. As we have pointed out through this book, many of the problems experienced by people arise from loss. Nurses often are directly involved with people who are experiencing a wide range of losses, whether from physical problems or through death of a loved one. Of all psychiatric and medical professionals, nurses probably have access to more people in a direct way at times when they are most vulnerable. If nurses were to incorporate some of the principles of crisis intervention into their daily work, not only in psychiatric practice, but in all realms of nursing, they could perhaps be the most effective interveners and helpers. Nurses who practice within the community have access to a wide range of social networks and could be effective interveners in these community systems. By and large, nurses are identified by people in all socioeconomic strata as "helpers," and from this perspective they can most effectively help people grapple with their common human problems to reach better resolutions than they could achieve by themselves. The important thing to bear in mind is that not only do nurses deal with the physical problems of patients, but they also have a responsibility for being available to help people who seek to solve their problems.

HOW SHALL TREATMENT BE FINANCED?

The position of this book has been that all matters of behavior and health are embedded in the social system. A further example of this is the question of financing and health services. Societies differ one from another in whether health services are regarded as basic rights to which all citizens are entitled or as privileges that can be afforded by those wealthy enough to pay for such services. The United States seemingly is of two minds about this matter. Since some attempt is made to provide certain health services for the indigent, it may be argued that we view health services as a basic right. But closer examination shows a wide divergence in the types and quality of services made available, as well as considerable controversy over whether health services should be provided free or should be paid for. There are many instances where receiving free services involves the acceptance of second-class status.

Perhaps the manner in which varying forms of health care are financed is the best indicator of prevailing social values and views. In the field of mental health, the preponderance of funding is for treatment or custody of the mentally ill, with limited funds available for crisis intervention or other types of preventive programs. Financing of general health care is devoted mainly to those who are sick rather than directed toward efforts or programs to keep people well. While recent years have evidenced some attempts to reverse this order, such attempts are generally abandoned when the economy slumps or in an election year. One program that is an exception to this general attitude is aimed toward the establishment of a system of comprehensive community mental health centers.

LEGISLATION FOR COMMUNITY MENTAL HEALTH

The community mental health movement developed following World War II, stimulated by the number of psychiatric casualties resulting from the war. It was difficult to classify these servicemen in the same way the mentally ill had previously been classified, and treatment other than the custodial care seemed necessary. Interest turned to finding new types of intervention that would be particularly related to their crisis experiences and effective in working with the large number of men who needed treatment. In response to these concerns, new modes of psychotherapy such as group therapy and later family therapy were developed. Development of psychotropic drugs also contributed to experimentation with new treatment forms, particularly in community settings rather than in the hospital. It was noted that people who were treated outside institutional settings were more likely to regain their mental health than those who were hospitalized. Hospitalization was regarded as promoting chronicity.

Throughout the 1950s these new forms of treatment and attitudes about the desirability of avoiding or minimizing hospitalization were becoming increasingly popular. They were given impetus by several legslative acts:

1. The National Mental Health Act of 1946 provided funds for research, treatment, training, and community services.

2. The National Institute of Mental Health was established in 1949.

3. In 1955 the Mental Health Study Act provided for the establishment of the Joint Commission on Mental Illness and Health. *Action for Mental Health,* published in 1961, made wide-ranging recommendations for the adult mentally ill and particularly recommended improvement of mental hospitals through decreasing their physical size.

4. The Community Mental Health Centers Act of 1963 authorized 150 million dollars in federal aid to states for the construction of comprehensive mental health centers.

Under the Community Mental Health Centers Act, each comprehensive center, to qualify for funds, was required to provide five essential services: (1) inpatient care, (2) outpatient care, (3) partial hospitalization, (4) emergency care, and (5) consultation and education. Special consideration was given to those centers that also included, in addition to the basic services, diagnostic service, rehabilitative service, pre-care and after-care, training, and research and evaluation. This legislation provided the impetus for changing the emphasis from treatment in a large-scale mental hospital, far removed from the person's home setting, to treatment available within the individual's community.

Each comprehensive community mental health center was to serve a particular geographic area, called a catchment area. To qualify for federal funding, the applicant organization was required to demonstrate community control and citizen participation in the planning and programming of the community mental health centers.

Accompanying these legislative acts, a new model was proposed for the organization and treatment of psychiatric patients. Instead of the traditional medical model, the public health model of prevention was advocated. Primary prevention programs were to be established to lower the rate of mental disorder in the community. Three major groups became targets for primary prevention activities: children and adolescents, young adults, and the elderly. Early identification of emotional problems to prevent chronicity is the goal of secondary prevention. For those who were mentally ill, tertiary prevention was proposed to attempt to reduce the residual effects of mental illness. These organizing concepts are commonly used to provide the direction for program planning.

SUMMARY

Nurses in psychiatry are confronted by a number of ethical dilemmas. On the one hand, they have been socialized into and are oriented toward a medical model of treatment. On the other, most of what they deal with is a wide range of social, personal, and ethical dilemmas that confront people. Nurses first are confronted with an issue of who should be treated, the person or the wider societal network. To what end should nurses work? Toward maintaining the status quo by working to help patients "fit in" to the predominant social structure? Or toward the alternative of changing constricting societal forces?

If nurses engage in therapeutic work, another set of issues confronts them. Who makes the decision as to the direction of treatment? Establishing a contract agreed to by the patient is a necessary part of the treatment process. The issue of who is qualified to treat also bears consideration. The psychiatric professional may be knowledgeable about human behavior but not about the person's social networks or support systems. while, conversely, the community workers may not have the necessary knowledge of human behavior to help people in some of their personal dilemmas. Nurses are in a unique position because they work with people at points of personal crisis. Through a broad range of knowledge and experience with people, they may be vital in assisting individuals to achieve more personally satisfying and productive lives. The move toward Community Mental Health Programs provides a new set of opportunities for nurses in helping people cope with a broad spectrum of human problems.

FURTHER READINGS

Bulbulyan, Ann, et al. "Nurses in a Community Mental Health Center." *American Journal of Nursing* 69 (Feb. 1969): 328-331.

Cullen, Agnes. "Labeling Theory and Social Deviance." *Perspectives in Psychiatric Care* 12, no. 3 (1974): 123-125.

Drage, Elaine, and Lange, Blanche. "Ethical Considerations in the Use of Patients for Demonstration." *American Journal of Nursing* 69 (Oct. 1969): 2161-2165.

Duran, Fernando, and Errion, Gerald. "Perpetuation of Chronicity in Mental Illness." *American Journal of Nursing* 70 (Aug. 1970): 1707-1709.

Murray, Jacquelyn. "Patient Participation in Determining Psychiatric Treatment." *Nursing Research* 23 (July-August 1974): 325-333.

Ramshorn, Mary. "The Use of the Indigenous Non-Professional in Community Mental Health Services." *ANA Clinical Sessions* (1966): 157-163.

Schmieding, Norma. "Institutionalization: A Conceptual Approach." *Perspectives in Psychiatric Care* 6, no. 5 (1968): 205-211.

Ujhely, Gertrud. "The Nurse in Community Psychiatry." *American Journal of Nursing* 69 (May 1969): 1001-1005.

———. "The Nurse as Psychotherapist: What Are the Issues?" *Perspectives in Psychiatric Care* 11, no. 4 (1973): 155-160.

Accidental (or **situational**) **crisis** — A crisis initiated by some unanticipated hazardous event that involves a threat to the individual.

Achieved status — Societal position attained through individual accomplishments, e.g., college graduate, medical doctor.

Acting out — The expression of conflicts, urges, or fantasies through uncontrolled action.

Addiction — Dependence on the use of certain substances to a degree that the person experiences withdrawal symptoms if he or she abstains from their use. This term is currently not used as much as in the past.

Addictive coping style — One in which a person short-circuits his or her experiencing of anxiety through the use of some substance such as alcohol.

Affect — Any experience of feeling or emotion.

Alcoholics Anonymous — A voluntary organization of alcoholics and former alcoholics who seek to control their compulsive urge to drink through the group process.

Ambivalence — Simultaneous presence of opposite feelings toward some person or goal.

Amnesia — A sudden inability to recall one's identity or any aspects of the past.

Amphetamines — A group of related antidepressant drugs that produce a temporary feeling of well-being through stimulating the brain and central nervous system.

Antabuse — A drug used in the treatment of alcoholism that produces intense discomfort if one also takes any alcoholic beverage.

Anticipatory counseling — A form of preparation for persons who can be expected to experience a traumatic or stressful experience, in which they are led through a problem-solving sequence before they encounter the crisis situation; a form of psychological immunization.

Anxiety — A diffuse feeling of apprehension and of impending doom.

Anxiety neurosis — One in which the person suffers acute episodes of anxiety that he or she cannot relate to any specific cause.

Ascribed status — Societal position granted by virtue of certain givens, e.g., sex, age, race.

Autism — A form of thinking dominated by fantasies that have little relation to reality.

Behavior therapy — A type of psychotherapy based on conditioning.

Catatonic schizophrenia — A form of schizophrenia characterized by two extremes of behavior, stupor and excitement.

Catharsis — The expression of emotionally charged feelings that underlie anxiety or other symptoms.

Compensation — The development of strength in one area to make up for weakness in another.

Compulsion — An uncontrollably persistent urge to perform a certain behavior.

Conflict — Opposing desires, feelings, goals, etc., that are of importance to the person.

Conversion reaction (hysteria) — A neurotic reaction in which anxiety is unconsciously transformed into a physical symptom.

Coping ability — The capacity to handle problem situations with some degree of success.

Coping style — One's characteristic way of contending with problems.

Crisis — A turning point at which the person experiences loss or a threat of loss or fails to achieve a goal that is of personal significance. The way in which a person handles a crisis sets a trend for either improved or diminished coping abilities.

Crisis intervention — A form of therapy in which the therapist attempts to assist the person to handle a crisis in a way that increases his or her ability to cope successfully.

Culture — Total patterns of living and values of social groups that are transmitted from one generation to another.

Cyclazocine — A narcotic antagonist with low abuse potential, which blocks the effect of heroin and makes the user sick, much like the action of Antabuse with alcohol.

Defense mechanism — A characteristic response developed to protect oneself from anxiety, potential loss of self-esteem, or guilt.

Delusion — False, irrational beliefs that are not culturally shared. Usually they are of three types: (1) persecutory, (2) grandeur, and (3) reference. *Delusion of persecution:* Belief that the person has been singled out for persecution.

Delusion of grandeur: Beliefs that the person has some special power. *Ideas of reference:* Individual beliefs that certain happenings relate to oneself.

Denial — A mechanism of defense in which one denies the existence of painful facts.

Depersonalization — A state in which one subjectively detaches oneself so that he or she no longer perceives either himself or herself or the environment as real.

Depression — An emotional state of dejection and sadness; depressions range from mild transitory states to feelings of all-pervasive hopelessness and despair.

Depressive coping style — A style developed out of repeated experiences in which the person suffers a loss (of love, status, or self-esteem) and directs his or her activities toward reducing these losses. Persons with this pervasive style experience any security as conditional, and they must have constant direct signs that they are approved and loved. Not attaining this approbation results in feelings of worthlessness and hopelessness.

Descriptive psychiatry — A systematic approach based on observation, classification of symptoms, and diagnosis made from assumptions of underlying drives and forces.

Desensitization — A form of behavior therapy in which a person with strong fears of certain things is led by the therapist through an exploration of the things he or she fears, from the weakest to the strongest; through this process the anxiety-generating potential of the objects the patient fears is dissipated.

Detoxification – The treatment of withdrawal symptoms.

Developmental stages – Stages of life in which certain developmental tasks predominate. Accomplishment of the tasks of each developmental stage is important if the person is to move progressively forward to increasingly sophisticated problem-solving.

Deviance – A pattern of veering from acceptable societal norms and values.

Disequilibrium – Any deviation from normal patterns or relationships causing a disruption in usual roles and relationships.

Displacement – Transfer of emotion from the object with which it was originally experienced to a replacement.

Disturbance of affect – A distortion of emotion so that the expected emotional response to stimuli is not forthcoming.

Disturbance in association – A lack of logical connections in the person's thoughts.

Dissociative hysteria – Gross disturbance of awareness and memory.

Double-bind communication – A form of communication in which conflicting messages are simultaneously transmitted by a person of great significance. The person receiving the message feels obliged to respond or suffer severe consequences. He or she cannot escape from the situation.

Drives – Basic tension states that impel people to action.

Drug dependence – A person's need to rely on drugs to function both physically and psychologically.
Physical dependence: The body has so accommodated to the presence of drugs that the drug is required to maintain normal functioning. If the drug is stopped, withdrawal symptoms occur.
Psychological dependence: Reliance on the drug for solely nonphysical reasons; the psychologically dependent person feels he or she cannot get along without the effects of the drug.

Drug use – Ingesting, in any manner, a chemical substance that has an effect upon the body.

Emergency psychotherapy – Short-term therapy directed toward solving a current problem; it does not attempt reconstitution of the personality.

Empathy – The attempt to understand another person and his or her perceptions of experiences.

Existentialism – A school of philosophy that emphasizes the experiential realm of existence as having its own reality. When applied to psychiatry, existentialism views schizophrenia, for example, as an outgrowth of episodes when it is impossible for the person to conduct his life within the stream of existence surrounding him or her. Not being able to mesh life appropriately in the experiential realm leads to a shattering of the sequential ordering of experience. The symptoms of schizophrenia develop out of the person's attempts to manage the attendant anxiety. Existential analysis focuses on an attempt to discern new modes of relating so that the person's existence may proceed in an orderly fashion.

Family theme – Particular patterns of feelings, fantasies, and understandings developed within a family and shared by family members, giving them a unified view of "reality" and ways of dealing with it.

Family therapy — Treatment of the family as a group rather than as individual family members.

Grief — Typical response to situations of loss; an emotional state of intense sadness.

Group — A set of people, characterized by certain features that hold the members together in a common purpose.

Group dynamics — The study of the underlying features of group behavior, interactions that take place between persons, and the relationship of group members within a social field.

Hallucination — A false sensory perception without basis in reality.

Hebephrenic schizophrenia — Massive disturbance of behavior that is clearly regressed, fragmented, and silly.

Hysteria — A form of neurosis in which anxiety from the original conflict is transformed into specific physical manifestations.

Ideas of reference — A type of delusion in which an individual believes falsely that certain happenings relate to himself or herself.

Insight — A sudden grasp of a relationship that brings understanding or leads to the solution of a problem.

Insight therapy — Treatment focused on bringing to awareness relationships buried in the unconscious that affect current behavior. It is believed that by understanding the unconscious basis, the person can be freed of these repetitive patterns in his or her current modes of behavior.

Integration — Bringing together all the parts of personality organization into an integrated whole.

Intellectualization — A defense mechanism in which feelings are hidden through intellectual activity.

Involutional depression — A form of depression occurring during middle or late middle life, usually of two forms: (1) agitated, in which the predominant feature is gross motor activity and anxiety; and (2) paranoid, in which the person tends to have delusions of a persecutory nature.

Labeling — A sociological theory of mental illness that holds that as persons are designated as having a certain type of mental illness, others begin to react to them on the basis of these labels, and they in turn reciprocate by producing the expected behavior. In this view, mental illness is created by society.

Loss — Anything that a person once had, or had aspirations for, and now has no possibility of acquiring.

Manic-depressive psychosis — A cyclic, reoccurring pattern of a relatively short manic phase and a relatively longer depressed stage.

Methadone — A synthetic narcotic that produces addiction but one that, in the opinion of its proponents, has fewer deleterious effects on the social functioning of its users.

Milieu therapy — A form of treatment in which patients are treated primarily through individual psychotherapy, with the therapist outlining a treatment regime to be followed on the unit.

Need-fear dilemma — A situation in which, because of faulty ego development, the person has inordinate needs for others with whom he or she can be close and who will perform some of the ego functions the person lacks. At the same time he or she has just as strong a fear about the dire consequences of getting into these relationships.

Neurotic coping style — A characteristic pattern of dealing with anxiety by overuse of common defensive mechanisms. Anxiety from originating concepts is transformed into neurotic symptoms.

Obsession — Preoccupation with thoughts usually distressful and always strange; never perceived by the person as reasonable, they always create anxiety but cannot be banished from his or her consciousness.

Obsessive-compulsive neurosis — A form of neurosis in which anxiety from the originating conflicts is handled by fixation upon certain thoughts or certain actions.

Organ vulnerability — A theory that specific body organs are particularly vulnerable to certain types of stress.

Organic (endogenous) depression — A depression caused by biological factors, e.g., arteriosclerosis of the brain.

Panic — An acute reaction of confusion and overwhelming fear arising out of a situation perceived to be of extreme danger.

Paranoid schizophrenia — A form of personality disorganization whose main distinguishing feature is delusions, usually persecutory in nature.

Pejorative label — A label that carries with it negative connotations, e.g., "welfare mother."

Perceptual field — The established frame of reference in which current experience is perceived; the background against which current situations are organized.

Personality disorganization — Interruptions in the life style of the individual where behavior loses its usual coherence and connectedness to his or her cognitive experience.

Phobia — Persistent fear of a specific place or thing which one is unable to banish from one's mind.

Pleasure principle — The point of view that behavior is designed to produce pleasure and avoid pain.

Primary process thinking — An infantile mode of thinking in which unsocialized, primitive, magical kinds of symbol manipulation predominate.

Projection — The defense mechanism in which the blame for certain shortcomings is shifted to another person; the imparting of one's own faults to another.

Pseudomutuality — A family style in which all areas of conflict are masked, so that on the surface the family mirrors all the stereotypes of the "happy family."

Psychic determinism — A view that all behavior has meaning and never happens randomly, and that current behavior is built on past experiences.

Psychoanalysis — Oldest formalized type of psychotherapy, focused on the person's gaining insight into the basic conflicts of the early period of his or her life that have resulted in certain current patterns. Symptoms seen as manifestations of unconscious conflicts.

Psychogenic (exogenous) depression — A depression produced by environmental or psychological factors; sometimes called reaction.

Psychosomatic — Describing a group of physical disorders whose etiology is related to psychological factors.

Rationalization — A defense mechanism in which the person justifies or makes something seem reasonable that otherwise would be irrational.

Reaction-formation — A defense mechanism in which urges unacceptable to the person are transformed into their opposites; for example, a person who has an urge to be dirty becomes compulsively clean.

Repression — Automatic forgetting.

Role — A configuration of behaviors people carry out in respect to one another in a given social situation.

Role expectations — The set of behaviors expected from a person occupying a certain role set, e.g., mother, teacher.

Role model — An individual whose particular behavior in a role serves as a model to be copied by another who aspires to a similar role.

Role obligations — Those behaviors a person is obligated to perform by virtue of his or her societal position.

Role performance — The way a person actually performs his or her role in a given situation.

Role reciprocity — Social roles that are defined by typical interaction between two individuals, e.g., husband-wife, mother-child. [A typical type of behavior, for instance, crying because of hunger is reciprocated by feeding.]

Role-taking ability — The capacity to imagine oneself in the position of another.

Scapegoating — A process in which one member of a family or a group acts out the conflict in the system and becomes the focal point of interaction.

Schismatic families — A family pattern in which there is continuing overt conflict between spouses, with each undercutting the worth of the other to their children.

Schizophrenia — A form of personality disorganization in which the person does not make what are considered to be appropriate social responses; he or she engages in behavior that is considered to be abnormal.

Simple schizophrenia — Characterized by apathy, flat affect, withdrawal from social relationships, and associative looseness.

Schizophrenogenic mother — One who is characterized as being impervious to the needs of other family members and is extremely intrusive into her child's life.

Sequential (or maturational) crisis — A naturally occurring crisis involving the loosening of previous personality structures so that the person may move to a new developmental stage.

Skewed families — A family pattern in which one parent is overinvested in a child as a fulfillment of things he or she feels were denied him or her while the parental partner withdraws from involvement in the relationship. The most usual pattern described is between mother and son.

Social norm — A rule of behavior defined by the shared expectations of two or more people about what behavior is considered socially acceptable.

Social system — A set of interacting persons or groups perceived as an entity distinct from the individuals who compose the social network.

Socialization — The learning of behavior appropriate in a certain social context.

Sociometric patterns — Patterns of association established between group members.

Sociopathic behavior — Behavior in which a person disregards the usual social rules and violates normative constraints.

Status — A person's position in a given social structure.

Supportive therapy — Treatment that encourages and promotes the person's current assets; objectives are to strengthen existing defenses.

Suppression — Forgetting as a result of a person's conscious effort to put some anxiety-provoking experience out of his or her memory.

Symbolic interaction — A theoretical view that focuses upon the interactive aspects of human behavior, e.g., communication, language, symbolic gestures.

Therapeutic community — A treatment setting in which emphasis is placed on group treatment, and decision-making is shared by patients and staff.

Universality — A process operating in groups by which a person learns that his or her experience is not unique, that others share the same dilemmas.

Value — An abstract, generalized principle of behavior to which the members of a group have a strong commitment.

Withdrawal — Cessation of drug use.

Working through — Process in which a person gains new insights about the way in which he or she interacts with others and begins to change his or her behavior.

LEARNING
ACTIVITY
PLANS

Some users may wish to adapt the Learning Activity Plans (LAP) on the following pages as a method of mastering the content of this text. For those who choose this approach, this section contains Learning Activity Plans that follow the content of the book. These LAP's are written so they may be used directly by students or teachers in guiding their learning. It is our hope that even readers who are not interested in following this learning approach will benefit from selecting some of the exercises as a means of reinforcing major points of the text. The exercises suggested are by no means exhaustive. They do, however, give an indication of the kind of abilities the authors feel should be developed by beginning nurses.

Each LAP lists the objectives to be accomplished for a unit of study and presents learning activities to attain these objectives. Most LAP's are divided into several lessons, with objectives and learning activities for each. In most cases, alternative learning activities are given; that is, you may choose whichever activity best suits your particular learning style. Some students prefer to study independently, others in a group; some like attending lecture-discussion classes, while others gain more from simply reading (and perhaps outlining) the material.

Most of the activities can be either reported individually in writing or handled as a group discussion. The instructor should see all individual activity reports. The options for learning activities may be used in other ways, too, if the teachers and students prefer. For example, the entire group might decide which activities to do, rather than individuals making this choice. Also, the teachers and students might think of learning activities that are not included here, but that would, for them, be equally or more effective in attaining the objectives. This is encouraged. The authors value flexibility and variety and did not intend the LAP's to be followed rigidly or to be the only source of ideas.

In addition to objectives and learning activities, each lesson in the LAP's contains a self-test. With these, you can evaluate your own attainment of the objectives.

The final element in each LAP is suggestions for independent study if you want to pursue a particular area in depth.

CONTENTS

LEARNING ACTIVITY PLANS

CHAPTER

1   The Patterning of Behavior: A Societal Perspective 460

2   The Patterning of Behavior: A Developmental Model 468

3   Life Crises, Defensive Mechanisms,
        and the Evolution of Coping Styles 474

4   Psychosomatic and Neurotic Coping Styles 481

5   Drug Dependence 486

6   Depressive Coping Styles 493

7   Retreat as a Form of Coping 499

8   Types of Treatment Intervention 505

9   The Nurse in the Treatment Process 508

10 Anticipatory Counseling and Crisis Intervention 516

11 The Family System: Normality, Disturbance, and Intervention 521

12 The Group: Dynamics, Therapeutic Potential, and Intervention . .527

13 The Therapeutic Community 532

14 Ethical Issues 536

CHAPTER ONE:
THE PATTERNING OF BEHAVIOR: A SOCIETAL PERSPECTIVE

OBJECTIVES

1. To understand the sociological concepts of social systems, socialization, role, status, and norms as related to personality development.

    1.1 To define the concepts of social systems, socialization, role, status, and norms.

    1.2 To explain the relationship of these concepts to personality development.

2. To assess the sociological factors of social systems, socialization, role, status, and norms as they affect the personality development of an individual.

3. To analyze interpersonal situations using the concepts of social systems, socialization, role, status, and norms.

CHAPTER ONE: LESSON 1

OBJECTIVES

1. To understand the sociological concepts of social systems, socialization, role, status, and norms as related to personality development.

1.1 To define the concepts of social systems, socialization, role, status, and norms.

1.2 To explain the relationship of these concepts to personality development.

LEARNING ACTIVITIES

1. Read Chapter 1 of the textbook. You may also want to outline the main points as you read and take part in a lecture/discussion on this material.

2. This activity may be reported individually in writing or in a group discussion. It entails observing for examples of the concepts being studied in this lesson; that is, social systems, socialization, role, status, and norms.

Go somewhere where a group of people interact on a regular basis and observe their interactions without their being aware you are doing so. Some of the places you might make observations are the dorm or cafeteria in your school, a unit or department in your school or a hospital, or a business, court, or other institution. Another source of examples, though it does not provide an experience of direct observation, is the newspaper.

Describe at least one example of each concept, explaining why your example represents the concept.

LESSON 1: SELF-TEST

Without consulting your notes, answer the following questions. If you find you cannot answer one or more parts, study your notes until you are able to answer them.

1. Define these concepts: social systems; socialization; role; status; norms.

2. Explain the relationship of these concepts to personality development.

CHAPTER ONE: LESSON 2

OBJECTIVE

2. To assess the sociological factors of social systems, socialization, role, status, and norms as they affect the personality development of an individual.

LEARNING ACTIVITIES

Choose either activity for individual reporting or group discussion.

1. Read the situation below and discuss the factors of social systems, socialization, role, status, and norms as they affect the personality development of the main character.

This is the story of Peter, a warm, friendly, considerate, but rather uptight young man who suffers frequent headaches and gastric upsets. Peter is twenty-nine year old and has been married four years. He and his wife, June (age twenty-seven), have a son, Henry, two months old.

Peter and June had not planned to begin their family for several more years, but succumbed to subtle and not-so-subtle pressure from Peter's parents. Peter's father, also named Henry, reminded Peter periodically of his (Henry's) advancing age and his wish to have a grandchild before he "passed on."

Peter is an only child, born to his parents after sixteen years of marriage. His parents easily provided for all his material needs, but, though they loved him, they were strict disciplinarians and tempered their love with many limits.

Peter was a frail child, suffering from asthma and frequent colds that limited his participation in active games and sports. His mother also tended to be oversolicitous about his health and physical needs. His health improved, however, when he went to college, and he is now in good health.

In college, Peter majored in history. After graduation, he taught for two years, but disliked the work because of constant friction with the principal. He now works in the historical research department of a publishing company and is successful and happy. His father had offered to recommend him for a position as a department supervisor, but Peter preferred to "make it on his own."

Peter met June at the high school where they both taught. They agree their marriage is, for the most part, happy and good for both of them. They have many interests in common, the most recent being their baby son. They find they are extremely pleased with him, even though financially they would have preferred to wait a few years.

Early in their marriage, Peter had gastric upsets whenever he and June disagreed. Gradually, though, with her encouragement, he learned to talk about his problems and feelings, and his physical symptoms have diminished considerably. At the present time, they are experiencing a conflict because June misses teaching and wishes she were back at work, while Peter feels she should stay home and take care of the baby. They are discussing the situation and trying to resolve it.

2. If you choose to attend a group discussion on this activity, come prepared to present a situation for discussion. The group should assess several situations as time allows.

Examine the personality development of a patient you are presently working with or an acquaintance of yours, assessing the influence of the factors of social systems, socialization, role, status, and norms on his or her development.

Gather as much information as possible about the individual you are assessing, particularly information on his or her childhood and family.

LESSON 2: SELF-TEST

Assess the factors of social systems, socialization, role, status, and norms as they contribute to the personality development of the individual in the following situation.

David, born in the Netherlands, was just one year old when his parents were arrested by the Nazis and taken from their home to a concentration camp, where they died. David's existence for the next two years was somewhat precarious. He stayed with three different families, friends of his parents. The last family managed to send him to safety in England, where he stayed in an orphanage for six months. At that point, he was found by his mother's sister, who had come to England earlier and had not known of David's whereabouts or the fate of his parents.

David, then three, was adopted by his aunt and uncle. He was very much wanted and loved by them, and over time he changed from a pathetic, sad little boy to a smiling, mischievous one. He considered his aunt and uncle as his parents. The family immigrated to the United States, where they found more difficulty than they had anticipated in finding work. During these first few years David's aunt hired herself out as a domestic day-worker to help the family's finances, and David's reaction to this was explosive. He was terrified of being left with anyone except his uncle or aunt, and carried on so that the aunt arranged jobs where she could take David with her. This arrangement seemed to work, and though she worried about spoiling him by giving in to him, the aunt continued this practice until he was in school. David's behavior improved, and he could be described as a docile, quiet child who had occasional nightmares.

David did not look forward to going to school, but did so because he had no choice. He managed the school routine and did quite well with the work becaues of his interest in numbers and his exposure to books and children's programs on TV.

Making friends was another matter, and David was considered shy and a "loner." He turned out to have considerable dexterity, however, and through his latency, was a sought-after partner in sports and making models. He was still shy, but was responsive to other boys' friendly overtures. He was known for being orderly and for keeping his belongings in both his desk and locker just so, a quality which stood out in contrast to the general messiness of most of his classmates. In the fifth grade, he had a fistfight with a boy who had borrowed his art things without asking and had returned them in bad condition, messing up David's desk in the process.

By the time David was in high school, his family was secure financially, and David had found a niche for himself in school. Some years earlier, he had found a best friend who also attended the same high school. With Jim, his friend, he managed a situation that had troubled him—he got up enough nerve to take a girl to one of the school dances, double-dating with Jim. Since then, he has engaged in group situations with both sexes and has developed some ease and skill in dealing with girls. His scholastic abilities were sufficient for him to be admitted with no difficulty to a good local college, where he planned a career in banking. He also thought he might like real estate development, but saw that as a future stage of his career. During his senior year, Jim moved to another city, and David found himself more let-down than he expected. He was quite moody and irritable for a long while and dropped out of his extracurricular clubs. One of the deciding factors in his choice of college is that he expects Jim and several other members of his high school group to be there. David wanted to go somewhere that would not be entirely new.

David is now twenty-one and a junior, having a successful college career and living at home. He feels less certain about his choice of banking as a career and is very drawn toward choosing something adventurous that would require traveling. He also feels that his relationship with his family has deteriorated during these college years; he feels they are unjustifiably critical of some of his friends and activities. He has one special girl with whom he has considered a more stable liaison, but fears she would not be orderly enough for him; it is the one issue that always leads to heated words between them—she accuses him of being "picky," and he regards her as "sloppy." David worries about their chances of maintaining a good relationship. Sometimes, David wonders why, at age twenty-one, he has all these worries; he feels that, somehow, all these issues should have been settled by now.

CHAPTER ONE: LESSON 3

OBJECTIVE

3. To analyze interpersonal situations using the concepts of social systems, socialization, role, status, and norms.

LEARNING ACTIVITIES

1. Take a situation familiar to both the students and the instructor (e.g., school of nursing, classroom, hospital unit, other health setting) and examine the factors of social systems, socialization, role, status, and norms as they operate in the setting.

The following questions will serve as a guide in this activity:

(a) In what way is the setting a special system?

(b) What socialization processes are in operation?

(c) What roles do different individuals have?

(d) What status is associated with these roles? Is it ascribed or achieved?

(e) What are the norms of behavior in the setting?

2. Examine roles, status, and norms in your present student group, using the following questions as a guide.

(a) What roles do different individuals have in the group?

(b) What roles do these individuals have outside the group?

(c) What status is associated with the roles of different individuals in the group?

(d) Is this status ascribed or achieved?

(e) What are the norms of behavior in the group?

(f) Which norms existed prior to this experience and which ones started with it?

3. This activity emphasizes the interactive nature of role behavior, i.e., the fact that a role enacted in a particular way is likely to elicit certain behavior in response. Begin with some role-playing; then the participants and the group are to discuss how the way in which the roles were portrayed affected the response of the other person involved.

Some roles suggested are patient and nurse, physician and nurse, parent and child, or teacher and student. The group can decide which ones it wants to enact. It is recommended that the roles be played in different ways, perhaps by different participants, to illustrate that different kinds of behavior elicit different responses. For example, if the role of an irritable patient is being enacted, two or more different approaches can be tried by the nurse to see how these affect the patient's response.

Some examples of behavior that might be portrayed are an irritable, crying, or withdrawn patient; an authoritarian or democratic physician; a critical or inconsistent parent; an authoritarian, democratic, or insensitive teacher; an anxious or hostile student.

Before you portray a role, spend some time putting yourself in the person's position and imagine how he or she feels and how he or she would act. In your role-playing, portray the role as you imagined it.

LESSON 3: SELF-TEST

Analyze the following situation by answering these questions:
(a) In what way is this setting a social system?
(b) What evidence of socialization do you see?
(c) What roles do different individuals have?
(d) What status is associated with these roles? Is it ascribed or achieved?
(e) What are the norms of behavior in the setting?

> Ward C is an orthopedic unit of General Hospital. Most of the nursing staff are young and transient, except for the head nurse, Sarah Burke, who has worked at General Hospital for eighteen years. The patients, many of whom are in good health except for fractures, enjoy watching TV late in the evening to help relieve the boredom of their often lengthy hospital stays. Ms. Burke tells the evening nurses that all TV's and lights must be out by 11:00 P.M., however, because patients are awakened at 6:00 A.M. and do not get sufficient rest if they are up late. Some of the nurses and physicians have been trying for six months to change the hospital routine of awakening patients early. Ms. Burke resists, saying the day's activities (hygiene, meals, physiotherapy, etc.) could not be satisfactorily carried out or completed if patients were not awakened at 6:00 A.M.

CHAPTER ONE: OPTIONS FOR INDEPENDENT STUDY

If you wish to study more about societal influences on personality development and behavior, choose one or more of the following activities.

1. Discuss (in writing or in a group) an experience in which you violated the norms of a specific group. You may choose to create such a situation, for example, by going to class in clothes markedly different from the usual student garb or your usual dress. Observe and report the responses of others to you and the feelings you experienced.

2. As an individual or a group, make a plan to change a norm (of the classroom, school of nursing, hospital unit, or other health setting), discussing the following:

How would you go about this?

Whom would you involve? Why?

What arguments would you present?

What would be the worst way to proceed?

3. Using theory from Chapter 1 of the textbook, debate the question: Can one be labeled mentally ill without actually being so?

4. Write a short story about how someone becomes mentally ill, explaining the societal factors influencing his or her present state.

CHAPTER TWO: # THE PATTERNING OF BEHAVIOR: A DEVELOPMENTAL MODEL

OBJECTIVES

1. To understand personality development according to Erikson.

    1.1 To list the eight stages of personality development with positive and negative outcomes, as set forth by Erikson.

    1.2 To explain the consequences to the individual of the accomplishment or lack of accomplishment of the central task of each stage of development.

    1.3 To explain the influence of physical attributes, family, socioeconomic level, and culture on personality development.

2. To assess the extent to which a given individual has completed the central task of each stage of development.

3. To assess the influence of physical attributes, family, socioeconomic level, and culture on personality development.

GENERAL INFORMATION

This LAP has three lessons, with the option to do Lessons 1 and 2 or Lesson 3. As usual, there also are options for learning activities within the lessons.

CHAPTER TWO: LESSON 1

OBJECTIVES

1. To understand personality development according to Erikson.

1.1 To list the eight stages of personality development with positive and negative outcomes as set forth by Erikson.

1.2 To explain the consequences to the individual of the accomplishment or lack of accomplishment of the central task of each stage of development.

1.3 To explain the influence of physical attributes, family, socioeconomic level, and culture on personality development.

LEARNING ACTIVITIES

1. Read Chapter 2 of the textbook. Supplement your reading by outlining the main points and /or taking part in a lecture-discussion.

2. Read a short story, biography, or novel, or view a film about a person who interests you. He or she may be someone of historical interest or current fame or a fictional character.

From the present behavior or description of the person, speculate as to what some of his or her developmental experiences were. (Remember that this is a speculative activity, in that one cannot say for certain what these experiences were. Use your imagination in trying to link present behavior to past experiences, but be consistent in what you conclude.)

(a) What present behavior might be linked to the stages of trust, autonomy, and so on?

(b) What factors do you think influenced the person in his or her developmental years?

LESSON 1: SELF-TEST

Without consulting your notes, answer the following questions. If you find you cannot answer one or more parts, study your notes until you are able to answer them.

1. List the eight stages of personality development according to Erikson, stating the positive and negative outcomes of each stage.

2. Explain the consequences to the individual of the relative accomplishment or lack of accomplishment of the central task of each stage of development.

3. Explain the influence of physical attributes, family, socioeconomic level, and culture on personality development.

CHAPTER TWO: LESSON 2

OBJECTIVES

2. To assess the extent to which a given individual has completed the central task of each stage of development.

3. To assess the influence of physical attributes, family, socioeconomic level, and culture on personality development.

GENERAL INFORMATION

In this lesson, you will be assessing particular individuals to determine their relative success in completing the stages of personality development.

Such a study is necessarily speculative; that is, one cannot say with certainty that the conclusions are correct and so must maintain an open mind to new information. It is a useful exercise, nevertheless, as it will help you focus on significant behavior and better understand human needs.

LEARNING ACTIVITIES

Choose 1 or 2 below. Use the following questions as a guide. As you discuss each question, explain the reasoning that led to your conclusions. (These may be done individually or as a group.)

—At what stage of personality development is the individual at this time?

—To what extent has he or she successfully completed the central task of each stage?

—How does the relative success at each stage affect the individual's present behavior?

—What has been the effect of physical attributes, family, socioeconomic level, and culture on this person's personality development?

1. Read the situation on page 462 (Chapter 1, Lesson 2) and assess the extent to which the main character, Peter, has progressed through the stages of personality development. Note: The emphasis now is on developmental factors in this situation, rather than sociological ones as in Chapter 1. (If you need assistance in assessing personality development, reread Chapter 2 in the text, noting particularly the assessment of Peg and her family.)

2. Assess a patient with whom you are now working or an acquaintance of yours, trying to determine the extent to which he or she has progressed through the stages of personality development. (You may want to reread Chapter 2, noting particularly the assessment of Peg and her family.)

Gather as much information as possible about the individual you are assessing, particularly information on his or her childhood and family.

If you choose to attend a group discussion for this activity, come prepared to present a situation for discussion. The group will assess several situations as time allows.

LESSON 2: SELF-TEST

Reread the case situation in the self-test of Chapter 1, Lesson 2 (pages 463-464). Assess the extent to which David, the central character in the situation, has successfully completed the task of each level of personality development.

CHAPTER TWO: LESSON 3

This lesson is an alternative for Lessons 1 and 2 and has the same objectives. The self-test for this lesson combines those following Lessons 1 and 2.

LEARNING ACTIVITY

In this lesson, you and the other students who choose this option will present a seminar on the stages of personality development.

One or two students should present each stage, depending on the number of participants. (If there are more than sixteen students, it is advisable to form two or more groups to ensure everyone adequate opportunity for discussion.) The instructor and the students will decide upon the length of time for each presentation.

In your presentation:

(a) Explain the central task to be accompanied in the stage you are discussing, with its positive and negative outcomes, as well as what factors influence the outcomes.

(b) Give examples and situations illustrating positive and negative outcomes of the stage of development you are discussing. Explain what you think contributed to this outcome. You may use for situations patients you have worked with or people you have known, or you may use examples from your reading.

Recommended references for this activity, besides Chapter 2 in the textbook are:

> Erikson, Erik. *Childhood and Society.* 2nd ed. New York: W. W. Norton & Company, Inc., 1963. Chapter 7 is particularly recommended. This book also contains many examples.
>
> Maier, Henry. "The Psychoanalytic Theory of Erik Erikson." In *Three Theories of Child Development*, pp. 12-74. New York: Harper & Row, Publishers, 1965.

CHAPTER TWO: OPTIONS FOR INDEPENDENT STUDY

Students who wish to study more about the stages of personality development may do one or both of the following activities.

1. Assess your own personality development and the extent to which you have completed the tasks of each stage. You may find it beneficial to discuss this with some of your friends who are also doing self-assessments.

2. Write a short story about how someone becomes mentally ill, explaining what happened during the person's developing years that contributed to his or her present condition. (If you chose to do this option after Chapter 1, you may use the same story, adding to it.)

CHAPTER THREE: # LIFE CRISES, DEFENSIVE MECHANISMS, AND THE EVOLUTION OF COPING STYLES

OBJECTIVES

1. To understand crisis theory.

 1.1 To define crisis.
 1.2 To describe the four phases of a crisis.
 1.3 To explain the two types of crisis.
 1.4 To distinguish positive and negative outcomes of a crisis.
 1.5 To define anxiety.
 1.6 To explain the role of anxiety in the development and resolution of crisis.

2. To identify times in the life cycle when an individual is vulnerable to crisis.

3. Given a situation, to identify the evidence that an individual is experiencing a crisis.

4. To plan nursing activities based on crisis theory.

5. To understand the concept of coping style.

 5.1 To review the mechanisms of defense against anxiety.
 5.2 Explain the role of significant others in the development of a coping style.
 5.3 To differentiate the concepts of coping style and crisis.
 5.4 To explain various unhealthy coping styles, such as focusing on physical symptoms, neurotic coping style, passiveness, and avoidance of involvement.
 5.5 To explain the concept of mental illness as a deviant coping style.

CHAPTER THREE: LESSON 1

OBJECTIVES

1. To understand crisis theory.

   1.1 To define crisis.

   1.2 To describe the four phases of a crisis.

   1.3 To explain the two types of crisis.

   1.4 To distinguish positive and negative outcomes of a crisis.

   1.5 To define anxiety.

   1.6 To explain the role of anxiety in the development and resolution of a crisis.

2. To identify times in the life cycle when an individual is vulnerable to crisis.

3. Given a situation, to identify the evidence that an individual is experiencing a crisis.

LEARNING ACTIVITIES

1. Read pages 52-63 of Chapter 3. To supplement your reading, outline the main points and/or take part in a lecture-discussion.

2. Reread the situation on page 462 (Chapter 1, Lesson 2) and identify times that you think the characters did experience or could have experienced a maturational or situational crisis. Consider each person individually and answer the following questions. (Note: The purpose in using the same situation in these three LAP's is to help you understand the interrelationship of sociological, developmental, and crisis factors in the patterning of behavior in a given individual.)

(a) List the maturational crises each experienced. What are the evidences that these events are crises?

(b) List the situational crises each experienced. Why do you view these events as a crises?

(c) Select two crises from your lists in (a) and (b) and describe the positive and/or negative outcomes of each crisis. [You may use the same crises for (d) and (e) below.]

(d) Select two crises from your lists in (a) and (b) and explain which phase the crisis is currently in.

(e) Select two crises from your lists in (a) and (b) and explain the relationship of anxiety to these crises.

LESSON 1: SELF-TEST

Without consulting your notes, answer the following questions. If you find you cannot answer one or more parts, study your notes until you are able to answer them.

1. Define crisis.

2. What are the four phases of a crisis? Describe each briefly.

3. Explain the two types of crisis.

4. What are some possible positive and negative outcomes of a crisis?

5. Define anxiety.

6. What is the role of anxiety in the development and resolution of crisis?

7. Reread the case situation in the self-test of Chapter 1, Lesson 2 (pages 463-464). For this lesson, identify the maturational and situational crises that David, the main character, has experienced or is likely to experience in the next several years.

CHAPTER THREE: LESSON 2

OBJECTIVE
4. To plan nursing activities based on crisis theory.

LEARNING ACTIVITIES

1. Read pages 52-63 of Chapter 3. To supplement your reading, outline the material and/or take part in a lecture-discussion.

2. In this activity, you are to discuss what situations might be crisis-producing for patients and what might help them to cope. Think of a health care setting in which you have worked (hospital, clinic, etc.) and identify three or four situations that might be crisis-producing for patients (e.g., chronic illness, diagnostic tests, unemployment, being confined to home). There are many such situations with which patients must deal. Put yourself in the patient's shoes and imagine how you would feel if you had his or her problems.

Discuss how crisis theory might be used to assist the patient(s), using the following questions as a guide.

(a) What help is the patient likely to receive in dealing with his or her crisis? Who will provide this help?

(b) As a nurse or nursing student, what could you do to help this patient cope with his or her situation?

(c) Are there factors in the way this particular health care setting operates that tend to promote rather than mitigate patients' crises?

LESSON 2: SELF-TEST

Imagine you have just been named head nurse in a prenatal clinic where you have worked for three months and that you see a number of ways in which patient services might be improved through the application of crisis theory. It disturbs you that the clinic is so busy and you must rush from patient to patient. Patients complain about waiting hours to be seen and then being seen by a different physician on every visit. You realize, though, that the chief of service is proud of this efficiently operated clinic and not likely to accept easily the idea that some improvements might be made.

1. List two nursing activities appropriate for such a clinic that are applications of crisis theory.

2. What reasons would you present to the chief of service for wanting to implement these activities?

CHAPTER THREE: LESSON 3

OBJECTIVES

5. To understand the concept of coping style.

5.1 To review the mechanisms of defense against anxiety.*

5.2 To explain the role of significant others in the development of a coping style.

5.3 To differentiate the concepts of coping style and crisis.

5.4 To explain various unhealthy coping styles, such as focusing on physical symptoms, neurotic coping style, passiveness, and avoidance of involvement.

5.5 To explain the concept of mental illness as a deviant coping style.

GENERAL INFORMATION

The general intent of this lesson is to help you see the relationships between the concepts of the first three chapters.

LEARNING ACTIVITIES

1. Read pages 63-81 of Chapter 3 of the text. Attending a discussion or outlining the material can supplement your reading.

2. Reread the situation on page 462 and discuss Peter's coping style, using the following questions as a guide for your written report or group discussion:

(a) What are the positive and negative aspects of Peter's style of coping?

(b) What role have significant others (past and present) had in the development of his coping style?

(c) How do you think he will fare in the future? Why?

---

*Because many students take a prior course in basic psychology that includes study of the defense mechanisms, this objective focuses on review. If you want to do more than review, a learning activity related to defense mechanisms is included as Option 4 in the Independent Study Options at the end of the LAP.

3. Read this case situation and discuss crisis and the individual's coping style, using the questions below as a guide for either a group discussion or written report.

> George is a 32-year-old man who was brought to the mental health clinic by his parents; they complained that he hears voices, broke some furniture, and was staying up all night. They said he had been hospitalized for similar behavior three times before. George, they said, is usually a very quiet, polite person. He is home alone all day while his parents work and spends his time doing a little housework and walking around downtown looking in the stores. He has no friends except his dog, who disappeared two weeks ago.

(a) Distinguish between this individual's crisis and his coping style.
(b) What role have the significant persons in his life played in the past? What do you think they might do now and in the future?
(c) Compose two endings for this situation, one in which the individual's usual functioning improves and one in which it deteriorates. Describe what happened to bring about the improvement or deterioration.

LESSON 3: SELF-TEST

Without consulting your notes, answer the following questions. If you find you cannot answer one or more parts, study your notes until you are able to answer them.

1. What is the role of significant others in the development of a coping style?

2. What is the relationship of coping style to crisis?

3. Explain how some individuals cope with life's problems through the use of physical symptoms, a neurotic coping style, passiveness, or avoidance of involvement.

4. Explain the concept of mental illness as a deviant coping style.

CHAPTER THREE: OPTIONS FOR INDEPENDENT STUDY

Students who wish to study more about life crises and coping styles may do one or more of the following activities.

1. Think of your own life and the developmental and situational crises you have experienced. Take one or more of these and describe what happened and how the crisis was resolved. You may find it beneficial to exchange information with some of your friends.

2. Write a short story about how someone becomes mentally ill, explaining what situational and developmental crises the character experienced that helped or hindered his or her adjustment. If you chose this option in Chapters 1 and 2, add to the story already begun.

3. Discuss in a small group the definition of the psychiatric nurse in this chapter as being a person who promotes a productive life style for each individual. Do you agree with this conception of the nurse's role? Why or why not?

4. Read the following situation and add to it by explaining how the individual involved would cope with her anxiety using different defense mechanisms. (See Chapter 3 in the text for a list and description of defense mechanisms.) Try writing different endings using different defense mechanisms.

> Susan, a nursing student, was waiting anxiously for her evaluation conference with her instructor. She felt jumpy and slightly nauseated. Finally, the time came, and Susan went in for her conference. She and the instructor talked and agreed on all major points except one, the grade. Susan wanted an A, and the instructor had given her a B. Intellectually, Susan agreed with the B grade, but she felt upset and disappointed because she had wanted the A very badly. She left the instructor's office and returned to her room.

CHAPTER FOUR: PSYCHOSOMATIC AND NEUROTIC COPING STYLES

OBJECTIVES

1. To understand theories about the relationship between stress and psychosomatic illness.

    1.1 To explain the physiological, learning, psychological, and sociological theories related to the general effects of stress.

    1.2 To give examples of theories that relate specific conflicts to specific psychosomatic disorders.

2. To integrate the concept of neurotic coping style with the various types of neurosis.

    2.1 To explain how an individual develops a neurotic coping style.

    2.2 To describe the behavior seen in anxiety, phobic, obsessive-compulsive, and hysteric neuroses.

    2.3 To identify the functions a neurosis serves in a person's life.

    2.4 To explain the necessity of treating neurosis within the social network.

CHAPTER FOUR: LESSON 1

OBJECTIVES

1. To understand theories about the relationship between stress and psychosomatic illness.

1.1 To explain the physiological, learning, psychological, and sociological theories related to the general effects of stress.

1.2 To give examples of theories that relate specific conflicts to specific psychosomatic disorders.

LEARNING ACTIVITIES

1. Read pages 87-93 of Chapter 4. Supplement the text reading by outlining the main points or attending a lecture-discussion.

2. Think of a patient on a general hospital ward whom you formerly cared for or are now caring for who has a psychosomatic disorder. Examine the patient's situation in light of the theories about the relationship between stress and psychosomatic illness, and present a discussion or written report. As sources of information you might use the patient's chart, the nursing and medical staffs, and the patient and his or her family. If you talk to the patient and/or the family, do it with consideration for their feelings.

(a) In what way do the theories about the general effects of stress relate to this person's situation?

(b) What specific conflicts might be related to his or her disorder?

LESSON 1: SELF-TEST

Without consulting your notes, answer the following questions. If you find you cannot answer one or more parts, study your notes until you are able to answer them.

1. Explain these theories related to the general effects of stress: (a) physiological; (b) learning; (c) psychological; (d) sociological.

2. Give some examples of theories that relate specific conflicts to specific psychosomatic disorders.

CHAPTER FOUR: LESSON 2

OBJECTIVES

2. To integrate the concept of neurotic coping style with the various types of neuroses.

2.1 To explain how an individual develops a neurotic coping style.

2.2 To describe the behavior seen in anxiety, phobic, obsessive-compulsive, and hysteric neuroses.

2.3 To identify the functions a neurosis serves in a person's life.

2.4 To explain the necessity of treating neurosis within the social network.

LEARNING ACTIVITIES

1. Read pages 93-109 of Chapter 4, outlining the main points or attending a lecture-discussion to supplement your reading.

2. Read the following situation and discuss (with a group or in writing) the individual's neurosis and neurotic coping style, using the following questions as a guide.

(a) What neurotic behavior does this person exhibit?

(b) What past and present factors in her life have contributed to her neurotic style of coping?

(c) What functions does her neurosis serve for her?

(d) Speculate as to her family's contribution to her neurotic coping style (e.g., what factors besides economic ones might have prompted their taking her out of the hospital?).

(e) What alternate methods of treatment might have been more effective in treating this individual within the context of her social network?

> Carol Phillips is a 32-year-old single woman admitted to a private psychiatric hospital for treatment of a severe obsessive-compulsive neurosis. She has complicated rituals that consume several hours a day. Her morning bathing takes about two hours, and she has open sores on her ankles from excessive scrubbing. She is over-meticulous about all aspects of her per-

sonal care; for example, she insists on eating her meals alone in her room, and she will not take medication touched by anyone else.

Her social history indicates that she lives with her father. Her mother died when she was nineteen. Carol worked as a secretary for two years after high school, but has worked very little since then. She had another job in a secretarial pool that she enjoyed, but quit because her brother pressured her to do so. The family state that her condition is chronic, but worsened recently when her father retired.

Carol related to the staff her history of gradually worsening compulsive behavior, which began about the age of fourteen. She spoke of a strict upbringing, where the "virtues" of cleanliness and control were valued and outward shows of affection were rare.

During her hospital stay, Carol's anxiety and her rituals decreased. The nursing staff worked intensively with her and she participated in group therapy. After six weeks of hospitalization, she was eating in the dining room with other patients, and her morning bathing ritual had decreased to an hour. She seemed relaxed and at times even appeared happy. She had made several visits home, and she began to talk about wanting her own apartment.

One day, without warning, her brother announced that she must leave the hospital because the family could no longer afford treatment. The hospital staff tried to convince her to stay, saying they would help her explore alternate means of financing treatment, but she was unable to go against her brother's wishes and went home with him.

LESSON 2: SELF-TEST

Without consulting your notes, answer the following questions. If you find you cannot answer one or more parts, study your notes until you are able to answer them.

1. Explain how one develops a neurotic coping style.

2. Describe the behavior seen in these various types of neuroses: (a) anxiety; (b) phobic; (c) obsessive-compulsive; (d) hysteric.

3. What functions does a neurotic coping style serve in a person's life?

4. Explain the necessity of treating neurosis within the person's social network.

CHAPTER FOUR: OPTIONS FOR INDEPENDENT STUDY

If you wish to study more about psychosomatic and neurotic coping styles, choose one or both of the following activities.

1. Read the following, according to your interest:

Angyal, Andras. *Neurosis and Treatment: A Holistic Theory.* New York: John Wiley & Sons, Inc., 1965.

Shapiro, David. *Neurotic Styles.* New York: Basic Books, Inc., 1965.

2. Read the psychiatric history of a patient who uses a neurotic coping style and show how the development of this coping style may be better explained from a sociological rather than a psychological point of view. If you want to read more about the sociological point of view, the following are recommended:

Becker, Howard. *Outsiders.* London: Collier-Macmillan Ltd., 1963. Pp. 1-18.

Rubington, Earl, and Weinberg, Martin. *Deviance: The Interactionist Perspective.* 2nd ed. New York: The Macmillan Company, 1973. Pp. 1-30, especially pp. 11-15.

CHAPTER FIVE: # DRUG DEPENDENCE

OBJECTIVES

1. To understand the use of drugs as a coping style.
   1.1 To explain group and cultural influences on a person's use of drugs to cope.
   1.2 To define terms related to drug use, i.e., use and abuse, medicinal and recreational use, physical dependence (addiction) and psychological dependence.

2. To assess causes and consequences of the abuse of various drugs.
   2.1 To explain psychological, sociological, and physiological theories about the causes of heroin addiction.
   2.2 To identify the effects of heroin addiction upon the life of the addict.
   2.3 To explain the psychological, sociological, and physiological theories about the causes of alcoholism and alcohol abuse.
   2.4 To identify the effects of excessive alcohol intake upon the alcohol abuser.
   2.5 To describe the effects of the use of barbiturates, nicotine, amphetamines and cocaine, hallucinogens, marijuana and hashish, and inhalants.

3. To analyze treatment issues related to the use of drugs as a coping style.
   3.1 To describe the psychosocial and pharmacological aspects of the treatment of heroin addiction.
   3.2 To describe various approaches to the treatment of the alcohol abuser, i.e., detoxification and physical care, Alcoholics Anonymous, family treatment, and primary and secondary prevention.
   3.3 To identify several important aspects of the treatment of abuse of the following drugs: barbiturates, hypnotics, tranquilizers; amphetamines and cocaine; hallucinogens.
   3.4 To explain different roles the nurse can play in the treatment of drug abuse.

CHAPTER FIVE: LESSON 1

OBJECTIVES

1. To understand the use of drugs as a coping style.

1.1 To explain group and cultural influences on a person's use of drugs to cope.

1.2 To define terms related to drug use, i.e., use and abuse, medicinal and recreational use, physical dependence (addiction) and psychological dependence.

LEARNING ACTIVITIES

1. Read pages 112-117 of Chapter 5. Attending a lecture on this material or outlining the main points will supplement your reading.

2. The following group discussion activity may be done in groups in class or in independent groups outside class time. If you work in an outside group, summarize your discussion and give it to your instructor for feedback.

Think of different people you know and what kinds of drugs, including alcohol, they use. Try to select persons your age and both older and younger than yourself. The following questions may be used to guide the discussion.

(a) What drugs are used by different age groups?

(b) How do you think these people first started using these drugs?

(c) Why do you think they continue to use them?

(d) How do people's peer groups affect what drugs they use?

(e) What is the effect of the American culture on drug use?

(f) Would you classify drug use for other than the control of disease as simply use (for recreation) or abuse? Why?

LESSON 1: SELF-TEST

Without consulting your notes, answer the following questions. If you find you cannot answer one or more parts, study your notes until you are able to answer them.

1. How does group identity influence the use of drugs?

2. Explain the influence of culture on drug use.

3. Define and distinguish between the following terms as they relate to drugs: (a) use and abuse; (b) medicinal use and recreational use; (c) physical dependence (addiction) and psychological dependence.

CHAPTER FIVE: LESSON 2

OBJECTIVES

2. To assess causes and consequences of the abuse of various drugs.

2.1 To explain psychological, sociological, and physiological theories about the causes of heroin addiction.

2.2 To identify the effects of heroin addiction upon the life of the addict.

2.3 To explain the psychological, sociological, and physiological theories about the causes of alcoholism and alcohol abuse.

2.4 To identify the effects of excessive alcohol intake upon the alcohol abuser.

2.5 To describe the effects of the use of barbiturates, nicotine, amphetamines and cocaine, hallucinogens, marijuana and hashish, and inhalants.

LEARNING ACTIVITIES

1. Read pages 117-142 of Chapter 5 of the textbook; you may also want to outline the main points as you read—or attend a lecture-discussion.

2. Imagine you are the school nurse at a local high school and are asked to speak to a parents' group about "The Drug Problem." You decide to conduct the session by responding to questions from the group. What would your answers be to the following questions and comments?

(a) "My son said marijuana is a harmless drug, but I read that it can damage chromosomes and cause birth defects."

(b) "Well, our son told me that marijuana should be legalized because it does less harm than the two martinis my husband has every day when he comes home from work."

(c) "Last year one of the senior boys died from a heroin overdose. Why would such a young person be using heroin?"

(d) "Which drugs are most harmful to the body?"

(e) "Can drugs cause mental illness?"

(f) "I read recently that alcohol is used more often by teen-agers than drugs. Why do these kids drink?"

LESSON 2: SELF-TEST

Without consulting your notes, answer the following questions. If you find you cannot answer one or more parts, study your notes until you are able to answer them.

1. Explain the different theories about the causes of heroin addiction: (a) psychological; (b) sociological; (c) physiological.

2. What are the effects of heroin addiction on the life of the addict?

3. Explain the different theories about the causes of alcoholism and alcohol abuse: (a) psychological; (b) sociological; (c) physiological.

4. What are the effects of excessive alcohol intake upon the alcohol abuser?

5. What are the effects of each of these drugs? Barbiturates, nicotine, amphetamines and cocaine, hallucinogens, marijuana and hashish, inhalants.

CHAPTER FIVE: LESSON 3

OBJECTIVES

3. To analyze treatment issues related to the use of drugs as a coping style.

3.1 To describe the psychosocial and pharmacological aspects of the treatment of heroin addiction.

3.2 To describe various approaches to the treatment of the alcohol abuser, i.e., detoxification and physical care, Alcoholics Anonymous, family treatment, and primary and secondary prevention.

3.3 To identify several important aspects of the treatment of abuse of the following drugs: barbiturates, hypnotics, tranquilizers; amphetamines and cocaine; hallucinogens.

3.4 To explain different roles the nurse can play in the treatment of drug abuse.

LEARNING ACTIVITIES

1. Read pages 142-155 in Chapter 5 of the text, outlining the main points or attending a lecture if you wish.

Choose one of these projects.

2. Debate with fellow students some of the issues surrounding the treatment of alcohol and drug abuse. Using one or more of the following questions and comments as a guide, different individuals can present different points of view. Support your ideas with evidence, including search studies, reports, and other references. (Note: Some of the statements that follow are opinions, not necessarily facts.)

(a) Our country's narcotic problem began with the Harrison Act of 1914, which resulted in the criminalization of nonmedical narcotic use.

(b) Considering the point of view that when public attention is focused on the abuse of various substances (e.g., speed, marijuana, airplane glue), the number of users increases rather than decreases, would it not be preferable to ignore such problems?

(c) Is the abuse of alcohol, heroin, and other drugs a psychological, sociological, medical, moral, or legal problem?

(d) Persons who abuse heroin and alcohol should be treated by other persons who have had the same problem, i.e., ex-addicts or former alcoholics, because these persons have a better understanding of the problems and have had more success in treatment than professional persons.

(e) Why are some drugs legal (e.g., alcohol, tobacco), while others are illegal (e.g., heroin, marijuana)? Should they not all be legal or all be illegal?

(f) Should drug abuse treatment programs focus primarily on pharmacologic (e.g., Methadone) or psychosocial (e.g., therapeutic community) treatment approaches?

(g) How do you view the nurse's role in the treatment of drug and alcohol abuse in the hospital? In specialized treatment programs? In relation to primary prevention?

3. Arrange for some people involved in the treatment of drug abuse and of alcoholism to come as guest speakers. If possible, have both professional and nonprofessional persons (ex-addict staff, Alcoholics Anonymous members). Ask the speakers briefly to present their ideas about treatment and then to spend the remainder of the time discussing questions from the group. You might consider asking the visitors their ideas about some of the questions and comments from Activity 2 above.

LESSON 3: SELF-TEST

Without consulting your notes, answer the following questions. If you find you cannot answer one or more parts, study your notes until you are able to answer them.

1. Describe the psychosocial and pharmacological approaches to treating heroin addiction.

2. Describe these various approaches to the treatment of alcoholism: (a) detoxification and physical care; (b) Alcoholics Anonymous; (c) family treatment; (d) primary and secondary prevention.

3. Identify one or two important aspects of the treatment of abuse of the following groups of drugs: (a) barbiturates, hypnotics, and tranquilizers; (b) amphetamines and cocaine; (c) hallucinogens.

4. Explain three roles the nurse can play in the treatment of drug abuse.

CHAPTER FIVE: OPTIONS FOR INDEPENDENT STUDY

If you wish to study more about alcohol and drug abuse, choose one or both of the following activities.

1. Prepare a report on the extent of the use of drugs and alcohol in your community (or another community) and what treatment resources are available for these problems. If a group works together on this, different individuals can concentrate on different aspects of the report. If you are doing this alone, you may want to limit the problem studies in some way, as the project could become quite extensive.

(a) Assess the extent of the use of various substances by contacting the Board of Health, police, local newspapers, schools, stores selling alcohol and tobacco, and so on.

(b) Determine whether the extent of use is average, above average, or below average. What factors in the community affect the extent of use?

(c) What programs are available to help persons who use drugs and alcohol to cope? (Such as Alcoholics Anonymous, drug treatment center, alcoholic treatment program, crisis telephone line or walk-in service, teen center, mental health clinic.)

2. Visit a facility involved in treating drug or alcohol abuse to see firsthand what the treatment encompasses. Small groups of students might visit different agencies and later exchange impressions. (Many programs view public education as one of their functions and welcome visitors. Some have public education programs already arranged.)

CHAPTER SIX: DEPRESSIVE
COPING
STYLES

OBJECTIVES

1. To recognize depression as a coping style.
1.1 To explain the development of this coping style.
1.2 To explain grief as a type of normal depressive reaction.
1.3 To identify manifestations or characteristics of depression.

2. To understand the theories about types of depressive illness.
2.1 To explain the physiological, psychological and developmental, and sociological theories about the cause of depression.
2.2 To describe the different types of depression—normal and neurotic, manic-depressive, and involutional.

3. To plan nursing intervention for suicidal persons.
3.1 To investigate the incidence of and clues to suicide.
3.2 To describe settings in which a nurse might encounter suicidal persons.
3.3 To assess an individual's suicide potential.
3.4 To explain the factors of relationship, observation, protection, and crisis intervention in nursing intervention with suicidal persons.

CHAPTER SIX: LESSON 1

OBJECTIVES

1. To recognize depression as a coping style.

1.1 To explain the development of this coping style.

1.2 To explain grief as a type of normal depressive reaction.

1.3 To identify manifestations or characteristics of depression.

LEARNING ACTIVITIES

1. Read pages 158-163 of Chapter 6. In addition, you may want to outline the text material or attend a lecture-discussion.

2. This activity is to assist you in identifying the manifestations of depression. Think of one or two depressed persons you have known (as patients or otherwise). What symptoms or characteristics of depression did they manifest? Remember to include physical, mental, and emotional manifestations in your report or discussion.

3. Imagine you are the nurse caring for Mrs. Porter, a 55-year-old woman injured in an automobile accident last night. She sustained a head injury with extensive brain damage when she was thrown from the car, and she is not expected to live. Her husband, who was driving the car when it skidded on the ice and went off the road, received only minor injuries. He has been sitting at her bedside since the accident, just looking at his wife and holding her hand. He says little and remains calm despite the grave prognosis. In the afternoon, their daughter arrives by plane. She cries in anguish when she sees her mother and is sustained by Mr. Porter, who holds and comforts her. She is grateful that her father is such a strong person and that she has him to lean on.

Discuss the grief experienced by Mr. Porter and his daughter, using the following questions as a guide.

(a) Considering their behavior at this time, who would you expect to pass through the grieving process more easily?

(b) What problems might each encounter in grieving their loss?

(c) What steps would you take to facilitate their grieving process?

LESSON 1: SELF-TEST

Without consulting your notes, answer the following questions. If you find you cannot answer one or more parts, study your notes until you are able to answer them.

1. Explain the factors that contribute to the development of depression as a coping style.

2. In what way is grief considered to be a normal depressive reaction?

3. What are some manifestations or characteristics of depression?

CHAPTER SIX: LESSON 2

OBJECTIVES

2. To understand the theories about types of depressive illness.

2.1 To explain the physiological, psychological and developmental, and sociological theories about the cause of depression.

2.2 To describe the different types of depression—normal and neurotic, manic-depressive, and involutional.

LEARNING ACTIVITIES

1. Read pages 163-177 in Chapter 6. Outlining the text or attending a lecture-discussion will supplement your reading.

Choose one of the following activities.

2. Conduct a panel discussion with different members of the class presenting different points of view about the cause of depression. The points of view can be sociological, biochemical, genetic, psychological, and developmental. Use about half the time for presentation and half for questions and discussion from the class.

3. Invite persons to class who hold differing points of view about the cause of depression, asking them to present a panel discussion and explain their points of view. You might, for instance, invite a sociologist, a biochemical researcher, a developmental expert, and so on. Use about half the time for presentations and half for questions and discussion from the class.

4. Read the case study of Mary on pages 162 and 187-191 of the text and discuss the factors leading to her depression. How would a sociologist describe the factors contributing to her depression? A biochemical researcher? A geneticist? A psychologist? A developmentalist? Put your analysis in a written report that you turn in to your instructor.

LESSON 2: SELF-TEST

Without consulting your notes, answer the following questions. If you find you cannot answer one or more parts, study your notes until you are able to answer them.

1. Explain these different theories about the case of depression: (a) genetic; (b) neurohormonal; (c) psychological and developmental; (d) sociological.

2. Explain the distinguishing characteristics of neurotic, psychotic, manic-depressive, and involutional depression.

CHAPTER SIX: LESSON 3

OBJECTIVES

3. To plan nursing intervention for suicidal persons.

 3.1 To investigate the incidence of and clues to suicide.

 3.2 To describe settings in which a nurse might encounter suicidal persons.

 3.3 To assess an individual's suicide potential.

 3.4 To explain the factors of relationship, observation, protection, and crisis intervention in nursing intervention with suicidal persons.

LEARNING ACTIVITIES

1. Read pages 177-187 of Chapter 6. To supplement the text, outline the main points and/or attend a lecture-discussion.

2. Discuss the four situations below, first in relation to each person's suicide potential, and second, in terms of what nursing interventions you think are indicated in each situation. Use these questions as a guide:

(a) How suicidal is this person? Support your assessment with facts related to the incidence of and clues to suicide.

(b) What interventions would you initiate for each person? Consider the different aspects of intervention—relationship, observation, protection, and crisis intervention—and what is appropriate in each situation.

1. Alfred is a 79-year-old man admitted with numerous cuts over his body. He was transferred from the nursing home where he is a resident after giving his wife a fatal overdose of medication (she was senile and bedridden) and cutting himself in an apparent suicide attempt. He sits in his room most of the time and sobs deeply when he talks about his deceased wife. He said to a nurse, "Why am I still here? I should be dead."

2. Bernice is the younger sister of a friend of yours who has been having numerous problems lately with her family, her boyfriend, and school. She has a prescription for Librium obtained from her private physician, and she takes them to calm down and to help her sleep. She says she sometimes takes six or eight pills in an attempt to relieve her feelings of distress. She is concerned about failing in school, and her parents refuse to let her see Charlie, her boyfriend, until her grades improve.

3. Connie is a young woman (age twenty-eight) who, though not suicidal in the sense of wanting to die or end her life, acts impulsively when she is angry and occasionally injures herself. For example, twice she swallowed some thumbtacks, and once she left the hospital and was caught by a policeman as she was climbing over a fence to get onto some commuter-train tracks. She had had a disagreement with the nursing staff and said she hoped a train would hit her so they would be sorry.

4. Drew is a 57-year-old man hospitalized with chronic kidney disease. He is thin and pallid, and he hardly speaks at all. He does nothing but lay in bed all day staring out the door.

LESSON 3: SELF-TEST

Without consulting your notes, answer the following questions. If you find you cannot answer one or more parts, study your notes until you are able to answer them.

1. Explain and describe incidence of suicide and clues to suicide.

2. What are the settings in which the nurse might encounter suicidal persons?

3. Explain the following factors in nursing intervention with suicidal persons: (a) relationship, (b) observation, (c) protection, (d) crisis intervention.

CHAPTER SIX: OPTIONS FOR INDEPENDENT STUDY

If you wish to study more about depressive coping styles, you may do one or both of these projects.

1. Some studies have been done regarding the "survivors" of suicide, that is, the family and friends of a person who has committed suicide. If you are interested in investigating this aspect of suicide, reread the situation of Mary on pages 162 and 187-191 of the text, and discuss what might be done to help her family and her boyfriend cope with the loss they have experienced. What reactions would you expect each to have? What help would you suggest for them?

If you need more information upon which to base your analysis, refer to *Suicide: Prevention, Intervention, Postvention,* by Earl Grollman (Boston: Beacon Press, 1971), pp. 107-117.

2. Discuss the feminist movement and its effect upon women in relation to their self-concepts and their roles in society. Think of different aspects of this phenomenon: the depression of some women resulting from limited role options and from society's view of their role, which they have incorporated into their self-concept; the possible effects upon individual women when they realize they can make choices and change their situation; the fact that any changes that occur within individuals will affect those around them.

CHAPTER SEVEN: # RETREAT AS A FORM OF COPING

OBJECTIVES

1. To understand the nature of schizophrenia.

    1.1 To explain retreat from societal norms as a coping style.

    1.2 To explain the historical development of the concept of schizophrenia.

    1.3 To describe various manifestations of schizophrenia—associative disturbances and autism, delusions and hallucinations, affective disturbances and ambivalence, and loss of ego boundaries.

    1.4 To define different types of schizophrenia—process and reactive, simple, paranoid, hebephrenic, catatonic, and schizoaffective.

2. To understand theories about the origin of schizophrenia.

    2.1 To describe some biological theories about the cause of schizophrenia.

    2.2 To explain psychological theories about the cause of schizophrenia: the need-fear dilemma and family theories.

    2.3 To describe some sociological theories about the origin of schizophrenia.

3. To analyze treatment issues related to schizophrenia: hospitalization, isolation, and family and group treatment.

CHAPTER SEVEN: LESSON 1

OBJECTIVES

1. To understand the nature of schizophrenia.

1.1 To explain retreat from societal norms as a coping style.

1.2 To explain the historical development of the concept of schizophrenia.

1.3 To describe various manifestations of schizophrenia—associative disturbances and autism, delusions and hallucinations, affective disturbances and ambivalence, and loss of ego boundaries.

1.4 To define different types of schizophrenia—process and reactive, simple, paranoid, hebephrenic, catatonic, and schizoaffective.

LEARNING ACTIVITIES

1. Read pages 195-212 of Chapter 7. To supplement your reading, attend the lecture-discussion or outline the material.

2. Read the situation on pages 226-234 and discuss (as a group or in writing) the following questions related to it.

(a) What manifestations of schizophrenia were exhibited by the main character?

(b) Why did they occur?

(c) Would you describe his coping behavior as process or reactive schizophrenia? Why?

3. Discuss the following three situations, with their questions and comments, in relation to schizophrenia. Do you agree with them? Why or why not? (Think of the meaning of the various manifestations of schizophrenia.)

1. Ellen, who is recovering from an acute schizophrenia reaction, had a noisy argument with her parents last evening. During morning report, one of the night staff comments that Ellen slept poorly and was irritable when told she would have to stay in bed. The nurse cannot understand Ellen behaving this way because she is always so even-tempered. She suggests that perhaps the parents should not be allowed to visit. What do you think of this suggestion? How else might arguments between Ellen and her parents be dealt with?

2. Howard is a third-year engineering student admitted two weeks ago with a diagnosis of acute paranoid schizophrenia. He seems to be quite an intelligent person and enjoys discussing science, philosophy, and politics. He was explaining to one of the nursing students about the relationship between the planets and the electromagnetic forces of the earth. The student later says to her classmates, "He is so bright I can't follow him. I really don't see why he is here. It's true he doesn't have much to do with the other patients, but then he is so much more intelligent than they are." What would you say to her comment?

3. Sam is taken from his college dorm and admitted to a psychiatric unit with an acute schizophrenic reaction. He is hallucinating, confused, and somewhat combative. He is unable to sleep and paces the hall all night. One of the attendants, who is a student at the same college as Sam, says: "Sam is really bad off. I don't think he's going to make it. What a shame, being so close to graduation and all." Do you agree with the attendant? Why or why not?

LESSON 1: SELF-TEST

Without consulting your notes, answer the following questions. If you find you cannot answer one or more parts, study your notes until you are able to answer them.

1. Explain how retreat from societal norms develops as a coping style.

2. How did the concept of schizophrenia develop historically?

3. Explain the following manifestations of schizophrenia as set forth by the descriptive school: (a) associative disturbances; (b) autism; (c) delusions; (d) hallucinations; (e) affective disturbances; (f) ambivalence; (g) loss of ego boundaries.

4. Define the different types of schizophrenia: (a) process and reactive; (b) simple; (c) paranoid; (d) hebephrenic; (e) catatonic; (f) schizoaffective.

CHAPTER SEVEN: LESSON 2

OBJECTIVES

2. To understand theories about the origin of schizophrenia.

2.1 To describe some biological theories about the cause of schizophrenia.

2.2 To explain psychological theories about the cause of schizophrenia: the need-fear dilemma and family theories.

2.3 To describe some sociological theories about the origin of schizophrenia.

3. To analyze treatment issues related to schizophrenia—hospitalization, isolation, and family and group treatment.

LEARNING ACTIVITIES

1. Read pages 212-234 and 234-238 of Chapter 7. To supplement the text, attend the lecture-discussion or outline the main points.

2. This activity relates to the origins and treatment of schizophrenia. Read the situation on pages 226-234 of the text and discuss the questions below. For a group activity, different members of the class should address themselves to different questions, trying to convince others of their views. Those in the class who do not present material can ask questions for clarification and later, based on the presentations, write what they believe to be the origin of the main character's schizophrenia and what treatment seems indicated. Both presenters and reactors should provide a rationale for their views.

(a) Explain the origin of schizophrenia in the main character from a biological point of view.

(b) Explain the origin of schizophrenia in the main character based upon the need-fear dilemma.

(c) Explain the origin of schizophrenia in the main character using family theories.

(d) Explain the origin of schizophrenia in the main character using sociological theories.

(e) Based upon the points of view presented above, what treatment measures do you feel are indicated? In making your decision, consider the consequences of each treatment approach; for example, what are the possible consequences of hospitalizing or not hospitalizing someone?

3. Discuss (in class or in a written report) issues of treatment and how they might be dealt with in the following problematic situations.

(a) A schizophrenic person who is socially isolated, that is, who has no family or friends.

(b) A chronic schizophrenic person who is to be returned to the community after fifteen years of hospitalization: How can this person be helped to build a social network?

(c) A child or young adolescent schizophrenic in an unhealthy (for him or her) family situation—for example, with a schizophrenic mother and an alcoholic father.

LESSON 2: SELF-TEST

Without consulting your notes, answer the following questions. If you find you cannot answer one or more parts, study your notes until you are able to answer them.

1. What are some biological theories about the cause of schizophrenia?

2. Describe the need-fear dilemma and some family theories as causes of schizophrenia.

3. What are some sociological theories about the origin of schizophrenia?

4. Discuss the following issues related to the treatment of schizophrenia: (a) hospitalization; (b) isolation; (c) family and group therapy.

CHAPTER SEVEN: OPTIONS FOR INDEPENDENT STUDY

If you wish to study more about retreat as a form of coping, choose one or more of the following activities.

1. Read one of these accounts of a personal experience with schizophrenia:

> Green, Hannah. *I Never Promised You a Rose Garden.* New York: New American Library, 1964.

> Sechehaye, Marguerite. *Autobiography of a Schizophrenic Girl.* New York: Grune & Stratton, 1951.

2. Reread the situation of Girard and his family on pages 226-234 of the text. Discuss, individually in writing or in a group the crises the members of this family experienced and how these related to their development of coping styles. At what points might intervention have improved their coping styles?

3. This activity combines concepts from Chapters 7 and 9 ("Retreat As a Form of Coping," and "The Nurse in the Treatment Process"). It is a group discussion among students who are involved in one-to-one relationships with schizophrenic patients. Discuss the issues or problems that have come up in relating to schizophrenic patients, and what you have done about them. Also discuss the effect on your relationship with the patient of other staff members' involvement (nursing staff, physicians, occupational therapists, etc.).

TYPES OF TREATMENT INTERVENTION

CHAPTER EIGHT:

OBJECTIVES

1. To understand different types of treatment interventions.

1.1 To explain psychoanalysis and brief psychotherapy as examples of "talking" therapies.

1.2 To describe the different types of behavior modification.

1.3 To explain intervention through the use of chemotherapy and electroconvulsive therapy.

LEARNING ACTIVITIES

1. Read Chapter 8. To supplement it, attend the lecture-discussion and/or outline the text material.

Choose one of these activities.

2. Interview different persons who give treatment or make decisions about it, trying to determine what factors they consider in deciding on treatment methods. Different members of the class can interview different persons and exchange information. The following questions can be used as an interview guide.

(a) What treatment methods do you usually use? Why?

(b) How do you involve the person's social network (family, friends)?

(c) How do the person's past and present coping styles affect what treatment is used?

3. Invite to class a panel of persons who give or make decisions about treatment. Select persons who use different types of treatment interventions and ask them to discuss what factors they consider in deciding which method(s) of treatment to use. The class can ask the panelists questions about treatment decisions, using some of the questions from Activity 2.

SELF-TEST

Without consulting your notes, answer the following questions. If you find you cannot answer one or more parts, study your notes until you are able to answer them.

1. Compare psychoanalysis and brief psychotherapy in terms of the principles and goals of each.

2. Describe the different types of behavior modification as applied in treatment.

3. How are drugs used in treatment?

4. How is electroconvulsive therapy used in treatment?

CHAPTER EIGHT: OPTIONS FOR INDEPENDENT STUDY

If you wish to study more about treatment interventions, you can choose one or both of the following activities.

1. Select a particular method of treatment and discuss the pros and cons of its use. Some of the methods suggested are psychoanalysis, Behavior modification, and electroconvulsive therapy.

2. Read one or more of the books listed below and write a critique of the treatment interventions used. Several students might read different books and exchange views.

Beers, Clifford. *A Mind That Found Itself.* New York: Doubleday, 1953.

Green, Hannah. *I Never Promised You a Rose Garden.* New York: Holt, Reinhardt & Winston, 1964; New York: New American Library, 1964.

Parker, Beulah. *A Mingled Yarn; Chronicle of A Troubled Family.* New Haven: Yale University Press, 1972.

Plath, Sylvia. *The Bell Jar.* New York: Harper & Row, 1971; New York: Bantam, 1972.

Ruben, Theodore. *Lisa and David.* New York: Ballantine Books, 1962.

Sechehaye, Marguerite. *Autobiography of A Schizophrenic Girl.* New York: Grune & Stratton, 1951.

Ward, Mary Jane. *The Snake Pit.* New York: The New American Library, 1973.

CHAPTER NINE:

THE NURSE IN THE TREATMENT PROCESS

OBJECTIVES

1. To use oneself in a therapeutic way in relating to an individual patient.

1.1 To explain qualities that facilitate the use of self in a therapeutic way.
1.2 To distinguish a therapeutic from a social relationship.
1.3 To identify the influence of the nurse's feelings in the nurse-patient relationship.
1.4 To identify therapeutic and nontherapeutic responses in relating to patients.

2. To utilize the nursing process in relating to an individual patient.
2.1 To plan, implement, and evaluate nursing intervention for a patient.
2.2 To integrate nursing intervention with the treatment plan for a patient.

3. To analyze the characteristics of the three phases of a nurse-patient relationship with an individual patient.

GENERAL INFORMATION

This LAP has just one lesson because the three objectives, as well as the learning activities, are so interrelated that it is not feasible to separate them.

One difference you will notice about this LAP is that, because of the nature of some of the learning activities, they will extend throughout most or all of your experience in psychiatric nursing; that is, your relationship with an individual patient will last for a period of time, and the activities related to this relationship, as explained in this LAP, will also last for that period of time.

LEARNING ACTIVITIES

Activity 1 of the lesson will give you the knowledge necessary to achieve the objectives of the lesson, that is, knowledge of the therapeutic use of self, the nursing process, and the phases of the nurse-patient relationship. Activities 2, 3, and 4 are applications of this knowledge.

1. Read Chapter 9 of the text. Attend the lecture-discussion and, if you wish, outline the text material.

2. *Process Recordings*
Choose a patient for a one-to-one relationship and write daily process recordings of your interactions with him or her, including analysis and interpretation of the interaction as well as your own feelings and reactions. Refer to your notes from Activity 1 of this lesson as you need, to analyze and interpret the interactions.

Your process recordings are to be given to your instructor periodically, for feedback and assistance as necessary.

A sample process recording is included on pages 512-514 of this LAP as an example of one way to write them. You may use this format or one recommended by your instructor.

3. *Nursing Care Plan*
The steps in the nursing process are observation, analysis and interpretation of data, defining goals, developing interventions, and evaluating the effectiveness of the intervention. From your interactions with the patient as detailed in your process recordings, define the patient's needs, determine your goals, and plan your interventions. At frequent intervals (for example, each week), evaluate the effectiveness of your intervention and revise your

goals and intervention as necessary. A sample nursing care plan is included on pages 512-515 of this LAP.

4. *Nurse-Patient Relationship Paper*

As you write process recordings during the course of your relationship with the patient, note when the relationship is in the initiating, working, and terminating phases, and explain what you observe that leads to your conclusions.

At the end of the course, or when your relationship with the patient is terminated, write a paper on your relationship with the patient in which you discuss:

(a) each phase of the relationship and its characteristics;

(b) the goals, interventions, and evaluation carried out in each phase;

(c) how you integrated your intervention with the treatment plan for the patient;

(d) your feelings and reactions during each phase, how you dealt with them, and how they affected your relationship with the patient.

This paper will summarize and solidify what you have learned about relating to individual patients. In writing it, you will need to reflect on how you used yourself in relating to the patient, your application of the nursing process in giving nursing care, and the phases of the nurse-patient relationship as you experienced them.

SELF-TEST

Without consulting your notes, answer the following questions. If you find you cannot answer one or more parts, study your notes until you are able to answer them.

1. What qualities in the nurse facilitate using oneself in a therapeutic way?

2. What qualities distinguish a therapeutic relationship from a social one?

3. How did your feelings affect your relating to your patient?

4. What are some therapeutic responses you found helpful in relating to patients? What nontherapeutic responses did you notice in analyzing your interactions?

5. How did you utilize the nursing process in relating to an individual patient?

6. How did you integrate your intervention with the treatment plan for the patient?

7. What characteristics of the three phases of the nurse-patient relationship did you experience in your relationship with an individual patient?

CHAPTER NINE: OPTIONS FOR INDEPENDENT STUDY

Students who want to study more about the nurse in the treatment process may wish to read further about relating to individuals. The following books are suggested:

Fromm-Reichmann, Frieda. *Principles of Intensive Psychotherapy.* Chicago: University of Chicago Press, 1950.

Gendlin, Eugene. "Client-Centered: The Experiential Response." In *Use of Interpretation in Treatment,* edited by Emanuel Hammer, pp. 208-227. New York: Grune & Stratton, 1968.

Holmes, Marguerite, and Werner, Jean. *Psychiatric Nursing in a Therapeutic Community.* New York: The Macmillan Company, 1966. Pp 75-95.

Rogers, Carl. *Client-Centered Therapy.* Boston: Houghton-Mifflin, 1951.

SAMPLE PROCESS RECORDING

NURSE: VERBAL AND NONVERBAL	PATIENT: VERBAL AND NONVERBAL	PRINCIPLES THAT EXPLAIN BEHAVIOR AND INTERVENTION; FEELINGS AND OBSERVATIONS
Date:	Interaction Number 12	Goals: To help patient identify situations arousing discomfort and how he handles them.
Mr. E. had just returned from a home visit. He came over to me and said he had to check his clothes and would be right back. I said I would wait for him in the usual place. He returned ten minutes later at 8:10 A.M.		I was a little irritated that Mr. E. would be late; even though I knew it was ward policy that his clothes be checked at once. However, I waited in the usual place. Reinforcing trust by being on time and remaining there for patient. Maintaining terms of contract.
	How was your weekend?	
Fine, and yours?		Focus conversation back to patient.
	Well, I was out on pass. I had a good time. I spent a lot of time straightening things up—putting summer clothes away and sorting out things. I could only work a few hours and then had to take a snooze.	Fatigue may be emotional as well as physical. Sleep can be a defense against a trying situation.
	We had company too. My sister had just told people that I wasn't feeling well. She didn't tell them what was wrong and they expected to see me with casts or something. She left it to me to tell them what was wrong.	Patient's anxiety rose here, shown by much moving around in his chair, embarrassed laughter, and lack of eye contact. Sister probably gave responsibility to patient because of her own feelings.
How did you feel about telling them?		
	Oh, I had no feelings about it at all. They're friends and they understand. They've seen me upset and angry. They understand.	Denial of feelings as a protective mechanism. Hopes friends understand but not sure.
What do you do when you get angry?		
	Well, I count to ten. Mostly I keep it in. My friends all realize that. I don't get violent like some people.	Helping patient to be aware of his behavior in reaction to stress.

SAMPLE PROCESS RECORDING (Continued)

NURSE: VERBAL AND NONVERBAL	PATIENT: VERBAL AND NONVERBAL	PRINCIPLES THAT EXPLAIN BEHAVIOR AND INTERVENTION; FEELINGS AND OBSERVATIONS
Does what you do help?		
	I've seen the other way to react in the shop. The boys get pretty upset. (Patient went into detail about the problems in the printing plant and the tensions among the employees.)	Helping patient to evaluate the effectiveness of his coping mechanism.
What do you do when you're angry?		
	Well, really I don't get angry.	The patient uses protective defenses here by focusing on factual discussion of printing plant and the feelings of others rather than his own.
	(Silence.)	
	If you have to have an answer, I guess I walk away from it. (Goes on to talk about the job and how anger leads to firing someone which causes sorrow, not himself but others at the plant.)	Factual discussion and focus on others decreases anxiety.
		Again, easier to talk of others' anger than his own.
Can you focus on your own anger?		
	Well, I can't display my anger in front of the employees. Usually it doesn't have to do with them and I work it out with the back office. (Again goes on to give examples having to do with the technology of printing.) *Do you think you understand?*	The need to support his self-image forces him to hide his feelings. He wants acceptance by others and suppresses his feelings to get it. ("They won't like me if I get angry.")
Yes, I believe I follow you. Do you think I don't?		
	Well, it might be too technical; maybe we shouldn't discuss all that technical stuff.	Avoidance of discussion of feelings which increases his anxiety.
I thought I understood you. However, you have only discussed anger in connection with your job. What about your personal life?		
	Oh, I never have any anger with my friends. I don't express it violently. I like to assert myself in an argument, but I don't get angry with my friends.	Here again there is immediate denial; then he reverses himself and begins to let me see that he does get angry.

SAMPLE PROCESS RECORDING (Continued)

NURSE: VERBAL AND NONVERBAL	PATIENT: VERBAL AND NONVERBAL	PRINCIPLES THAT EXPLAIN BEHAVIOR AND INTERVENTION; FEELINGS AND OBSERVATIONS
Are you ever angry with me?		
	No. You may think so when I'm silent or when I seem upset. You make a comment about me looking nervous or upset. When we are silent and sit here and stare at each other, it makes me nervous. It seems we have nothing to say sometimes.	Relating to here and now. This question helped the patient to ventilate some feelings about last week. He gave me a lot of feedback. It also increased his anxiety.
Does that make you upset?		
	Well, we're sitting here. I think I'm acting cool, not nervous or anything, and you come up with those statements like, "You seem upset."	His comments made me feel quite anxious, but I thought it was important to pursue this topic.
Do my statements about seeing you as upset make you upset?		
	Well, sort of. It makes me wonder what you are thinking of me. You seem to think my little habits show that I'm nervous. Could we stop at 8:25 A.M.? I have to be at O.T. and she yells if I'm late. Sometimes I'd like to clout her. (Laughs) Enough said for today?	Eliciting further discussion by restating what patient has said. Change of subject to decrease anxiety. Displaces anger at me to O.T.?
I'll listen to whatever else you'd like to say.		
	You're cute that way. Always making me say everything.	Again showing his anger toward me for making him assume some responsibility for working during the meetings.
Goodbye, Mr. E. I'll see you here tomorrow at 8:00 A.M.		

SAMPLE NURSING CARE PLAN

Background Information

The patient is a 40-year-old man who lives at home with his parents. He has been hospitalized several times for psychotic behavior. Six weeks ago, he was brought to the hospital because he was agitated and destroying the household furnishings. His behavior upon admission was extreme withdrawal; he spoke to no one and seemed to be hallucinating. Since admission, he has shown considerable improvement. He now communicates verbally and no longer hallucinates.

A nursing student has been working with him since admission. Early in the relationship, her goals and intervention concentrated on developing trust and orienting the patient to reality. After that, she gave the patient opportunities to talk about his feelings and problems, but since this seemed too threatening to him at the time, she planned other ways to meet his needs. At the time the following care plan was written, plans were being made for his transfer to a day-care program in about two weeks.

Goals	*Intervention*
Increase socialization.	Continue meeting with him daily, but respect his need for distance and do not force eye contact. Try to engage in more group activity. Point out games he can plan with others and suggest that he ask others to join.
Increase self-esteem.	Provide experiences in which he can achieve satisfaction and success (e.g., playing checkers, occupational therapy). Encourage him in his desire to ask for more privileges (to go off the unit alone and to the cafeteria for meals).
Prepare for termination.	Discuss with him how things will be in the day program. Tell him my feelings about termination and help him express his. Reinforce idea of coming to the clinic if he ever feels the need in the future to talk to someone.

CHAPTER TEN:

ANTICIPATORY COUNSELING AND CRISIS INTERVENTION

OBJECTIVES

1. To apply principles of anticipatory counseling.

1.1 To review the theory relating to situational and developmental crises.

1.2 To describe the phases of anticipatory counseling; vivid anticipation of the event, providing information, and follow-up.

1.3 To identify target groups for anticipatory counseling.

2. To apply principles of crisis intervention.

2.1 To describe the stages of crisis intervention: assessment of the problem, identifying supports and coping mechanisms, and resolution of the crisis.

2.2 Given a situation, to plan activities applying the principles of crisis intervention.

CHAPTER TEN: LESSON 1

OBJECTIVES

1. To apply principles of anticipatory counseling.

1.1 To review the theory relating to situational and developmental crises.

1.2 To describe the phases of anticipatory counseling: vivid anticipation of the event, providing information, and follow-up.

1.3 To identify target groups for anticipatory counseling.

LEARNING ACTIVITIES

1. Read pages 308-319 of Chapter 10. Also attend the lecture-discussion and, if you wish, outline the text material.

2. If necessary, review the types of crises by rereading Chapter 3 of the text or your class notes.

3. In a group discussion or individual report, discuss how the process of anticipatory counseling might be helpful to a patient you are working with or one whose situation you know well. Select a particular event the patient is anticipating in the near future that is problematic to him or her and discuss the following questions. (Note: Some examples of events are a weekend pass, a visit from the family, a job interview.)

(a) How would you assist the patient in vividly anticipating the event?

(b) How would you assess what information the patient needs, and how would you provide it?

(c) What follow-up would you do after the event?

4. Think of a group in your local community that would benefit from anticipatory counseling regarding specific problems they face. The kind of group you choose will depend on the character of the community and the particular problems of the people living there. Some examples are minority groups, the unemployed, the poor, the elderly, those about to retire.

Devise a plan to do anticipatory counseling with the group you select, incorporating the three phases. Write either an individual report on your plan or one to be used in a group discussion.

LESSON 1: SELF-TEST

Without consulting your notes, answer the following questions. If you find you cannot answer one or more parts, study your notes until you are able to answer them.

1. Explain what is meant by situational and developmental crises.

2. Describe the three phases of anticipatory counseling.

3. List three groups for whom anticipatory counseling would be helpful.

CHAPTER TEN: LESSON 2

OBJECTIVES

2. To apply principles of crisis intervention.

2.1 To describe the stages of crisis intervention: assessment of the problem, identifying supports and coping mechanisms, and resolution of the crisis.

2.2 Given a situation, to plan activities applying the principles of crisis intervention.

LEARNING ACTIVITIES

1. Read pages 319-340 of Chapter 10, attending the lecture and outlining the main points if you wish.

2. Turn back to the LAP for Chapter 3, Lesson 2, on Life Crises, and review the situations you discussed that might be crisis-producing for patients. Consider again how you might help patients cope with these crises, using the following questions as a guide:

(a) In light of the theory presented about the different aspects of crisis intervention, what steps would you go through in helping these patients cope with their crises?

(b) What problems do you think you might encounter in carrying out your plan from (a)?

(c) Would doing crisis intervention with patients involve any change in your role in the health care setting?

(d) Does the daily operation of the health care setting facilitate or interfere with helping people with crises? In what way?

3. Examine your local community for points at which crisis intervention might prevent further development of problems. Think, for example, of different facilities and agencies that have contact with people who may be in crisis, such as schools, churches, courts, social service agencies, banks and loan companies, bars, and hairdressers. Visit one or two of these places and assess the extent to which people receive help there with their crises. Use the questions below as a guide. If you are doing this activity with a group, different members of the group can visit different places and compare experiences.

(Note: The way in which you gather data will depend upon the situation. If possible, observe what goes on for a period of time and draw your own conclusions. If you interview people at the agencies, ask questions indirectly to obtain the necessary information. For example, instead of asking what is done to help people in crisis, ask what a typical day is like, who comes in, what is done.)

(a) What is done to help people who may be in crisis?

(b) What nonhelpful reactions do people in crisis receive?

(c) Try to determine what happens to people who do not resolve their crises. (Do they become "mentally ill," "social misfits," alcoholics, criminals, or what?)

LESSON 2: SELF-TEST

Without consulting your notes, answer the following questions. If you find you cannot answer one or more parts, study your notes until you are able to answer them.

1. Review the situation described in the self-test of Chapter 3, Lesson 2 (page 477).

(a) Did you, at the time, suggest any nursing activities that would be applications of anticipatory counseling?

(b) What activities would you now suggest, recalling the elements of anticipatory counseling?

2. Describe the activities at each stage of crisis intervention:

(a) Assessment of the problems.

(b) Identifying supports and coping mechanisms.

(c) Resolution of the crisis.

CHAPTER TEN: OPTIONS FOR INDEPENDENT STUDY

Students wishing to study more about anticipatory counseling and crisis intervention can choose from the following activities.

1. Carry out the plan you made for anticipatory counseling in Learning Activity 3 or 4 of Lesson 1 (page 517). Ask your instructor for supervision as you carry out the plan, writing process notes of what occurs and discussing them. Secure the necessary clearance, if any, before proceeding.

2. Carry out the plan you made for doing crisis intervention with a patient in Learning Activity 2 of Lesson 2 (page 518). Ask your instructor for guidance as you do the intervention, writing process notes and then discussing them. Secure the necessary clearance, if any, before proceeding.

3. Review the types of psychotherapy described in Chapter 10, and note the difference between psychotherapy and crisis intervention. How does the focus differ? The time involved? The role of the helping person?

CHAPTER ELEVEN:

THE FAMILY SYSTEM: NORMALITY, DISTURBANCE, AND INTERVENTION

OBJECTIVES

1. To identify normal family processes.
1.1 To explain the relationship of individual freedom and connectedness to the development of family members.
1.2 To explain the meaning of congruent images in a family system.
1.3 To give examples of family themes.
1.4 To describe some boundaries a family gives its members.

2. To identify disruptive patterns in a family system.
2.1 To describe how loss disrupts a family system.
2.2 To describe the process of scapegoating within a family.
2.3 To explain the connection between problems with intimacy and patterns of the schismatic family and pseudomutuality.
2.4 To explain the elements of double-bind communication.

3. To apply principles of intervention to disturbed family systems.
3.1 To identify a family problem.
3.2 Given a situation, to plan interventions to promote change within the family system.

GENERAL INFORMATION

In addition to two regular lessons, this LAP provides several options for independent study. The first of these can be used as an alternate to the two lessons (see page 526).

CHAPTER ELEVEN: LESSON 1

OBJECTIVES

1. To identify normal family processes.

1.1 To explain the relationship of individual freedom and connectedness to the development of family members.

1.2 To explain the meaning of congruent images in a family system.

1.3 To give examples of family themes.

1.4 To describe some boundaries a family gives its members.

LEARNING ACTIVITIES

1. Read pages 342-350 of Chapter 11. To supplement the text, attend the lecture-discussion; you may want to outline the main points.

2. Select a family to study family processes. Try to select one that appears normal, that is, one in which there are no apparent behavioral problems among the members. (Note: This does not mean the family has no problems or crises; all families have these.) You might select the family of a patient you are caring for on a pediatric, obstetric, or medical-surgical unit, or a family you are visiting in the community. (Do not select the family of a patient in a mental health facility.) You might also select a family you know in your community.

Discuss, as a group or in a written report, the following questions in relation to family processes, supporting your conclusions with examples.

(a) What sense of connectedness do you perceive among the family members?

(b) What freedom is allowed individual members to develop their own identities?

(c) How do the members perceive each other? How does this compare with how you think each individual perceives himself or herself and with how you perceive each member?

(d) What are some of the family themes? For example, how does the family perceive itself? What themes do you notice in relation to the world outside the family?

(e) What boundaries does the family set for its members? For example, how invested are members expected to be in the family? What experiences are allowed each member outside the family?

(f) If a family member is ill, how has the illness changed the family? How is the fact of illness incorporated in the family system? How will it alter role perceptions? If there is a new member in the family, how will role perceptions change?

LESSON 1: SELF-TEST

Without consulting your notes, answer the following questions. If you find you cannot answer one or more parts, study your notes until you are able to answer them.

1. How do the factors of individual freedom and connectedness within a family affect the development of its members?

2. What is meant by congruent images within the family system?

3. Give some examples of family themes.

4. What are three boundaries a family might give its members?

CHAPTER ELEVEN: LESSON 2

OBJECTIVES

2. To identify disruptive patterns in a family system.

2.1 To describe how loss disrupts a family system.

2.2 To describe the process of scapegoating within a family.

2.3 To explain the connection between problems with intimacy and patterns of the schismatic family and pseudomutuality.

2.4 To explain the elements of double-bind communication.

LEARNING ACTIVITIES

1. Read pages 350-356 of Chapter Eleven. Also attend the lecture-discussion and/or outline the text material.

2. In this activity, you will be discussing disruptive patterns in a family. Select a family in which one of the members is identified as having some behavioral problem, such as a family in which a member is receiving inpatient or outpatient psychiatric treatment, one engaged in family therapy, or one with a child who is referred because of behavior problems. (If you are working with a patient in a one-to-one relationship, studying his or her family will add to your understanding.)

Use as many means as possible to gather information about the family; that is, talk to the family, the identified patient, and other professionals involved, read any available records, and so on.

Another option for studying a family is to view family therapy in session or on videotape, if such experiences are available.

Discuss the following questions in relation to disruptive patterns in the family, supporting your conclusions with examples.

(a) Has the family suffered any losses recently? What are these?

(b) What role does the identified patient play in the family? Is he or she being scapegoated? What reciprocal roles do family members play?

(c) Do family members have problems with feeling intimate or close to one another? How is this manifested? In conflict and splits in the family? In different members feeling inadequate or overadequate? In pseudo-mutuality?

(d) Are there problems in communication patterns, such as double-bind communications?

(e) What conflicts in the family does the identified patient express or resolve?

LESSON 2: SELF-TEST

Without consulting your notes, answer the following questions. If you find you cannot answer one or more parts, study your notes until you are able to answer them.

1. How might losses experienced by a family disrupt the family system?

2. How does the process of scapegoating operate in a family?

3. How are problems with intimacy related to the schismatic family and pseudomutuality?

4. Explain the elements of double-bind communication.

CHAPTER ELEVEN: LESSON 3

OBJECTIVES

3. To apply principles of intervention to disturbed family systems.

3.1 To identify a family problem.

3.2 Given a situation, to plan interventions to promote change within the family system.

LEARNING ACTIVITIES

1. Read pages 356-362 of Chapter Eleven. To supplement the text, attend the lecture-discussion; you may also want to outline the material.

2. In this activity, you will apply principles of intervention to the family you studied in Lesson 2, using the following questions as a guide.

(a) What do you identify as the family's problem(s)? (Data from Lesson 2 should assist you in determining this.)

(b) In what ways will the entire family have to change in order for the identified patient to change?

(c) Describe two or three interventions you would attempt if you were doing therapy with this family.

LESSON 3: SELF-TEST

Without consulting your notes, answer the following questions. If you find you cannot answer one or more parts, study your notes until you are able to answer them.

1. Describe the stage of assessment or problem identification in family therapy.

2. Describe two interventions that are helpful in resolving family problems.

CHAPTER ELEVEN: OPTIONS FOR INDEPENDENT STUDY

Students wishing to study more about family systems may do one or both of the following activities.

1. The following activity, in addition to being an independent study option, may be used as a substitute for Lessons 1 and 2, if certain individuals or the class as a whole so chooses.

Two students will each describe a family to the class, one a normal family and one a family with disruptive patterns. Consult Learning Activity 2 in both Lessons 1 and 2 for help in selecting families and for guide questions in collecting data on the families.

Participants in this activity will compare and contrast the two families in regard to both the normal and the disruptive patterns that are observed.

2. After obtaining the necessary clearances and with guidance from your instructor, plan for some involvement of the family of a patient you are working with. Apply the principles of anticipatory counseling in assisting the family to deal with a particular issue they face, for example, a home visit or discharge.

Plan to discuss with the family, including the patient (if feasible), how they think the event will go and to provide them with any necessary information.

As you discuss the issue, observe the family's pattern of interacting. Who is the family spokesman? How does the family relate to the patient?

Write some process notes on the session and discuss them with your instructor. If possible, convene the family again, after the event, to discuss how things went and to plan further for the future.

CHAPTER TWELVE:

THE GROUP: DYNAMICS, THERAPEUTIC POTENTIAL, AND INTERVENTION

OBJECTIVES

1. To identify group processes.

1.1 To explain the features that characterize a group: membership, group consciousness, shared purpose, interdependence, interaction, and unity.

1.2 To explain properties of a group: background or history, participation, communication, cohesion, atmosphere, standards or norms, sociometric patterns, structure and organization, and procedures.

1.3 To explain how a group promotes change in its members.

2. To identify the curative factors in a group; that is, sharing of information, instilling of hope, universality of experience, altruism, recapitulation of prior experiences, development of social skills, imitative behavior, interpersonal behavior, cohesiveness, and catharsis.

3. Given a situation, to apply principles of intervention to a group.

3.1 To explain functions of the leader in a therapeutic group.

3.2 To identify goals for the initial session of a group.

3.3 To identify the stages of conflict and cohesiveness in a group.

3.4 To identify reactions of group members to termination.

CHAPTER TWELVE: LESSON 1

OBJECTIVES

1. To identify group processes.

1.1 To explain the features that characterize a group: membership, group consciousness, shared purpose, interdependence, interaction, and unity.

1.2 To explain properties of a group: background or history, participation, communication, cohesion, atmosphere, standards or norms, sociometric patterns, structure and organization, and procedures.

1.3 To explain how a group promotes change in its members.

LEARNING ACTIVITIES

1. Read pages 365-373 of Chapter 12. You can also attend the lecture-discussion and/or outline the main points.

2. Select a group, with the approval of your instructor, that you will observe and analyze in terms of group processes. You can work alone or in groups of two or three. Some suggestions for groups are community groups such as church or neighborhood groups, youth clubs, men's or women's groups; local clubs such as J.C.C., Kiwanis, Eastern Star, garden clubs, auxiliaries; a nursery school group; a group of expectant parents; an Alcoholics Anonymous group; a faculty group.

Observe the group as many times as necessary to analyze the group process, using the following as a guide:

(a) Give examples of how this group manifests the features that characterize a group (listed in Objective 1.1).

(b) Give examples of the properties of a group manifested in this group (listed in Objective 1.2).

(c) What changes does the group promote in its members? How does the group bring about these changes?

3. As part of learning about group process, review your clinical group several times during the term. Do this in a group, with members sharing their observations of group process. Use questions (a), (b), and (c) in Learning Activity 2 above as a guide.

LESSON 1: SELF-TEST

Without consulting your notes, answer the following questions. If you find you cannot answer one or more parts, study your notes until you are able to answer them.

1. List and explain the features that characterize a group.

2. Explain the following properties of a group:
(a) Background or history.
(b) Participation.
(c) Communication.
(d) Cohesion.
(e) Atmosphere.
(f) Standards or norms.
(g) Sociometric pattern.
(h) Structure and organization.
(i) Procedures.

3. How does a group promote change in its members?

CHAPTER TWELVE: LESSON 2

OBJECTIVES

2. To identify the curative factors in a group; that is, sharing of information, instilling of hope, universality of experience, altruism, recapitulation of prior experiences, development of social skills, imitative behavior, interpersonal behavior, cohesiveness, and catharsis.

3. Given a situation, to apply principles of intervention to a group.

   3.1 To explain functions of the leader in a therapeutic group.

   3.2 To identify goals for the initial session of a group.

   3.3 To identify the stages of conflict and cohesiveness in a group.

   3.4 To identify reactions of group members to termination.

LEARNING ACTIVITIES

1. Read pages 374-388 of Chapter 12. Also attend the lecture-discussion and/or outline the text material.

2. Observe (and participate in if possible) a therapeutic group and identify curative factors and interventions in the group. You can observe an actual group, such as a community, award or team meeting, a therapy group, or videotapes of a group. (Your instructor will help you arrange this experience.)

Use the following questions as a guide in observing and analyzing the group:

(a) Give three or four examples of curative factors in the group. (Curative factors are listed in Objective 2.)

(b) Study the role of the leader(s) or therapist(s) in the group: How do they build cohesiveness in the group? How do they promote growth in the members? If you were a leader, what would you do differently?

(c) Describe the initial meetings of the group. What did the therapists and the members say and do? How did the initial session differ from later sessions?

(d) Give examples of conflict and cohesiveness observed in the group. Was hostility expressed toward the leaders? How did they react to it?

(e) Describe the process of termination in the group. What did the leaders say and do at this time? How did the members react to termination?

LESSON 2: SELF-TEST

Without consulting your notes, answer the following questions. If you cannot answer one or more parts, study your notes until you are able to answer them.

1. Explain the following curative factors of a group:
(a) Sharing of information.
(b) Instilling of hope.
(c) Universality of experience.
(d) Altruism.
(e) Recapitulation of prior experiences.
(f) Development of social skills.
(g) Imitative behavior.

(h) Interpersonal behavior.

(i) Group cohesiveness.

(j) Catharsis.

2. Explain the function of the leader in a therapeutic group.

3. What are the goals of the initial session of a therapy group?

4. Explain the stages of conflict and cohesiveness in the life of a group.

5. What are some common reactions of group members to termination of a group?

CHAPTER TWELVE: OPTION FOR INDEPENDENT STUDY

If you wish to study more about group process, you can do the following activity. It is suggested that two students do this together.

With the supervision of your instructor, and after obtaining the necessary clearances, conduct a group. Depending upon the institution and the patient population, your group might be, for example, an activity group, a group convened to discuss particular issues (e.g., discharge), or a learning group (e.g., sex education groups).

Discuss with your instructor what the focus of your group will be and plan for this, including selecting members and initiating the group. Keep process notes on the group and tape-record the sessions, reviewing these weekly with your instructor to obtain the help you need.

CHAPTER THIRTEEN:

THE THERAPEUTIC COMMUNITY

OBJECTIVES

1. To analyze treatment issues in the therapeutic community.

1.1 To describe how admission to a hospital constitutes a crisis.

1.2 To explain elements in a therapeutic community that help a person deal with problems in living.

1.3 To explain problems of re-entry from a hospital into the family, community, and work.

2. To apply principles of relating to patients in the therapeutic community.

2.1 To describe problems occurring in the therapeutic community.

2.2 To explain principles of intervention related to specific problems encountered in the therapeutic community.

CHAPTER THIRTEEN: LESSON 1

OBJECTIVES

1. To analyze treatment issues in the therapeutic community.

1.1 To describe how admission to a hospital constitutes a crisis.

1.2 To explain elements in a therapeutic community that help a person deal with problems in living.

1.3 To explain problems of re-entry from a hospital into the family, community, and work.

LEARNING ACTIVITIES

1. Read pages 391-425 of Chapter 13. Also, attend the lecture-discussion and, if you wish, outline the text material.

2. This activity entails analyzing issues in an in-patient milieu where you are working as a student. It is preferable to do this activity in a mental health setting, which deals specifically with problems in living, but it may also be done in another type of unit. (Other units have many of the same problems.) You may do this activity in groups of two and three if you wish. In discussing the questions below, support your observations with examples. If possible, use the same patient in discussing (a), (b), and (c).

(a) Observe the admission of a patient to the unit. Does the admission constitute a crisis for the patient and/or his or her family? What are their reactions? What do the intake worker and/or person admitting the patient do to alleviate the crisis? What else might they do? What factors encourage the patient to adopt the "sick role"?

(b) Consider how the milieu operates as an agent of change for the patient. What is the treatment plan to help the patient learn to cope with his or her problems in living? How is the plan decided upon and carried out? (Give some examples.) How are patients involved in decision-making—for example, patient government, ward or team meetings, talking to staff? How are patients involved in formulating and carrying out ward rules and procedures? What factors in the milieu promote interaction among patients? What factors hinder such interaction? How are patients involved in making decisions about their own and others' treatment, for example, privileges and passes? Based upon your observations, what improvements would you suggest for the milieu to be an agent of change?

(c) Consider how the patient is assisted with re-entry into the family, community, and work. In what ways is the patient prepared for re-entry from the day of admission and throughout hospitalization? How is the family involved in treatment? What consideration is given to re-entry into the community and the work role? How might re-entry be better facilitated?

LESSON 1: SELF-TEST

Without consulting your notes, answer the following questions. If you find you cannot answer one or more parts, study your notes until you are able to answer them.

1. In what ways does admission to a hospital constitute a crisis?

2. Explain three elements of a therapetuic community that assist a person in dealing with his or her problems in living.

3. What are some problems a patient might encounter as he or she leaves the hospital milieu and re-enters a family, a community, and a work situation?

CHAPTER THIRTEEN: LESSON 2

OBJECTIVE

2. To apply principles of relating to patients in the therapeutic community.

2.1 To describe problems occurring in the therapeutic community.

2.2 To explain principles of intervention related to specific problems encountered in the therapeutic community.

LEARNING ACTIVITIES

1. Read pages 411-432 of Chapter 13. In addition, attend the lecture-discussion and, if you wish, outline the text material.

2. In this activity you apply the principles of relating to patients that were discussed in the text. Identify two or three problems that you notice occurring frequently on the unit and discuss them, using the questions below.

(a) Describe the problem. What happened? Who was involved?

(b) What is your explanation for why the problem occurs?

(c) How is the problem dealt with by staff?

(d) How might it be better dealt with? What principle(s) from Chapter 13 would you apply in intervening?

LESSON 2: SELF-TEST

Without consulting your notes, answer the following questions. If you find you cannot answer one or more parts, study your notes until you are able to answer them.

1. Describe two problems that occur frequently in the therapeutic community.

2. Explain the principles underlying intervention in these problems.

CHAPTER THIRTEEN: OPTIONS FOR INDEPENDENT STUDY

If you wish to study more about the therapeutic community, choose from the following activities.

1. Debate the issue of how much patients should decide about what takes place in a therapeutic community. Think of this in relation to rules and procedures, treatment decisions, roles and functions of staff.

2. Examine the issue of setting limits.

(a) What limits exist in the therapeutic community?

(b) What is the origin of these limits (legal restrictions, hospital rules, the need of the situation, the needs of the staff, of the patients)?

(c) By comparison, think of the relationship between student government and administration. What limits exist and what is their origin?

CHAPTER FOURTEEN: # ETHICAL ISSUES

OBJECTIVES

1. To evaluate ethical issues related to treatment in the mental health field.

    1.1 To identify issues of mental health treatment regarding what is treated, who is treated, and who gives treatment.

    1.2 To criticize mental health practices regarding these issues.

LEARNING ACTIVITIES

1. Read Chapter 14, attending the lecture-discussion and outlining the text if you choose.

2. Using your clinical experience in psychiatric-mental health nursing as a data base, discuss the ethical issues involved in what you observe. The following questions may be used as a guide.

    (a) What, in your opinion, do the professionals you have seen take as their focus of intervention (e.g., individuals, families, communities)? Do you agree or differ with this focus? Why?

    (b) Whom do you see receiving treatment? Were these persons brought into treatment by themselves or others? What do you think of persons being given "treatment" against their will?

(c) To what extent are patients informed of the treatment they receive and its effects? Are they free to accept or reject treatment measures?

(d) Whom do you see giving treatment? Where does most of this treatment take place? What improvements would you recommend in regard to the questions of who treats and where treatment occurs?

SELF-TEST

Without consulting your notes, answer the following questions. If you find you cannot answer one or more parts, study your notes until you are able to answer them.

1. Explain one issue related to mental health treatment in each of the following areas:

(a) The focus of treatment.

(b) Who receives treatment?

(c) Who does treatment?

2. What is your opinion about how the above issues should be resolved? Why?

CHAPTER FOURTEEN: OPTIONS FOR INDEPENDENT STUDY

For students wishing to study more about ethical issues in treatment, the following books are recommended.

Szasz, Thomas A. *Law, Liberty, and Psychiatry: An Inquiry into the Social Uses of Mental Health Practices.* New York: The Macmillan Company, 1963.

——. *Ideology and Sanity.* Garden City, New York: Anchor Books, Doubleday & Company, Inc., 1970.

——. *The Myth of Mental Illness: Foundations of a Theory of Human Conduct.* 2nd ed. New York: Harper & Row, 1973.

INDEX

Abrams, Arnold, 125
Abscesses, 151
Acetaphenazine, 273
Adapin, 270
Adaptation, 63
Addiction, 113-50
  biochemical theories on, 125
  causes of, 124
  definition of, 116
  treatment by ex-addicts, 146
Adolescence, 41-45
  delinquency in, 44
  varying length of, 42
Adolescents, unmarried pregnant, 312-17
Adrenal medulla, 88
Affect, 206-09
Aging, 49-50, 172, 335-39
  depression and, 173-4
Akathisia, 273
Akineton, 274
Alcohol, 126-32, 147-50
Alcohol abuse, 126
Alcohol dehydrogenase, 131
Alcoholics
  and religion, 128-29
  and suicide, 181
Alcoholics Anonymous (AA), 149-150
Alcoholism, 49, 126-32, 334
  definition of, 127
  physical symptoms of, 130
  treatment of, 147-50
Ambivalence, 206-09
Amitriptyline, 270
Amnesia, 104
Amphetamines, 116, 135-38
  withdrawal from, 151
Anectine, 275
Angyal, Andreas, 95-96, 105
Anorexia, 160
Antabuse, 148
Anticipatory counseling, 311-18
Antidepressant drugs, 270-72
Anxiety, 57-63, 70, 300-01
  nurse's feelings of, 285-86
  physical symptoms of, 68
  using objects to allay, 112-15
  reasons for recurrence, 94
Anxiety neurosis, 97
Appetite, loss of, 137, 148
Arieti, Silvano, 175
Artane, 274
Assessment, 257-61, 322, 379
  of families, 356-59
Assessment interview, 258-61

Association, disturbance in, 203-06
Asthma, 92
Atarax, 268
Autism, 203-06, 207, 265
Autonomic nervous system, 89
Autonomy, 251-52
Aventyl, 270
Avoidance, 71, 216

Barbiturates, 132-34
  and alcohol, 133
Bardwick, Judith, 167-69
Beck, Aaron T., 160, 172
Behavior, 4
Behavior modification, 265-67
Benzedrine, 136
Benzodiazepines, 268
Benzotropine mesylate, 274
Bernard, Jessie, 173
Biofeedback, 92, 213
Biperiden, 274
Birth control, 317
Birth process, 315
Blacks, 173
Bleuler, Eugene, 201
Blood dyscrasia, 274
Boundaries, 347-50
Brecher, Edward M., 117, 120, 125
Butaperazine, 273
Butyrophenones, 272, 273

Cannabis sativa, 139
Cannon, W. B., 88
Caplan, Gerald, 54, 59
  on situational crisis, 57
Carphenazine, 273
Catchment area, 446
Catecholamines, 168
Character disorders, 199
Chemotherapy, 267-74
  for affective illness, 270-72
Chesler, Phyllis, 172-73
Child behavior
  bragging, 38-39
  phobia toward school, 99
Children
  alcohol consumption by, 132
  cultural influences on, 39
  depressive coping style in, 170-71
  treatment issues relating to, 440-41
Chlordiazepoxide, 119, 268
Chlorpromazine, 273, 274
  for LSD "bad trip," 139

Chlorprothixene, 273
Cocaine, 135
  effects of, 136
  withdrawal from, 151
"Cocaine bugs," 137
Cogentin, 274
Cohen, Charles, 125
Communication, 426-30
Community Mental Health Centers Act of 1963, 446
Community workers, indigenous, 443-44
Compazine, 273
Compensation, 66
Compliance, 243
Compulsions, 101
Compulsive behavior, management of, 101-02
Conflict, 69, 93, 352
  exploring, in therapy, 254
Congruent images, 344-45
Control, 100
Conversion, 67
Conversion hysteria, 103
Convulsions, 130
Coordination of treatment, 408
Coping, 63-64
Coping mechanisms, 322-23
Coping skills, 74
Coping styles, 53, 68-78, 241-44, 248-50
  changing (in hospital), 421-23
  individual development (diagram), 73
  neurotic, 93-107
  requiring hospitalization, 391, 404
  retreat, 195-98
  schizophrenic, 208-09
Crisis, 53-57, 244
  definitions of, 53, 308, 319
  family, 358-59
  requiring hospitalization, 392
  resolution of, 61-62
  stages of, 54-55
Crisis intervention, 186, 308, 319-35
  in hospital setting, 393-94
"Crutches," 70
Cyclazocine, 144, 146-47

Dartal, 273
Data on patients, 295-96
Death and dying, 310, 335-39
Decision-making, 438-39
  by patient, 396-98

Defenses
  See **Defensive mechanisms**
Defensive maneuvers, 261
Defensive mechanisms, 63-68
Delinquency, 44
Delirium, 175
Delirium tremens (DTs), 130, 148, 153
Delusional systems, 427-29
Delusions, 165, 204-05, 302
  major tranquilizers for, 273
Dementia praecox, 201
Denial, 65
Dependency, 90, 169
Depersonalization, 208-09
Depressants, 118
Depression, 157-93
  biochemical findings on, 168
  definition of, 158
  differentiating types of, 164, 166
  endogenous, 163
  exogenous, 163
  involutional, 176-77
  physiological factors in, 167-69
  psychological factors in, 169-71
  psychotic, 174
  sociological perspectives on, 172-74
  symptoms of, 161
  types of, 163-67
Depressive coping styles, 169-71
Depressive syndrome, 160
Desensitization, 265, 266-67
Desipramine, 270
Detoxification, 144-45
Deviance, 75, 77
  requiring hospitalization, 391-92
Deviant life styles, 197-200
Deviant roles, 56, 114
Deviant self-identity, 44
Diazepam, 119, 268
Differentiation, 214
Diphenylmethane derivatives, 268
Discontinuity in social roles, 22-24
Displacement, 66, 98
Dissociative hysteria, 104
Disulfiram, 148, 149
Divorce, 310
Double-bind communication, 220, 355-56
Doxepin, 270
Drives, 259
Drug abuse, 115
  See also **Addiction**
Drug-induced psychosis, 137, 151
Drugs
  antidepressants, 270-72
  physical dependence on, 116
  psychological dependence on, 116
  types of, 117-52, (*table*) 119
  See also **Chemotherapy**

Drug-taking culture, 114-15
Drug use, 70, 115, 242
  cultural context of, 141
  treatment of, 144
Drug withdrawal, 151
Durkheim, Emile, 260
Dyspnea, 148
Dystonia, 273

Ego boundaries, 208
Ego development, 214, 344
Ego impairment, 164
Elavil, 270
Electroconvulsive therapy, 274-75
Empathy, 283-84
"Empty nest syndrome," 181
Equanil, 268, 269
Erikson, Erik H., 29-51, 343
Erikson's Life Stages, 29-51
Eskalith, 271-72
Estrogen, 168
Ethical issues, 252-53, 267, 434-48

Family
  and schizophrenia, 217-21, 237
  assessment, 344, 356-59
  history, taking of, 351
  loss, 350-51
  structure, 35, 342-50
Family intervention and the aged, 337-38
Family system
  crisis in (hospitalization), 393
  disturbances in, 350-62
Family theme, 346-47
Fatigue, 98
Feedback, 429-30
  negative, 373
Female identity, 48
Financing of treatment, 444-45
"Flashback" (LSD), 139
Fluphenazine, 273
Formication, 137
Fugue, 104
Freudians, 161, 253-54
Freud, Sigmund, 88, 201, 255-56
  cocaine addiction of, 135
  nicotine addiction of, 134

Galvanic skin response, 213
Gastrointestinal complaints, 98
Glue sniffing, 140-41
Greenberg, Ruth L., 172
Grief, concept of, 160
Grief reaction, 161
Grieving process, 163
Group counseling, 312
Group history, 373
Group psychotherapy
  curative factors of, 374-78

intervention techniques, 378-87
  role of leader, 380-82
Groups
  cohesiveness in, 384-85
  dynamics of, 365-73
  membership in, 366-67
  properties of, 367-73
  sociometric patterns in, 371

Haldol, 273
Hallucinations, 137, 148, 224, 375
  in schizophrenia, 204-05
  major tranquilizers for, 273
  responses to, 428
Hallucinogens, 138-39
  treatment of use, 151-52
Haloperidol, 273
Harrison Act of 1914, 120-21
Hashish, 139-40
Hazardous life events, 311-12
Headaches, 98
Heiss, Jerold, 14, 15
Hepatitis, 151, 271
Heroin, 117, 119
  addiction to, 121-23
Homeostasis, 89
Homosexuals, 181, 244
Hope, instilling, 375, 397
Hospital attitudes, 409-11
Hospitalization of patient, 391-432
  admission to treatment unit, 399-406
  as crisis experience, 393-99
  emergency room experience, 394-99
  function of, 391-92
  initial interview, 402-06
  introduction to treatment unit, 411-13
  physical problems, 431
  reentering the community, 423-25
  staff role in decision-making, 419-21
  therapeutic community, 408-11
  ward living, 413-19
Hydroxyzine, 268
Hyperreflexia, 148
Hypertension, 92
Hypokinesis, 211
Hysteria, 103-04
  during hospital admission, 396

Identification, 67-68
Identity, 44-45, 342-44
Imipramine, 270
Impulses, 259
Inferiority feelings in children, 40
Informed consent, 441
Inhalants, 140-42
Insight, 263
Insight therapy, 253-57

Insomnia, 98, 160
Insulin therapy, 275-76
Intake interview, 327
Integration, 214
Intellectualization, 65
Interpersonal relationships, 282-83
Intervention plans, 296
Intervention, methods of, 245-46
Interventions, 244-77, 293, 302-03
    in groups, 378-87
    issues relating to, 436-47
    with families, 356-62
Interviews for groups, 379-80
Intimacy, 352-54
Introjection, 67
Involutional depression, 164,
    176-77
Isocarboxazid, 270

Jacobson, Edith, 161
Jaffe, Jerome, 124
Jaundice, 274

Kraepelin, Emil, 201
Kubler-Ross, Elizabeth, 339

Labeling, 234
    depressions, 165
    irreversibility of, 225
    of hospitalized patient, 399-400,
    431
Laing, R. D., 60, 61, 223-24
Learning theory, 89
Legal constraints, 420
Legislation, community mental
    health, 445-46
Librium, 119, 268, 269
Lidz, Theodore, 90, 218
Life history of patient, 262
Limit-setting, 430-31
Lindemann, Erick, 163
Lithane, 271-72
Lithium carbonate, 271-72
Lithonate, 271-72
Lofland, John, 55
Loss, 88-89, 310-11
    concepts of grief and, 160-61
    family, 350-51
    in childhood, 159-60
LSD, 115, 138-39
    "bad trip," 139

Manic depression, 275
Manic-depressive psychosis, 175
Manic-depressive state, 164
MAO, 168
MAOI's (drugs), 270-71
Marijuana, 113, 114, 119
    and hashish, 139-40
    and heroin use, 117

possible physical effects of, 140
Marijuana and Health: Second An-
    nual Report to Congress, 140
Marplan, 270
Maturational stage
    and crisis, 57
May, Rollo, 58
Mead, George Herbert, 4
Mellaril, 273
Menopause, 166
Mental Health Study Act of 1955,
    446
"Mental illness," 60, 62
    as excuse for rule-breaking, 76,
    77
    as myth, 435
    Szasz, Thomas, on, 224
Meprobamate, 119, 268
Mescaline, 115, 138
Methadol, 145
Methadone, 144-45, 153-54
Methamphetamine, 119, 136-37
Meyer, Adolf, 201
Middle age, 47, 176-77
Milieu therapy, 406-07
Miltown, 119, 268, 269
Minority groups, 166-67, 172
Minority status and depression, 173
Mirsky, I. A., 92
Monoamine oxidase. See MAO
Monoamine oxidase inhibitors. See
    MAOI's
Mulford, Harold, 128
Muscle aches, 98

Narcissim, 170
Nardil, 270
National Institute of Alcoholism
    and Alcohol Abuse (NIAAA),
    126, 128
National Institute of Mental
    Health, 446
National Mental Health Act of
    1946, 446
Navane, 273
Need-fear dilemma, 214-17
Neurosis, treatment of, 266
Neurotic anxiety, 95
Neurotic behavior
    characteristics of, 96-97
    compulsive, 96
    treatment of, 107-08
Neurotic coping styles, 69,
    93-107, 242
    anxiety neurosis, 97-98
    phobic neurosis, 98-101
    obsessive-compulsive neurosis,
    101-03
    hysteria, 103-04
Neurotic reactions, types of, 97

Nicotine, 134-35
    toxicity of, 134
Norms, 196, 198-99, 370-71
    breaking of, 440-41
    for hospitalized patient, 402
    See also Rule breaking; Social
    norms
Norpramin, 270
Nortriptyline, 270
Nurse-patient relationship, 283-304
    expectations, establishing, 405-06
    in anticipatory counseling,
    317-19
    in drug dependency situation,
    152-54
    in hospitalization, 394, 400-01
    nontherapeutic responses by
    nurse, 242-43
    phases of the, 297-304
    termination of the, 302-04
    with the aged, 337-39
Nurse role, 279-82
Nurse's managerial roles, 409
Nursing care plan, 297
Nursing process, 293-97

Observation of patients, 295-96
Obsessions, 260-61
    definition of, 101
Obsessive-compulsive behavior, 102
Obsessive-compulsive neurosis,
    101-03
Obsessive coping style, 94-95
Oedipal conflict, 108
Oedipal stage, 36
Old age, 49-50
    See also Aging
Operant conditioning, 265
Opiates, 118, 120, 142-46
    history of use, 118-20
    treatment of addiction, 142
Opium. See Opiates
"Oral" needs, 135
Organ specificity, 92
Orientation of hospitalized patient,
    402-03
Overemphasis on safety, 96
Oxazepam, 268

Panic, 59, 394
Paralysis, 103
Paranoia, 137-38, 150
Paranoid depression, 177
Paranoid schizophrenia, 211
Parenting, 310
Parents' groups, 317
Parkinsonian-like syndrome,
    273-74
Parnate, 270
Passive coping styles, 71

Patient contract, 299-300, 440
Patient government, 417-19
Patient role, 279-82
  in hospitalization, 401
Patterning of behavior, 27
Pentobarbital, 119
Permitil, 273
Perphenazine, 273
Personality disorganization, 74
Pertofrane, 270
Phenelzine, 270
Phenothiazines, 151, 272, 273
Phobia, case study of, 99-100
Phobic neurosis, 98-101
  characteristics of, 98
Physical problems of depressed
  persons, 431
Piperacetazine, 273
Plan, nursing care, 297
Pleasure principle, 255
Police as diagnosticians, 165
Postnatal adjustment, 315-17
"Pothead," 140
Power struggle between patient
  and nurse, 416-17
Pregnancy, 309
  in unmarried adolescents, 312-17
Prenatal groups, 317
Presamine, 270
Preventive work, 318-19
Primary process thinking, 203, 207
Problem solving, 53, 308, 311
Process recording, 297
Prochlorperazine, 273
Prohibition, 147
Projection, 67
  in schizophrenia, 205
Proketazine, 273
Prolixin, 273
Propanediols, 268
Protriptyline, 270
Pseudomutuality, 219-20, 354-55
Psilocybin, 119, 138
Psychiatric emergencies, 393
Psychiatric nursing, 250, 365
  role of nurse, 78-80
  treatment issues in, 436-47
  See also Nurse-patient relation-
    ship
Psychiatric patient, hospitalized,
  391-432
  reentering the community,
    423-25
Psychic determinism, 255, 256
Psychoanalysis, 87-88, 255-56
Psychodrama, 408
Psychosomatic coping styles, 88-92
  compared with neurotic coping
    style, 90
Psychosomatic illnesses, 68-69, 87

Psychosurgery, 213
Psychotherapy, brief, 257-65
  interpretations in, 263-65
  phases of, 262-63
  treatment goals in, 261
Psychotic behavior as response to
  crisis, 61
Psychotic depressions, 174

Quide, 273

Rationalization, 66
Ray, Oakley S., 115
Reaction-formation, 66-67
  and compulsive behavior, 102
Reciprocal inhibition, 266
Reciprocal roles. See Role
  reciprocity
Regression, 164, 203, 387
Reinforcement techniques, 265
Relating, principles of, 425-31
Repoise, 273
Repression, 63-64
Rogers, Carl, 283
Role consensus, 345
Role diffusion, 44-45
Role loss, 173, 321-22
Role performance, 248-49
Role relationships, 260
Role reciprocity, 91, 102-03, 348-50,
  354
  in hospitalization, 400
Roles
  family, 348-50
  marital, 328
  See also Norms; Social norms
Role shift, 259, 312, 326
  for hospitalized patient, 400,
    423-25
Role-taking, 4
Rule-breaking, 76, 198
Rules. See Norms

Scapegoating, 351-52
Schachter, S., 379
Scher, Jordan M., 409
Schismatic family configuration,
  218-19, 352-54
Schizophrenia, 200-38, 243
  anthropological theories on, 225
  biochemical factors in, 212
  biological theories on, 212-13
  catatonic, 211
  crises and, 215-16
  diagnosis of, 210
  and double-bind communication,
    355-56
  and epilepsy, 274-75
  family theories on, 217-21
  genetic factors in, 212

hebephrenic, 211
hospitalization for, 234-35
and MAOI's, 271
paranoid, 211
pseudomutuality and, 219-20
psychoanalytic theories of, 201-02
  as organic problem, 201
reactive, 210
schizoaffective, 211
simple, 210-11
sociological theories on, 221-26
symptoms of, 202-09
  affect and ambivalence, 206-09
  association and autism, 203-06
treatment issues, 234-38
types of, 209-11
undifferentiated, 211
Schizophrenic "break," 62
Schizophrenic coping style, 208-09
Schizophrenic life styles, 197, 200-38
Schizophrenics
  communicating with, 206, 428-29
  developing a relationship with,
    236
Schizophrenogenic condition, 60,
  218
Schreiber, Flora R., 104
Seconal, 119
Secondary gains, 103
Sedatives, 132-34
Seizures, 103
Self-esteem, 159, 168
Self-image, 345
  negative, 106
Seligman, Martin E. P., 160
Selye, Hans, 89
Separation (marital), 310
Serax, 268
Serotonin, 212
Sex roles in the family, 348, 349
Sexuality, 37, 105
  and the elderly, 336
  homosexuality, 181, 244
  loss of libido in depression, 160
  of manic-depressive person, 176
Shock treatment, 274-75
Sinequan, 270
Situational supports, 330
Skills, cultural values on, 40-41
Significant others, 74-75
Skewed family configuration, 218
Smoking, 115, 134-35
  See also Nicotine
Social control, 392
Socialization process, 8-12, 347,
  376-77
Social mobility, 19-22
  expectations, 20
  identity, 22
  labeling, 21

self-esteem, 21
status, achieved, 21
status, ascribed, 20
Social network, 72, 243
   and community mental health
      workers, 442
   and nursing interventions, 436,
      442
Social norms, 17-19
   correcting violations of, 18
   labeling, 19
Social position, 16-17
   status differentials and, 17
Social roles, 12-16
   role conflict, 15
   role-taking ability, 14
Social system, family as a, 342-50
Social systems, 4-8
Social workers, 441, 442-43
Societal norms, 244
Societal rule-breaking, 436
Sociopathic behavior, character-
      istics of, 199-200
Socio-psychological model of
      mental illness, 391
Solacen, 268
Somatic therapies, 274-76
"Speed," 137
Split personality, 201
Staff role in decision-making,
      419-21
Stelazine, 273
Stereotyping of behavior, 407
Steroids, 168
Stimulants, 135-38
Stimulant use, history of, 135
Stress, 88-92
Sublimation, 66
Succinylcholine, 275
Suicidal patient
   and tricyclic drugs, 271
   nursing care of, 182-87
   typical hospitalization case,
      395-99
Suicide, 177-91
   in aging population, 180, 183
   case study of, 187-91
   characteristics of persons
      attempting, 182-83
   chronic illness and, 179
   clues to, 178-82
   depression and, 158, 163
   evaluating the patient's poten-
      tial for, 259-60

and inability to express anger,
      243
incidence of, 177
verbal threats, 179, 185, 190-91
Suicide prevention centers, 186-87
Sullivan, Harry Stack, 71, 201, 203
Surgery and loss of bodily integ-
      rity, 310
Synanon, 142-44
Sybil, 104
Sympathetic nervous system, 68
Synthetic narcotics, 119
Synergistic effect of barbiturates,
      133
Szasz, Thomas, 224, 435
   on patient contracts, 440

Taractan, 273
Taraxein, 213
Termination, 301, 302-04
   for groups, 373, 386-87
Testosterone, 167-68
Therapeutic and nontherapeutic
      responses, 287-93
Therapeutic communities
   hospital, 390-433
   Synanon and others, 143
Therapies, "talking," 250-65
   brief psychotherapy, 257-65
   insight therapy, 253-57
Therapist
   role in groups, 378
   See also Nurse-patient relation-
      ship; Nurse role
Therapy, goals of, 244-45, 250
   See also Interventions
Thiopropazine, 273
Thioridazine, 273
Thiothixene, 273
Thioxanthenes, 272, 273
Thorazine, 152, 273, 274
Tindal, 273
Toddlers, emotional development
      in, 158
Tofranil, 270
Toilet training, 34
Toluene, 119
Tranquilizers, 133-34
   major, 272-74, (table) 273
   minor, 268-70, (table) 268
Transference, 256
Tranylcypromine, 270
Treatment
   of addiction by ex-addicts, 146

vs. custody, 409-11
of hospitalized patient, 391-432
of schizophrenia, 234-38
of suicidal patients, 182-86
   See also Interventions
Treatment issues, 252-53, 434-48
Treatment, psychiatric
   definition of, 279
Treatment roles, 441-44
   See also Nurse role
Tricyclics, 270, 271
   for suicidal patient, 271
Trifluoperazine, 273
Triflupromazine, 273
Trihexylphenidyl, 274
Trilafon, 273
Trust, developing, 32, 298-99
Tybamate, 268
Tybatran, 268

Ulcers, 87, 90, 92
Undoing, 67

Valium, 119, 268
Vesprin, 273
Victorian morality and opiates,
      118-21
Vision, lessening of, 103
Vistaril, 268
Vitamin-B deficiency, 130
Vivactil, 270
Vulnerability, 308, 310, 311

Will, Otto Allen, Jr., 429
Withdrawal, 301-02
Wolpe, Joseph, 266
Women
   and depression, 166-67
   and hormones, 167-68
   and role performance, 248-49
   and suicide, 177-78
"Word salad," 206
Working through, 256-57

X-ray, 412

Yalom, Irvin D., 374, 375, 376
   on termination of therapy, 387
Young adults and prevention pro-
      grams, 446
Youth
   See Adolescence